W9-CXM-320

THE
CARDIAC
CATHETERIZATION
HANDBOOK

THE CARDIAC CATHETERIZATION HANDBOOK

Second Edition

EDITED BY

Morton J. Kern, MD

Professor of Medicine
Director, The J. Gerard Mudd Cardiac
  Catheterization Laboratory
St. Louis University Health Sciences Center
St. Louis, Missouri

with 391 illustrations

Foreword by William Grossman

Mosby

St. Louis Baltimore Berlin Boston Carlsbad Chicago
London Madrid Naples New York Philadelphia
Sydney Tokyo Toronto

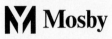

Mosby

Dedicated to Publishing Excellence

Editor: Stephanie Manning
Editorial Assistant: Colleen Boyd
Project Supervisor: Cindy Deichmann
Cover Design: Elizabeth Rohne Rudder

Printed in the United States of America
Editing and production by Spectrum Publisher Services, Inc.
Printing/binding by R. R. Donnelly & Sons Company.

Library of Congress Cataloging-in-Publication Data

The Cardiac catheterization handbook / edited by Morton J. Kern ;
   foreword by William Grossman. — 2nd ed.
      p.   cm.
   Includes bibliographical references and index.
   ISBN 0-8151-5036-9
   1. Cardiac catheterization—Handbooks, manuals, etc.
   [DNLM: 1. Heart Catheterization.   WG 1410.5.C2C2675
   1995]
RC683.5.C25C39   1995
616.1'20754—dc20
DNLM/DLC
for Library of Congress   94-19485
                                            CIP

94 95 96 97 98 9 8 7 6 5 4 3 2 1

CONTRIBUTORS

FRANK V. AGUIRRE, MD

Associate Professor of Medicine
The J. Gerard Mudd Cardiac Catheterization Laboratory
St. Louis University Health Sciences Center
St. Louis, Missouri

RICHARD G. BACH, MD

Assistant Professor of Medicine
The J. Gerard Mudd Cardiac Catheterization Laboratory
St. Louis University Health Sciences Center
St. Louis, Missouri

DIANE BROWN, RN, JD

Manager, Professional Liability Program
University of California
Office of the President
Office of Risk Management
Oakland, California

EUGENE A. CARACCIOLO, MD

Assistant Professor of Medicine
The J. Gerard Mudd Cardiac Catheterization Laboratory
St. Louis University Health Sciences Center
St. Louis, Missouri

UBEYDULLAH DELIGONUL, MD

Associate Professor of Medicine
Director, Cardiac Catheterization, Angioplasty and
  Atherectomy
University of Nebraska Medical Center
Omaha, Nebraska

THOMAS J. DONOHUE, MD

Assistant Professor of Medicine
The J. Gerard Mudd Cardiac Catheterization Laboratory
St. Louis University Health Sciences Center
St. Louis, Missouri

TED FELDMAN, MD

Associate Professor of Medicine
Hans Hecht Hemodynamic Laboratory
University of Chicago Hospital
Chicago, Illinois

MICHAEL S. FLYNN, MD

Clinical Instructor in Medicine
The J. Gerard Mudd Cardiac Catheterization Laboratory
St. Louis University Health Sciences Center
St. Louis, Missouri

M. CAROLYN GAMACHE, MD

Assistant Professor of Medicine
Electrophysiology Laboratory
St. Louis University Health Sciences Center
St. Louis, Missouri

DENISE JANOSIK, MD

Associate Professor of Medicine
Electrophysiology Laboratory
St. Louis University Health Sciences Center
St. Louis, Missouri

AILEEN O'ROURKE, JD, RN

Risk Manager, Professional Services
Cardinal Glennon Children's Hospital
St. Louis, Missouri

ROBERT ROTH, RN

Clinical Manager
The J. Gerard Mudd Cardiac Catheterization Laboratory
St. Louis University Health Sciences Center
St. Louis, Missouri

J. DAVID TALLEY, MD

Professor of Medicine
Associate Director, Division of Cardiology
University of Arkansas for Medical Sciences
Little Rock, Arkansas

CARL TOMMASO, MD

Associate Professor of Medicine
Chief, Cardiology
Northwestern Veterans Administration
Chicago, Illinois

To Margaret and Anna Rose

FOREWORD

The expansion and widespread application of cardiac catheterization throughout the world today could hardly have been imagined by Werner Forssmann when, in 1929, he was the first to pass a catheter into the heart of a living person—himself. For many years, cardiac catheterization remained primarily an investigative tool, but the precise information concerning anatomy and physiology in patients with heart disease that cardiac catheterization procedures yielded made possible the development of open heart surgery. Forssmann's initial intent, as stated in his historic article published in *Klinische Wochenschrift* in 1929, was to use cardiac catheterization as a therapeutic technique. In the last 15 years, cardiac catheterization has amply fulfilled Forssmann's dream, and each month sees the addition of new therapeutic innovations based on advanced catheter technologies.

Cardiac catheterization is practiced in every major university hospital throughout the United States, and is rapidly expanding to the point where even moderate-sized community hospitals have active programs of cardiac catheterization and angiography. This expansion of the field has led to increased demands for training of physicians, nurses, and technicians expert in the highly technical and demanding aspects of intravascular catheterization and angiography. Dr. Morton Kern's *The Cardiac Catheterization Handbook* provides an outstanding teaching manual for these individuals; this well-written and clearly focused book will be greatly enjoyed by all those who read it. So many aspects of cardiac catheterization and angiography cannot be explained simply through the use of description; this book has many excellent figures and diagrams that will help the reader to understand precisely what is meant in the text. Pressure tracings are presented, which are most helpful in the identification of specific conditions such as valvular stenosis, constrictive pericarditis, and cardiomyopathy. A section on high-risk cardiac catheterization defines the patient subgroups most likely to have complications during cardiac catheterization and angiography, and gives helpful suggestions as to how these complications might be avoided. A section on interventional techniques provides a highly concise and practical description of state-of-the-art aspects of coronary angioplasty including illustrations of application of the technique. Balloon valvuloplasty for aortic and mitral stenosis are two relatively new techniques that are discussed in very clear detail, with practical suggestions for their application. The use of thrombolytic agents in dealing with acute thrombotic states is discussed, with practical aspects (including dosages and routes of administration) described in detail. A unique section on medicolegal issues in the cardiac catheterization laboratory offers helpful hints as to common failings of documentation and record keeping, which must be avoided by the physician who wishes to protect himself against inappropriate malpractice suits. Finally, there are excellent sections dealing with the formulas for calculation of angiographic volumes, valve areas, and other hemodynamic parameters.

This handbook has become a valued companion for trainees entering into the cardiac catheterization laboratory, and Dr. Kern and his co-authors are to be congratulated on an impressive accomplishment.

William Grossman, MD
Dana Professor of Medicine
Harvard Medical School
Chief, Cardiovascular Division
Beth Israel Hospital
Boston, Massachusetts

PREFACE

One of the most satisfying events in academic medicine and cardiology is the acceptance of material to teach the fundamentals to individuals-in-training. This goal has been largely achieved in the first edition. We hope to continue the tradition by providing complete information in a basic format for the physician-in-training, noninvasive cardiologist, cardiovascular nurse, and technician within the cardiac catheterization laboratory. As indicated in the preface to the first edition, this practical guide and introductory framework is not intended to be all-inclusive, and the reader is referred to the excellent works of Drs. Grossman and Pepine and others, who provide enhanced detail and in-depth description, background, and methodology for the techniques indicated. This edition is notable for additions in many areas, especially interventional techniques. Catheterization laboratory environmental safety and OSHA precautions are added to Chapter 1. The complications of vascular access and new methods of hemostasis are discussed in Chapter 2. More hemodynamic examples (Chapter 3), an approach to electrophysiologic procedures (Chapter 4), how-to methods for coronary Doppler blood flow (Chapter 6), intraaortic balloon pump use in high-risk patients (Chapter 8), and descriptions of now standard atherectomy and coronary stent placement (Chapter 9) are also among the updated sections.

Again, I would like to acknowledge the J. Gerard Mudd Cardiac Catheterization Team. The encouragement of my wife, Margaret, and daughter, Anna Rose, was greatly appreciated. I would also like to acknowledge the support of

Dr. Frank Hildner in providing a forum for much of the hemodynamic material that has been published in *Catheterization and Cardiovascular Diagnosis* under the continuing series of hemodynamic rounds.

PREFACE

to the First Edition

This handbook is designed to provide the cardiovascular physician in training, noninvasive cardiologist, cardiovascular nurse, and other technical personnel unfamiliar with the cardiac catheterization laboratory a practical guide and basic introductory framework for the techniques used and care of the patient undergoing cardiac catheterization.

The handbook is not designed to be all inclusive. The comprehensive, complete, and detailed works (referenced at the end of Chapter 1) on cardiac catheterization are required reading. The introduction to the cardiac catheterization laboratory presented in this book discusses many seemingly obvious—but often overlooked—important points with regard to approach to the patient and routine angiographic and hemodynamic methodology. Practical points of patient care, handling intravascular equipment, evaluation of angiographic and hemodynamic data, and common errors and artifacts in data collection and interpretation are emphasized. Pertinent medical-legal aspects in catheterization laboratory management are reviewed. Where appropriate, examples are provided to help clarify confusing problems.

The invasive aspects of the practice of cardiology should not be undertaken by the uncommitted and not begun until the basics have been mastered. Although the safety of cardiac catheterization has improved greatly over the years, dedication to technique and patient safety must remain the highest priority of the operator and the cardiac catheterization team.

I want to thank the J. Gerard Mudd Cardiac Catheterization Team, Donna Sander for book preparation, and MMDK, ARDK.

Morton J. Kern

CONTENTS

I INTRODUCTION TO THE CATHETERIZATION LABORATORY I

Morton J. Kern, Robert Roth, and Ubeydullah Deligonul

Indications for the Procedure 1
Contraindications 5
Complications and Risks 5
Catheterization Laboratory Data 5
Preparation of the Patient 6
Special Preparations 13
The Team Approach to Cardiac Catheterization 17
Catheterization Laboratory Instruction 20
Equipment in the Catheterization Laboratory 22
Training Requirements 26

2 ARTERIAL AND VENOUS ACCESS 45

Ubeydullah Deligonul, Robert Roth, and Michael Flynn

Percutaneous Femoral Approach 46
Brachial Approach 60
Use of Heparin during Cardiac Catheterization 69
Problems of Vascular Access 69
Arterial and Venous Access: Nurse/Technician
  Viewpoint 80
Equipment and Instruments Used for Access 83

3 HEMODYNAMIC DATA 108

Morton J. Kern, Ubeydullah Deligonul, Thomas J. Donohue,
Eugene Caracciolo, and Ted Feldman

Pressure Waves in the Heart 108
Protocols for Right and Left Heart Catheterization 112
Computations for Hemodynamic Measurements 116
Computations of Valve Areas from Pressure Gradients
  and Cardiac Output 119

Use of Valve Resistance for Aortic Stenosis   123
Oxygen Consumption Measurement (Fick Method)   131
The Fick Oxygen Consumption Method   134
Indicator Dilution Cardiac Output Principle   135
Angiographic Cardiac Output   137
Differences Among Cardiac Output Techniques   138
Intracardiac Shunts   139
Equipment Used for Hemodynamic Study   149
Hemodynamic Recording Techniques   157
Hemodynamic Examples and Artifacts   161

**4   ELECTROPHYSIOLOGIC STUDIES AND
ABLATION TECHNIQUES   208**
Denise L. Janosik and M. Carolyn Gamache

Technical Aspects   209
Procedures   216
Utility of EPS for Specific Diagnosis   235
Catheter Ablation   243
Electrocardiography in the Cardiac Catheterization
   Laboratory   259
Components of the ECG   260

5   ANGIOGRAPHIC DATA   266
Ubeydullah Deligonul, Morton J. Kern, and Robert Roth

Coronary Arteriography   267
Problems and Solutions in the Interpretation of Coronary
   Angiograms   293
Ventriculography   304
Ascending Aortography   318
Pulmonary Angiography   321
Peripheral Vascular Angiography   325
Generation of the X-Ray Image   329
Digital Angiography   345
Comparison of Conventional Angiography and
   Subtraction   351
Radiation Safety   352
Injectors and Contrast Materials   355
Angiographic Catheters   364
Medications Used in Coronary Angiography   364
Pacemakers   370

6 RESEARCH TECHNIQUES 376

Morton J. Kern and Thomas J. Donohue

High-Fidelity Micromanometer-Tip
  Pressure Measurements 378
Quantitative Ventriculography and Wall Motion 379
Myocardial Blood Flow 381
Myocardial Metabolism 382
Coronary Sinus Catheterization 384
Doppler Coronary Flow Velocity Techniques 385
Angiographic Blood Flow Techniques:
  Videodensitometry 399
Combined Hemodynamic and Echocardiographic
  Methodologies 400
Physiologic Maneuvers in the Catheterization
  Laboratory 400

7 SPECIAL TECHNIQUES 414

Ubeydullah Deligonul, Richard G. Bach, Morton J. Kern, Michael S. Flynn, and Eugene A. Caracciolo

Transseptal Heart Catheterization 414
Direct Transthoracic LV Puncture 421
Endomyocardial Biopsy 422
CS Catheterization 429
Pericardiocentesis 430
Intravascular Foreign Body Retrieval 434
Special Conditions 438

8 HIGH-RISK CARDIAC CATHETERIZATION 444

Eugene A. Caracciolo, Thomas J. Donohue, Morton J. Kern, Richard G. Bach, Carl Tommaso, and Ubeydullah Deligonul

The High-Risk Patient 444
Management of Arrhythmias in the
  Catheterization Laboratory 452
Cardiac Support Devices 470
Technique for Elective Percutaneous
  Cardiopulmonary Support 479

9 INTERVENTIONAL TECHNIQUES 484

Ubeydullah Deligonul, Morton J. Kern, Richard G. Bach, Thomas J. Donohue, Eugene A. Caracciolo, Frank V. Aguirre, and J. David Talley

PTCA 484

Valvuloplasty   510
New Interventional Techniques   527
Stents   535

10 DOCUMENTATION IN THE CARDIAC CATHETERIZATION LABORATORY   541
Aileen O'Rourke and Diane Brown

Medical Malpractice   541
The Medical Record: General Points   542
Product Liability Issues in the Cardiac
   Catheterization Laboratory   550
Summary   554

GLOSSARY   555

APPENDICES

  I Patient Records, Orders, and Diagrams   559
 II Functional Anatomy of the Heart   564
III Coronary Artery Anatomy and Physiology   567
     Anatomy of the Arterial Wall   567
     Configuration of Lesions   568
 IV Normal Hemodynamic Value Tables   572
  V Units of Measure   574
     Conversion Factors and Constants   575
 VI Ventricular Volume and Mass   577
     Measurement of Ventricular Volume   577
VII Radiographic Identification of Prosthetic Valves   581
VIII PTCA and Other Interventional Equipment
     Specifications   587
 IX Electrocardiography in the Cardiac Catheterization
     Laboratory   598

INDEX   607

THE
CARDIAC
CATHETERIZATION
HANDBOOK

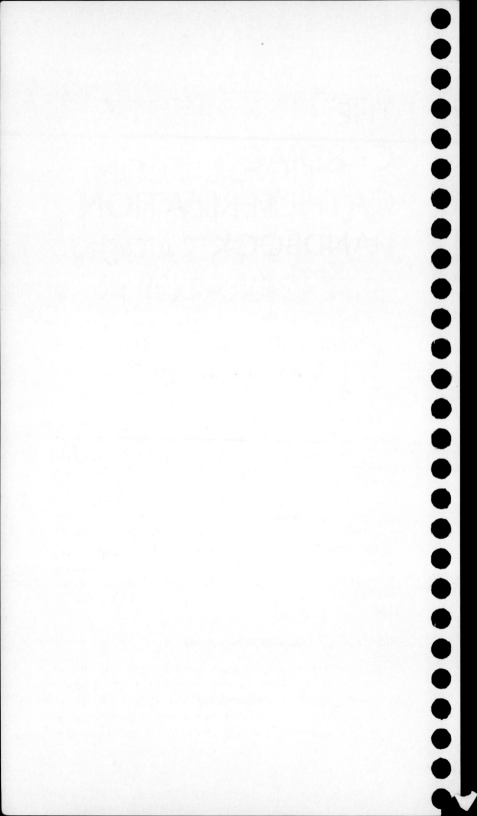

1

INTRODUCTION TO THE CATHETERIZATION LABORATORY

Morton J. Kern, Robert Roth, and Ubeydullah Deligonul

Cardiac catheterization is the insertion and passage of small plastic tubes (catheters) into arteries and veins up to the heart to obtain x-ray pictures of coronary arteries and cardiac chambers as well as to measure pressures in the heart (intracardiac hemodynamics). The cardiac catheterization laboratory also performs diagnostic angiography to obtain images and determine the function of the cardiovascular system for diseases of the aorta and pulmonary and peripheral vessels. Besides providing diagnostic information the cardiac catheterization laboratory also employs catheter-based therapies to intervene in the course of acute cardiovascular illness. The box on p. 2 lists procedures that can be performed with coronary angiography.

INDICATIONS FOR THE PROCEDURE

Cardiac catheterization is used to identify *structural* cardiac diseases such as atherosclerotic coronary artery disease, myocardial dysfunction (infarction or myopathy), and valvular or congenital heart abnormalities. In adults the procedure is used most commonly to diagnose coronary artery disease.

1

Procedures That May Accompany Coronary Angiography

PROCEDURE	COMMENT
1. Central venous access (femoral, internal jugular, subclavian)	Used as IV line for emergency medications or fluids, temporary pacemaker access (pacemaker not mandatory for coronary angiography)
2. Hemodynamic assessment	
a. Left heart pressures (aorta, left ventricle)	Routine for all studies
b. Right and left heart combined pressures	Not routine for coronary artery disease; mandatory for valvular heart disease; routine for congestive heart failure (CHF), right ventricular dysfunction, pericardial diseases, cardiomyopathy, intracardiac shunts, congenital abnormalities*
3. Left ventricular angiography	Routine for all studies; may be excluded with high-risk patients, left main coronary or aortic stenosis, severe CHF
4. Internal mammary artery selective angiography	Not routine unless used as coronary bypass conduit
5. Pharmacologic studies	
a. Ergonovine	Routine for suspected coronary vasospasm
b. Isoproterenol	Not routine, used to assess hypertrophic cardiomyopathy
c. IC/IV/sublingual nitroglycerin	Optionally routine for all studies
6. Aortic root angiography	Routine for aortic insufficiency, aortic dissection, aortic aneurysm, with or without aortic stenosis, routine to locate bypass grafts not visualized by selective angiography
7. Digital subtraction angiography	Not yet routine for coronary angiography; excellent for peripheral vascular disease
8. Cardiac pacing and electrophysiologic studies	Research or arrhythmia studies
9. Interventional and special techniques	Coronary angioplasty (PTCA)
	Myocardial biopsy
	Transseptal or direct left ventricular puncture
	Balloon catheter valvuloplasty
	Conduction tract catheter ablation

* See the box on p. 3 for indications.

Other indications depend on the history, physical examination, electrocardiogram (ECG), exercise treadmill test (ETT) results, echocardiographic results, and chest x-ray. Indications for cardiac catheterization have been presented in a special joint task force report from the American College of Cardiology/American Heart Association Subcommittee on Coronary Angiography summarized in the box that follows.

Indications for Cardiac Catheterization

INDICATIONS	PROCEDURES
1. Suspected or known coronary artery disease	
a. New onset angina	LV, COR
b. Unstable angina	LV, COR
c. Evaluation before a major surgical procedure	LV, COR
d. Silent ischemia	LV, COR, ERGO
e. Positive ETT	LV, COR, ERGO
f. Atypical chest pain or coronary spasm	LV, COR, ERGO
2. Myocardial infarction	
a. Unstable angina postinfarction	LV, COR
b. Failed thrombolysis	LV, COR, RH
c. Shock	LV, COR, RH
d. Mechanical complications (ventricular septal defect, rupture of wall or papillary muscle)	LV, COR, RH
3. Sudden cardiovascular death	LV, COR, R + L
4. Valvular heart disease	LV, COR, R + L, AO
5. Congenital heart disease (before anticipated corrective surgery)	LV, COR, R + L, AO
6. Aortic dissection	AO, COR
7. Pericardial constriction or tamponade	LV, COR, R + L
8. Cardiomyopathy	LV, COR, R + L, BX
9. Initial and follow-up assessment for heart transplant	LV, COR, R + L, BX

LV, left ventriculography; COR, coronary angiography; R + L, right and left heart hemodynamics; AO, aortography; BX, endomyocardial biopsy; ERGO, ergonovine provocation of spasm for normal COR; RH, right heart oxygen saturations and hemodynamics (e.g., placement of Swan-Ganz catheter).

Contraindications to Cardiac Catheterization

ABSOLUTE CONTRAINDICATIONS

Inadequate equipment or catheterization facility

RELATIVE CONTRAINDICATIONS

Uncontrolled congestive heart failure, high blood pressure,
    arrhythmias
Recent cerebral vascular accident (<1 month)
Infection/fever
Electrolyte imbalance
Acute gastrointestinal bleeding or anemia
Pregnancy
Anticoagulation (or known, uncontrolled bleeding diathesis)
Uncooperative patient
Medication intoxication (e.g., digitalis, phenothiazine)
Renal failure

Complications of Cardiac Catheterization

Death
Myocardial infarction
Cerebral vascular accident
Serious arrhythmia
• Ventricular tachycardia
• Fibrillation
• Atrial fibrillation
• Supraventricular tachyarrhythmia
• Heart block, asystole
Vascular injury
• Hemorrhage (local, retroperitoneal, pelvic)
• Pseudoaneurysm
• Thrombosis/embolus/air embolus
• Aortic dissection
Cardiac perforation, tamponade
Contrast reaction/anaphylaxis/nephrotoxicity
Protamine reaction
Infection
Congestive heart failure
Vasovagal reaction

Elective Procedures

In general, cardiac catheterization is an *elective* diagnostic procedure and should be deferred if the patient is not prepared either psychologically or physically.

Urgent Procedures

If the patient is unstable from a cardiac cause, such as crescendo angina or acute myocardial infarction, catheterization must proceed. In the event of congestive heart failure, rapid medical management is needed because inability to lie flat precludes easy catheter passage. However, acute cardiac decompensation may benefit more by aggressive management in the catheterization laboratory where intubation, intraaortic balloon pumping, and vasopressors can be instituted rapidly before angiography and revascularization.

CONTRAINDICATIONS (see the box on p. 4)

Contraindications include fever of unknown cause, anemia, electrolyte imbalance (especially hypokalemia predisposing to arrhythmias), or other systemic illness listed in the box on p. 4 needing stabilization.

COMPLICATIONS AND RISKS (see the box on p. 4)

Extensive analysis of the complications in more than 200,000 patients indicates the following risks: death <0.2%, myocardial infarction <0.5%, stroke <0.5%, serious ventricular arrhythmia <1%, and major vascular complications (thrombosis, bleeding requiring transfusion, or pseudoaneurysm) <1%. Vascular complications are more frequent when the brachial approach is used. Risks are higher in well-described subgroups (see the box on p. 6).

CATHETERIZATION LABORATORY DATA

Information gathered during the cardiac catheterization can be divided into two categories: hemodynamic (Chapter 3) and cineangiographic (Chapter 5). Cineangiography is the term used to describe the photographing of x-ray images onto movie film. The cineangiogram provides anatomic information about the chambers of the heart and the coronary arteries. Hemodynamic information recorded in the laboratory consists of pressure measurements, cardiac outputs, and blood oxygen saturation measurements.

Conditions That Predispose Patients to Be at Higher Risk for Complications of Catheterization*

Suspected or known left main coronary stenosis
Extensive three vessel coronary artery disease
Severe aortic stenosis
Severe congestive heart failure
Left ventricular dysfunction (left ventricular ejection fraction <35%)
Diabetes
Advanced age
Unstable angina
Acute myocardial infarction
Aortic aneurysm
Prior cerebral vascular accident
Renal insufficiency

* See also Chapter 8.

PREPARATION OF THE PATIENT
Consent for the Procedure

Consent is obtained by the operator or his or her assistant, usually a physician:

1. Explain in simple terms what procedure will take place and for what reason each step of the procedure will occur.
2. Explain the risks for routine cardiac catheterization.
   a. Major: Stroke
            Death
            Myocardial infarction
   b. Minor: Vascular injury
            Allergic reaction
            Bleeding
            Hematoma
3. Explain any portions of the study used for research and associated risks.
   a. "Hifi" transducer-tipped catheters—perforation, embolus <1:500
   b. Coronary sinus catheter—perforation, embolus <1:500

    c. Pharmacologic study—depending on drug

    d. Electrophysiologic study—perforation, arrhythmia
       <1:500

    e. Intracoronary Doppler study—spasm, MI, embolus,
       dissection <1:500

4. Provide the necessary information, but do not overwhelm
the patient.

There is no alternative to coronary angiography and often
the risk of "not knowing" the anatomy is greater than not
performing the test.

Communicate with the Patients: A Nonmedical Person's Understanding

Establish rapport and build the patient's confidence by listening and then explaining. The procedure should be discussed with the patient in terms he or she can understand.
The purpose of the procedure should be clear, e.g., "to look
at the coronary arteries" and "to examine the heart muscle
(ventricular function)." Simple terms are best so that the
patient can grasp the concepts. Explain what small catheters
are (plastic tubes like spaghetti) and that they will be used
to put x-ray contrast "dye" into the arteries supplying blood
to the heart. The heart "muscle" may be weakened (infarcted) in certain areas and that the way to identify this
"weakness" is to take x-ray "pictures." This example of a
simple, forthright explanation facilitates the operator team/
patient relationship so that confidence in the operator and
team performing the procedure is established.

Set the Laboratory Atmosphere: The Patient's Confidence Builder

1. In the laboratory a confident, professional attitude should
be assumed by all personnel at all times. Straightforward
routine communication should be performed quietly and
without alarming tones. When talking to patients, address them by name to let them know what their instructions are as opposed to requests or communications to
co-workers.

2. The circulating team members should be confident, reas-
suring, and businesslike in every respect. The patient
feels helpless and is "tuned in" to all types of stimuli
(especially verbal).

3. Extraneous conversation is distracting for both the patient and operators. In the laboratory all "players" should be in the game, that is, once in the room the patient's needs and safety become paramount.

4. Communication with the patient (and family) before, during, and after the procedure will ensure a satisfied and well-cared-for individual.

5. Avoid falling into the factory worker attitudes of "another coronary" or "another transplant." Each procedure is potentially life threatening and should be undertaken seriously and with concern as if each patient were a family member.

6. Cardiac catheterization is stressful to both the patient and operator team. Minimize this stress by thoughtful preparation and professional attention to detail.

7. Practical notes for the new operator include:

   a. Immediately preceding the catheterization in the laboratory, reexamination of the ECG is essential. A brief reiteration of the history will make sure that there has been no interval change since your last interview. A brief examination of the patient—checking heart sounds, breath sounds, and carotid and peripheral pulses—is also essential immediately before and after cardiac catheterization. No patient should be studied without full understanding of the clinical conditions and results of previous catheterizations and other pertinent laboratory data.

   b. Once on the catheterization table the patient remembers two major potentially painful points of a case: the initial introduction of the local anesthetic and any discomfort experienced after the study has been completed. Such discomfort usually occurs while the operator is holding the puncture site or closing the brachial arterial cutdown site.

   If the local anesthetic injection or the arterial closure or compression after the procedure is difficult or painful, the patient will remember that the doctor who performed catheterization "hurt me." The period between the two often is forgotten (thanks to premedication). These two points should be kept in mind as the major "take-home" messages. Patients cannot tell your skill or level of accomplishment during the procedure but judge you (and your team) on the manner and care at the beginning and end of the study. Obviously, skill and accomplishment during the procedure are essential, but these will be developed over the operator's training period.

8. Catheterization orders are as follows: Before catheterization, preferably the preceding night, precatheterization orders should be written. All medications, cessation of oral intake, and procedural premedications need to be tailored to the patient and timing of the catheterization; if the patient is using neutral protamine hagedorn (NPH) insulin, the dose should be reduced 50% and the patient should not eat breakfast. Watch carefully for later hypoglycemic reactions (e.g., shaking, confusion, and slurred speech). (Sample orders are shown in Appendix II.)

9. The patient shold be allowed to wear glasses and dentures to make communication easier.

In-Lab Preparations

The staff of the cardiac catheterization laboratory is responsible for patient preparation before the start of the procedure. Upon arrival in the laboratory a staff member should review a brief checklist to be sure that all preprocedural requirements have been met. A sample checklist follows:

_____ Check patient ID band
_____ Blood pressure and baseline ECG
_____ Known allergies?
_____ Recent anticoagulation therapy? If yes, prothrombin time (PT) _____ partial thromboplastin time (PTT) _____
_____ Consents for procedure signed and in chart? If not, obtain permits
_____ IV in if ordered? IV patent?
_____ NPO (nothing by mouth) since midnight or as ordered?
_____ Premedications given as ordered?
_____ Baseline check of peripheral pulses
_____ Assess patient's understanding of procedure/answer patient's questions
_____ Proper paperwork copied and filled out for procedure

_____ Check lab results (key labs: blood urea nitrogen [BUN], creatinine, PT, PTT, electrolytes)

_____ Document precatheterization condition and note any physical deficits

After all precatheterization requirements have been fulfilled the patient may be taken to the angiographic suite and the technical preparations for the procedure can be completed.

Catheterization Suite Preparations

Before the start of the catheterization procedure the staff will perform the following tasks:

1. *Establish ECG monitoring.* The ECG should be considered first of the two major "lifelines." The heart beat is monitored for rate and rhythm during the entire procedure. It is the responsibility of the staff to place the electrodes and lead wires in such a fashion that a quality trace is obtained. Care must be taken that the electrodes and lead wires do not interfere with the movement of the x-ray/cineangiographic unit. All leads should be secure and a clean trace present before the application of sterile drapes; it is very difficult to reach under the sterile drapes to reattach loose lead wires once the procedure has begun. Radiolucent leads permit complete 12-lead ECG monitoring but are more prone to breakage than heavier cable leads and are only used for specific procedures.

2. *Establish intravenous access for emergency medications or sedation.* The second lifeline is the IV access. Emergency drugs to counteract vagal or allergic reactions or other problems are often administered by this route. In most cases the patient is given an oral or IM sedative as premedication before arriving at the cardiac catheterization laboratory. Once the patient is in the laboratory, the nurse or physician may identify the need for additional sedation via the IV route before the start of the procedure. The IV is very important in preventing dehydration after cardiac catheterization.

PREMEDICATIONS: Benadryl 25 mg IV, Valium 2 to 5 mg IV; for PTCA (percutaneous transluminal coronary angioplasty) Demerol 25 mg IV is added; for agitation or pain during the procedure morphine 2 mg IV is used because the drug has a short half-life and its effect is easily reversible.

Exercise caution when premedicating elderly patients. If Demerol or morphine is used, a narcotic antagonist such as Narcan should be available. Flumazenil (mazieon, a benzodiazepine antagonist) should also be available if Valium or Versed is used.

Sterile Preparations

Prepare the vascular access site.   The most common vascular access site is the right or left groin for the femoral approach or the right (or occasionally left) antecubital fossa for a brachial approach. The usual sterile preparation is preceded by shaving the area and vigorously applying an antiseptic solution such as Betadine or Septisol solution. Shaving at the arterial entry site should be done carefully to avoid lacerations or abrasions.

During the period of patient preparation, the staff should always be aware of the patient's need for privacy. The patient should be kept covered as much as possible. Procedure rooms are typically cold; therefore, every effort should be made to keep the patient warm and comfortable.

Sterile field preparation and patient draping.   Cardiac catheterization is performed using aseptic technique. The staff member assigned to assist the physician in the procedure will do a surgical scrub and put on surgical gown, a hair cover, a face mask, and gloves. A sterile drape is placed, starting at the patient's upper chest and extending to the foot, to cover the entire examination table. A "Mayo" equipment stand is prepared in a sterile fashion and is used to hold all of the sterile catheters and other equipment for use during the procedure. At this time the circulating staff member will hand catheters and necessary equipment, not included in the sterile catheter laboratory pack, to the scrub nurse/technician.

It is important for all personnel to understand sterile techniques in order to avoid accidentally contaminating any sterile fields. As a basic rule, no unsterile objects may be passed over a sterile field. When moving around a crowded angiographic room, all personnel should be very careful to avoid bumping into or passing hands or arms over the sterile tray, table, or patient drapes. Also, avoid touching the end of any catheters, extension tubes, or syringe tips in a sterile field or the power injector syringe tip that is exposed.

NOTES FOR OBSERVERS IN THE LABORATORY: Any observers in the angiographic room always should wear a lead apron as protection against secondary and scatter radiation. Usually it will not be necessary for them to wear sterile gloves and gowns. Observers should also be aware of precautions necessary for protection from blood and body fluids.

Postprocedural Care

Postcatheterization checkup.   The operator should check on the patient several hours after the procedure. Vital signs should be stable. Low blood pressure usually is due to diuresis and will respond to normal saline. Tachycardia with low blood pressure indicates blood loss. Check arterial access for pain, hematoma, and loss of distal pulses. Urine output should be >30 ml/hr and will reflect satisfactory volume replacement or early onset of contrast-induced renal failure. A cold or cool extremity requires repeated attempts to assess whether thrombus, spasm, or vasoconstriction is responsible. If vascular injury or thrombus is suspected, aspirin 325 mg should be given orally and/or heparin 5000 U bolus plus 1000 U/hr. Limb ischemia requires urgent consultation with a vascular surgeon.

Angiogram review.   To provide the patient (and family) with an understanding of the coronary artery disease or other findings, a preliminary, schematic diagram can be provided in the catheterization laboratory, put in the chart, or carried back to the patient's room. A catheterization instruction book is often helpful and may contain a blank standard diagram. The booklet will explain the catheterization procedure and what the various findings on the coronary angiogram may mean. In our experience reviewing the coronary cineangiograms with the patient and family members has been especially helpful. This review at or after discharge provides the patient an opportunity to understand the pathology and to allow the patient to ask questions and receive answers specifically with regard to the future treatment (after discussing plans with the primary care physician). Patients have expressed a high degree of interest in this approach. "No one ever took time to explain my heart problem and now I understand what is wrong" is a frequent comment. The potential risk of a patient becoming alarmed or depressed after viewing the cineangiogram has not been borne out by experience with more than 20,000 patients in our laboratory since the late 1960s. The time commitment by the physician (for whom showing the films is not routine) is an additional burden but is certainly worth the effort.

SPECIAL PREPARATIONS (see the box on pp. 14–15)
Contrast Media Reactions

The Committee on Safety of Contrast Media of the International Society of Radiology report that in more than 300,000 patients the overall incidence of adverse reaction was ≤5%. Adverse reactions were found in 10% to 12% of patients with a history of allergy and in 15% of patients with reported reaction on previous examination. From these reports we can conclude that major life-threatening reactions do not tend to recur on reexamination, whereas minor reactions are more likely to be repeated.

There are three types of contrast allergies (see the box on p. 17): (1) cutaneous and mucosal manifestations; (2) smooth muscle and minor anaphylactoid responses; and (3) cardiovascular and major anaphylactoid responses. Management of contrast reactions is summarized in Fig. 1-1.

Major reactions involving laryngeal or pulmonary edema often are accompanied by minor, or less severe, reactions. Although some reactions to a pretest contrast dose may be violent (but rarely life threatening), pretesting has been found to be of no value in determining who will have an adverse reaction.

All procedures utilizing contrast media should be assessed for risk/benefit ratio and full emergency resuscitation equipment, as well as a trained team, should be avaliable for any patient receiving contrast.

If available, nonionic contrast media should be used to replace ionic contrast media for patients with prior allergic reactions.

PREMEDICATION: Patients reporting allergic reactions to contrast media should be premedicated with prednisone and diphenhydramine (Benadryl). Pretreatment with corticosteroids to alleviate reactions to IV contrast media has been found to be helpful in reducing all types of reactions except those characterized predominantly by hives. Premedication

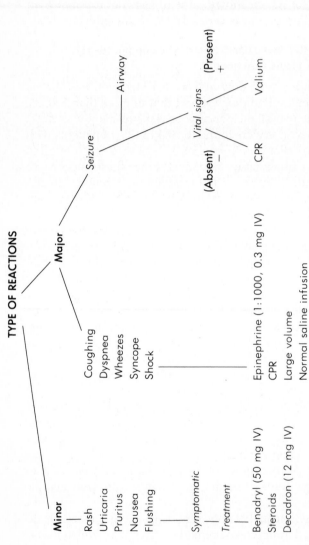

Fig. 1-1. Management of contrast reactions. Before contrast administration patient should be asked if he or she has a history of reaction during prior x-ray procedures of artery, kidney, or gallbladder or if patient has a known allergy to fish. After contrast administration, patient should be checked if a reaction is suspected; signs include hives, flushing, rash, and low blood pressure. EPI, Epinephrine; CPR, cardiopulmonary resuscitation.

may not prevent the occurrence of adverse reactions completely. The routine for the laboratory may vary, but common dosages include 60 mg prednisone the night before, and 60 mg of prednisone the morning of, along with 50 mg oral Benadryl given at the time of call to the catheterization laboratory.

Protamine Reactions

Although protamine is used widely for reversing systemic heparinization after cardiac catheterization, major reactions simulating anaphylaxis can occur, albeit rarely. Minor protamine reactions may appear as back and flank pain or flushing with peripheral vasodilation and low blood pressure. Major reactions involve marked facial flushing and vasomotor collapse, which may be fatal. Patients taking NPH insulin have an increased sensitivity to protamine. The incidence of major protamine reactions in NPH insulin–dependent diabetics is 27% compared to 0.5% in patients with no history of insulin use. It is recommended that diabetics on NPH insulin and patients with allergies to fish undergoing cardiac catheterization do so without use of protamine or, when necessary, that protamine be administered cautiously in anticipation of a major reaction.

Contrast-Induced Renal Failure

Patients with diabetes or renal insufficiency or those who are dehydrated as a result of any cause are at risk. Advanced preparations include adequate hydration and maintenance of large-volume urine flow ($\geq$200 ml/hr). These patients should be hydrated intravenously the night before the procedure. Lasix, Mannitol, and large-volume IV fluids also are administered during and following the contrast study.

After the study, monitor the urine output. If output falls and is not responsive to increased IV fluids, renal insufficiency is probable. A consultation with a nephrologist may be helpful.

Use of different types of contrast agents (ionic, nonionic, or low osmolar) does not reduce incidence of contrast-induced nephropathy.

The Insulin-Dependent Diabetic Patient

For patients taking subcutaneous insulin (NPH, regular), an overnight fast with their normal dose of insulin will cause

Conditions Requiring Special Preparations

CONDITION

1. Allergy
   a. Prior contrast studies
   b. Iodine, fish
   c. Premedication allergy
   d. Lidocaine
2. Patients receiving anticoagulation

3. Diabetes
   a. NPH insulin (protamine reaction)
   b. Renal function (prone to contrast-induced renal failure)
4. Electrolyte imbalance (K^+, Mg^{2+}, etc.)
5. Arrhythmias
6. Anemia

7. Dehydration
8. Renal failure

MANAGEMENT

1. Allergy
   a. Contrast premedication
   b. Contrast reaction reaction algorihthm (Fig. 1-1)
   c. Hold premedication
   d. Use Marcaine (1 mg/ml)
2. Defer procedure
   a. Vitamin K^+, 10 mequivalents/hr
   b. fresh frozen plasma
   c. Hold heparin
   d. Protamine for heparin
3. Hydration, Lasix, mannitol, urine output >50 ml/hr

4. Defer procedure, replenish electrolytes
5. Defer procedure, administer antiarrhythmics
6. Defer procedure
   a. Control bleeding
   b. Transfuse
7. Hydration
8. Limit contrast
   a. Maintain high urine output
   b. Hydrate

Anaphylactoid Reactions to Contrast Medium

CUTANEOUS AND MUCOSAL

Urticaria
Pruritus
Flushing
Angioedema
Laryngeal edema

SMOOTH MUSCLE

Bronchospasm
Gastrointestinal spasm
Uterine contraction

CARDIOVASCULAR

Vasodilatation
Hypotension (shock)
Arrhythmia

hypoglycemia. The dose of NPH insulin should be cut 50% for patients coming to the catheterization laboratory NPO in the early morning. Remember, patients receiving NPH insulin are at higher risk for protamine reactions.

THE TEAM APPROACH TO CARDIAC CATHETERIZATION
Physician Viewpoint

A new person in the cardiac catheterization laboratory should observe the variety of catheterization procedures for at least 10 consecutive cases. This observation period will give the new member of the catheterization team a chance to appreciate the timing, rhythm, and recurrent steps that are required of each member as an integral part of the laboratory. Each laboratory will have an "individual" routine that may vary among operators. There is no one laboratory routine that is best, but learning the routine and joining the team smoothly are important first steps.

Learn the "routine" overview

1. The patient is seen by a member of the cardiac catheterization team, indications for the procedure are discussed, risks explained, consent obtained, special preparations made, and orders and chart notes written.

2. The patient arrives in the laboratory, is greeted by the nurses, moved from a holding area into the angiographic suite, and prepared and draped in a sterile fashion. The doctor may or may not participate in the draping with the nurses.
3. Arterial and venous access is obtained depending on the needs of the patient's problem and routine of the laboratory.
4. Right heart catheterization, coronary angiography, and left ventriculography are performed as indicated by the clinical situation with the appropriate hemodynamic and angiographic measurements.
5. At the conclusion of the data collection and angiographic study, the catheters and sheaths are removed.
6. If a femoral or brachial percutaneous approach has been used, compression of the puncture site usually is performed in a holding area. After an appropriate period of compression the patient is returned to his or her room for observation and usually requires a minimum of 8 hours bed rest. For procedures in which a smaller catheter is involved, 4 to 6 hours of bed rest may be sufficient. If a brachial cutdown approach has been used, the operator repairs the arterial and venous access site with sutures. The patient is returned to the room for observation, but a strict period of prolonged bed rest is not required.
7. After the procedure, usually in the afternoon, a member of the catheterization team checks the patient's arterial access site(s), identifies and treats any problems that may have occurred, and presents the preliminary findings to the patient after discussion with the referring physician(s). Remember, unless the operator is the primary care physician, the catheterization team should discuss management options with the patient's primary physician first before taking the patient's treatment into their own hands.
8. Preparations for discharge (as an outpatient that day or as an inpatient on the following morning) or for further procedures will be made after the cardiac catheterization data has been reviewed by the attending physician.

The Catheterization Team: Nurse/Technician Viewpoint

The composition of a catheterization team varies among laboratories. The smallest functioning unit would consist of a physician, an assisting physician or nurse, a nurse circulator and/or recording technician assigned to the laboratory, and a nurse outside the laboratory able to assist. For more specialized procedures, the staff complement is increased appropriately.

Personnel are trained specifically to provide technical support necessary for the safe performance of cardiac catheterization procedures. Several disciplines are called upon to provide this support. Each member of the team assumes a very important role during the procedure.

Personnel and functions

1. A circulating nurse technologist is present who is capable of assisting the physician in all aspects of care of the cardiovascular patient including routine care and care in case of cardiovascular emergencies.
2. A scrub nurse is needed for assistance at the x-ray table to provide the operating physician with all the equipment and supplies needed in order to carry out the examination and to assist in the exchanging of catheters, and the like.
3. A radiologic technologist is trained in x-ray principles as they relate to cardiovascular procedures, cineangiography, and fluoroscopy and should have complete knowledge of use of power injectors, x-ray generators, cineangiographic systems, image intensifiers, and film processing equipment.
4. A monitoring and recording technologist is responsible for monitoring the ECG and the hemodynamic data. The technician keeps the physician appraised of changes in cardiac pressures and rhythms. The technician must be able to interpret pressure wave forms and operate all physiological recording equipment.

Optimal staffing. Every case of coronary arteriography does not require all of these people to be present. In most laboratories, three assistants usually are required for each catheterization procedure: one person is scrubbed and assists the physician at the table; one is not scrubbed and circulates in the room providing patient care and procuring any supplies that are needed during the procedure; and one performs the duties of recording technician and radiological technologist by selecting proper cineangiographic programs, field sizes, etc., as required.

Cross training. Cross training of the individuals in the laboratories is helpful in maintaining the morale and confidence in each job described. Cross training also means that each individual in the laboratory will be competent to start up the laboratory and assist in operation on an emergency 24-hour basis when needed.

Cardiopulmonary resuscitation (CPR). All members of the catheterization team should be trained fully in CPR and the use of defibrillators. An algorithm for CPR in the catheterization laboratory is shown in Fig. 7-1.

CATHETERIZATION LABORATORY INSTRUCTION
Patient Education

Teaching before the procedure.   In most cases patients undergoing cardiac catheterization have very vague and often confused ideas of how the procedure is performed. They know little as to what information will be provided about their cardiac status. Preoperative patient teaching is a very important part of the procedure to allay fears and obtain maximal patient care and cooperation.

The teaching should start at the time the patient enters the hospital. The nurse on the floor should provide information on what the patients should expect while being cared for on the floor, both before and after the cardiac catheterization. Topics such as the preprocedural diet, medications, IV therapy, and postprocedural bed rest should be discussed. Teaching by the staff of the cardiac catheterization laboratory should take place on two levels: the nurse's and the physician's.

The nurse should explain step-by-step how the procedure is performed, how long it will take, and what the patient should expect regarding sensations and discomfort associated with the procedure. A prepared booklet (with a videotape) explaining the procedure should be given to the patient to read before the procedure. This will reinforce the verbal teaching that has been done by the nurse (e.g., the steps of the catheterization, breath holding, etc., and types of equipment the patient will see). When possible, the nurse should see the patient first. The information given by the nurse may stimulate questions that the patient may ask when the physician arrives to speak to the patient. Some laboratories may not have the resources to send a staff member to do this type of teaching. If that is the case, the floor nurse needs to be well versed in invasive techniques in order to provide adequate patient teaching.

From the viewpoint of the catheterization laboratory staff, the physician's role in patient education should focus on four areas. First, the physician should make clear to the patient the reasons for which the procedure is being performed. Second, the patient should be told what information the cardiac catheterization is going to provide. Third, the patient should be told what treatment options are available once a diagnosis is made. The last point the physician should discuss with the patient is that of the possible risks and potential complications of the procedure. The issue of the risks versus benefits and alternatives to the catheterization should be discussed. After this teaching has been done, the physician then will obtain the written informed consent from the patient. Remember the physician is the person with final patient responsibility. It is not the nurse's/technician's job to obtain consent.

Teaching in the Laboratory

Teaching should continue once the patient has arrived in the catheterization holding area. The team members should introduce themselves and explain their jobs. A staff member should orient the patient to the x-ray suite and briefly explain the function of the various pieces of equipment. While in the laboratory, the patient should be encouraged to communicate freely with the staff and physician. It is important that the patient inform the staff of any pain or discomfort during the procedure.

Patient's Viewpoint

Because the patient often is overwhelmed by the mere thought of such an invasive procedure, it may be difficult for the patient to digest all of the information that will be given. Therefore teaching sessions should be limited to 10 to 15 minutes, with important points stressed two or three times. A well-informed patient is less anxious and this makes the procedure much easier and more comfortable for the patient, the physician, and staff members.

Team Teaching and Conferences

Educational experience is enhanced markedly by a daily cardiac catheterization conference. These conferences emphasize the relation of clinical data to the hemodynamic and angiographic data. Review of data and discussion of various therapies (medicine, surgery, angioplasty, and the like) provide an excellent opportunity to learn from colleagues who share cases of educational value.

EQUIPMENT IN THE CATHETERIZATION LABORATORY
(Figs. 1-2 to 1-5)

Fluoroscope

A high-resolution image-intensifying television system with cineangiographic and videotape capabilities are the "eyes" of the cardiovascular laboratory. The fluoroscope is mounted on a rotating C-arm that allows viewing from different x-ray angles (see Chapter 5). The C-arm is a semicircular support with the x-ray tube at one end and the fluoroscope on the other. The patient is placed in the center of the semicircle and the fluoroscope can be moved up to 180° around the patient as needed to visualize the heart. Two C-arms, side by side, are called "biplane" and with a double monitoring system can provide visualization of the heart at two different angles at the same time. Both the fluoroscopic and physiologic recorders will have display monitors. Other components of the fluoroscope include cineangiographic camera and film magazines, x-ray generator controls, and special patient table.

Physiologic Recorder

In addition to oberserving and recording images of the heart during catheterization, it is also necessary to observe and record the ECG and various blood pressures within the cardiovascular system. A reliable electrocardiographic and pressure monitoring system is essential for the safety of the patient and collection of diagnostic information (described in detail in Chapter 3).

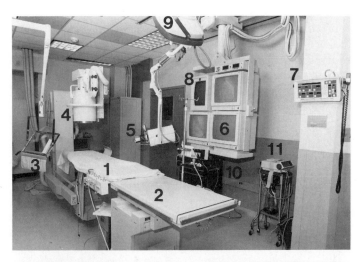

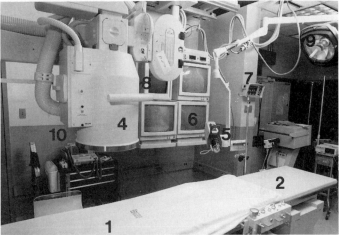

Fig. 1-2. Two views of the cardiac catheterization suite. *1*, Patient approximately where operator will stand, C-arm controls are shown on side of table; *2*, movable patient table; *3*, x-ray shield; *4*, C-arm with image intensifier on top and x-ray tube below table; *5*, ceiling-mounted contrast power injector; *6*, fluoroscopic monitorings; *7*, control panel for contrast power injector; *8*, physiologic monitor display; *9*, ceiling-mounted operating light; *10*, emergency cart; *11*, cardiac output thermodilution computer.

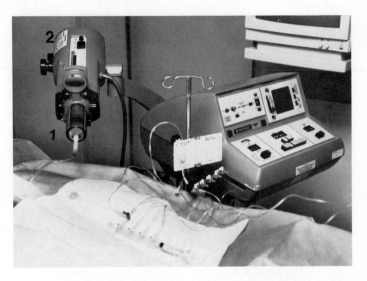

Fig. 1-3. Close-up view of the contrast power injector. *1*, The power injector; *2*, the syringe connection. Settings for contrast power injector are shown in Fig. 4-44.

Contrast Power Injector

A high-pressure contrast media injector is needed to administer the large bolus of contrast media into the left ventricle (30 to 50 ml), pulmonary arteries (20 to 50 ml), or aortic arch (40 to 60 ml). When properly set and flushed, the power injector can be used to inject contrast into the coronary arteries (3 to 8 ml).

"Crash Cart" and Defibrillator

In every cardiovascular laboratory you will also see an emergency "crash cart" near the x-ray table. The crash cart contains emergency drugs, oxygen, airways, suction apparatus, and other emergency equipment. The crash cart is equipped with a defibrillator that should be charged and ready for use during a procedure. The defibrillator must be tested daily and must be kept at close range for prompt use. Temporary pacemakers and electrodes should be on every cart.

Sterile Equipment and Supplies

The angiographer usually has a sterile pack or tray that contains the various supplies needed to perform the procedure.

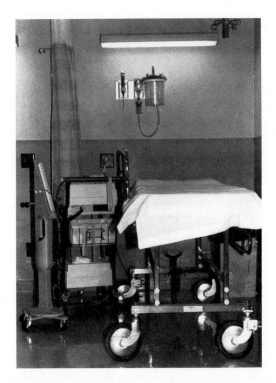

Fig. 1-4. View of the holding area for cardiac catheterization with an ECG machine, blood pressure sphygmomanometer, and wall suction. The patient can be comfortably observed in this area following the procedure.

The pack will contain syringes and needles, local anesthetic, basins for flushing solutions, small drapes and towels, towel clamps, scalpels, pressure manifolds and connecting tubings, and the like (see Fig. 1-5). These trays may be made up at the hospital or prepackaged by various suppliers.

Equipment for Sterilization

Steam autoclave sterilization uses superheated high-pressure steam to kill organisms. It is very effective, but most plastic items such as catheters and manifolds cannot withstand the intense heat.

Ethylene oxide sterilization, "gassing," is the most effective technique for heat-sensitive products. Pressures and temperatures used in the gas sterilizer are much lower than are

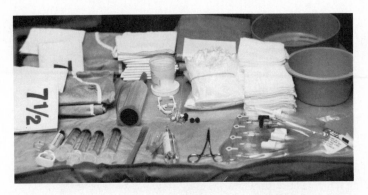

Fig. 1-5. Sterile supplies: syringes, needles, tubing, gauze, injection syringe, gown and gloves, and sterile towels and trays. See text for details.

those used in the autoclave. Gassing and properly ventilating an object take several hours longer than sterilizing with the autoclave method. Also, ethylene oxide is very toxic, and considerable care must be taken when it is used.

Chemical sterilization can be performed by several liquid antiseptic solutions. These chemicals are useful for soaking metal instruments or transducers that are reused frequently in the angiographic suite.

TRAINING REQUIREMENTS
Cardiovascular Technologist Training Requirements in Cardiac Catheterization

Cardiovascular technology is a field recognized by the American Medical Association.

Definition.   The cardiovascular technologist specializing in invasive cardiovascular technology is a health-care professional who, through the use of specific high-techology equipment and at the direction of a qualified physician, performs procedures on patients leading to the diagnosis and treatment of congenital and acquired heart disease and peripheral vascular disease. The technologist is proficient in the use of physiologic analytical equipment during diagnostic and therapeutic procedures. The cardiovascular technologist is trained in advanced life support techniques as the patient population under study is often at increased risk for cardiopulmonary arrest. The technologist, through established methodology of diagnostic examinations, creates a database from which a correct anatomic and physiologic diagnosis may be developed for each patient. The invasive cardiovascular technologist is therefore a highly specialized diagnostician of the various presentations of cardiovascular disease.

Area of practice.   The invasive cardiovascular technologist performs diagnostic procedures involving patients in the invasive cardiovascular laboratory (as well as coronary care and medical/surgical intensive care environments, if needed). The technologist also may assist a qualified physician in the performance of procedures in specialized clinics. The following are specific diagnostic examinations or procedures, but are not all inclusive (or exclusive) to the invasive cardiovascular technologist's scope of practice.

Invasive cardiovascular examinations and procedures

1. Selective vessel and heart chamber pressure recording
2. Selective vessel and chamber blood sampling
    a. Oximetry, carboxy, oxyhemoglobin
    b. Blood gas analysis (pH, Pco_2, Po_2)
    c. Electrolyte content (where suitable equipment is available)
    d. Blood sampling for other diagnostic determinations
        (1) Drug levels (digitalis, etc.)
        (2) Renin and angiotensin levels
        (3) Blood cultures
3. Cardiac output studies
    a. Thermodilution
    b. Dye dilution indicators (green dye, etc.)
    c. Fick determinations
4. Oxygen consumption
    a. Flow-through steady state
    b. Closed system steady state and/or exercise
5. Shunt detection studies
    a. Dye curves
    b. Right heart catheterization with multiple oxygen saturations, Qp/Qs determination
6. Selective contrast angiography
    a. Coronary artery studies

    b. Left ventriculogram (and planimetry of left ventricular volume)

    c. Selective heart chamber and vessel studies for congenital heart disease

    d. Peripheral vascular angiograms

NOTE: All of the above angiograms are performed in conjunction with radiographic film devices including single and biplane cinefluoroscopy, cut-film rapid sequence angiography and rapid sequence spot film cameras (70/105 mm) and are performed by, with the assistance of, or at the direction of a qualified physician.

  7. Electrophysiologic studies (EPS)

    a. Intracardiac atrial and ventricular pacing for zonal refractory periods, activation times, arrhythmia inducibility, arrhythmia and accessory bypass tract detection

    b. Intracardiac mapping

  8. Temporary and permanent transvenous pacemaker insertion

  9. Pericardiocentesis

10. Drug response studies

    a. Hypertension studies

    b. Pulmonary resistance studies

    c. 100% oxygen inhalation studies

    d. Arrhythmia suppression during EPS

    e. Ergonovine for coronary vasospasm

11. Pulmonary arterial wedge catheter placement

12. Balloon atrial septostomy

13. Percutaneous transluminal angioplasty (PTA)

    a. Coronary arteries and/or grafts (percutaneous transluminal angioplasty [PTCA])

    b. Peripheral arteries (PTA)

14. Retrieval of foreign body from the heart or great vessels

15. Transseptal puncture procedures

16. Left ventricular transthoracic punctures

17. Placement of arterial and/or central venous lines

18. Intracoronary thrombolytic infusion for acute myocardial infarction

19. Intraaortic balloon pump counterpulsation

20. Balloon valvuloplasty of pulmonary, mitral, or aortic valves

Any of the previous procedures may be combined with either diagnostic or supportive medications and therapeutic interventions.

Emergency life support.   The cardiovascular technologist is proficient in basic life support techniques as recommended by the American Heart Association.*

1. Techniques of CPR, cardioversion, or defibrillation
2. Management of airway including orotracheal and nasotracheal intubation and/or bag-mask ventilation
3. Proficiency in the preparation and delivery of emergency medications by means of IV line placement and transthoracic infusion, including the medications listed on Appendix II at the request of a qualified physician

Preparation,   inventory,   maintenance,   and   sterile techniques.   The invasive cardiovascular technologist is proficient in the preparation of the patient for all procedures and for the maintenance, inventory, stocking, and sterile preparations of all equipment, parts, catheter devices, and room preparations for each procedure.

1. Information and support to the patient before, during, and after each procedure, including sterile preparation of the patient
2. Cleaning, packaging, and sterilization of all sundry catheterization trays and ancillary area equipment
3. Maintenance of the sterile field during such procedures
4. Preparation, recording, interpreting, and filing of all procedural protocols and reports
5. Ordering of all disposable supplies necessary for each procedure
6. Retrieval of data regarding individual patients and disease entities for clinical and research purposes

Equipment   used   in   the   invasive   cardiovascular laboratory.   The invasive cardiovascular technologist is proficient in the operation and maintenance of all diagnostic and therapeutic equipment used for procedures, including electrical safety for each piece of equipment. The equipment listed below is neither all inclusive nor exclusive to the vari-

---

* American Heart Association: Basic Life support techniques: guidelines (1980 standards), *JAMA* 244(5):453–509, 1980.

ous types and brands of equipment used in the cardiovascular laboratory areas.

1. Physiologic equipment
   a. ECG/pressure recorder/analyzer (with or without computer interface)
   b. Pressure transducer
   c. Electrocardiography
2. Radiographic equipment
   a. Cineangiography magazine
   b. Image intensifier
   c. Television monitor and camera
   d. Photospot camera
   e. Cut film changer
   f. Digital subtraction interface
3. Film processor
   a. Cineangiographic processor
   b. Cut film/photospot film
4. Sensitometer and densitometer for film quality control
5. Cineangiographic film projector (including computer digitizer with left ventriculography analyzers)
6. Blood gas analyzer
7. Oxygen content/saturation analyzer
   a. Lex-O2-con
   b. Van Slyke
8. Cardiac output
   a. Thermodilution computer
   b. Dye dilution technique
      (1) Infusion/withdrawal pump
      (2) Cuvette
      (3) Densitometer
9. Spirometer
10. Contrast media pressure injector
11. Temporary pacemakers
    a. External
    b. Transvenous pacing catheters
    c. Pacemaker driver and connecting cables
12. Tape recorders
    a. Video
    b. FM
13. Intraaortic balloon pumps and consoles
14. Emergency (code) cart equipment including medications and defibrillator

15. Preparation equipment
  a. Cold sterilizers
  b. Gas and steam sterilizers
  c. Ultrasonic sterilizers

Patient and laboratory personnel safety. The invasive cardiovascular technologist is responsible for the radiation protection of patients and laboratory personnel in cooperation with the hospital radiation safety officer. Electrical hazard protection also is maintained through the technologist and the biomedical engineering department. The maintaining of sterility and cleanliness of the procedure equipment and supplies are the technologist's responsibility, including the following:

• Regular ground-fault checks of all electrical equipment
• Regular sterile-batch checks
• Infection control

Environmental safety in the catheterization laboratory. The cardiac catheterization laboratory is a potentially hazardous area if proper safety measures are not followed. There is the constant risk of exposure to radiation, blood and body fluids, and infectious diseases, such as hepatitis and tuberculosis. Laboratory-specific environmental safety plans reduce the risk associated with this environment.

Blood and body fluids. Occupational exposure to blood and body fluids is a serious concern for personnel working in the cardiac catheterization laboratory. The Occupational Safety and Health Administration (OSHA) published the bloodborne pathogen standards in the *Federal Register* (December 6, 1991). The standard outlines specific guidelines that must be followed to protect employees from occupational exposure and is highlighted in Table 1-1.

Bloodborne viruses. Hepatitis B (HBV) and human immunodeficiency virus (HIV) are two bloodborne viruses that pose a risk to health-care workers. These viruses have been found in blood, semen, vaginal secretions, tears, saliva, cerebrospinal fluid, amniotic fluid, breast milk, body cavity fluids, and urine. Blood and equipment contaminated with blood and bloody saline flush solutions pose the greatest risk to cardiac catheterization laboratory personnel.

Modes of transmission by occupational exposure. Transmission of bloodborne viruses can occur when contaminated

1-1.   Highlights of the OSHA standard

The catheterization laboratory should provide
• Information regarding the OSHA standards and the departmental
  exposure control plan
• An explanation of bloodborne diseases
• An explanation of the modes of transmission
• An explanation of the employee's risk category
• An explanation of environmental controls—benefit and limitations
• Rationale for selection of protective equipment being used
• Information on the hepatitis B vaccine
• Explanation of how to report an incident of exposure and the proper
  follow-up procedure

body fluids come in contact with the skin by needles or
through an open sore or small cut or contact with the eyes
or other mucous membranes.

Universal precautions. The goal of the exposure control
plan is to isolate the health-care worker from these hazards.
Universal Precautions is an infection control technique in
which *all* blood and body fluids are treated as if they are
contaminated. The Universal Precaution technique should
be incorporated in the specific exposure control plan for the
cardiac catheterization laboratory.

Environmental assessment. Assess the working environment before writing an exposure control plan. In the catheterization laboratory, procedure-specific hazards exist. Some
of these hazards and methods of protection are listed in
Tables 1-2 and 1-3.

1-2.   Catheterization laboratory hazards

Procedure	Exposure
IV therapy	Needle stick, blood to skin contact
Local anesthesia administration	Needle stick
Arterial puncture	Needle stick, splashing of blood
Catheter insertion/exchange	Splashing of blood to skin or mucous membrane contact
Catheter flushing	Splashing of blood to skin or mucous membrane contact
Catheter removal/groin compression	Splashing of blood to skin or mucous membrane contact
Contact with soiled linen/ equipment	Needle stick, splashing of blood to skin or mucous membrane contact

1-3. Methods of protection

Eye	Glasses with side shields or goggles
Nose/mouth	Masks
Skin	Gloves, fluid-resistant gowns
Parenteral	Proper methods of sharp instruments storage and disposal, do not recap or resheath needles

Eye, nose, and mouth protection. The eyes and nose should be protected from potential splashing of blood and contaminated fluids. Personnel at most risk are the operators and assistant, the circulating personnel, and the person removing the catheter/sheath and holding arterial puncture site pressure. Personnel performing these high-risk tasks should wear glasses or goggles, a face mask, or a face mask with an incorporated plastic eye shield if glasses/goggles are not worn (Fig. 1-6).

Skin protection. Gloves should be worn any time personnel are required to handle supplies or samples that are considered contaminated. Of course, anyone involved in the sterile

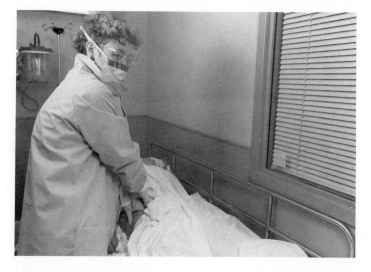

Fig. 1-6. A nurse/technician performing femoral artery compression wears protective gloves, gown, and face mask with shield (satisfying OSHA standards).

procedure would be wearing sterile gloves. Circulating personnel should wear gloves when accepting items being passed from the sterile field. Such items would include used catheters or wires, syringes containing blood for blood gas and saturation analysis, and biopsy specimens. Also, gloves should be worn if a pressure transducer is being flushed with saline that has been contaminated with blood during the case. This point is of particular concern because the saline may not appear to be contaminated. However, it may have been aspirated through the same manifold through which blood has passed, thus producing an invisible contamination.

Glove integrity should be monitored. If personnel are reporting holes or tears in gloves, double gloving or higher-quality gloves should be considered. Also, hand lotions containing petroleum products will compromise latex glove material and should not be used.

Exposed skin should be covered when removing catheters/sheaths and holding puncture site pressure. An inexpensive disposable gown such as an isolation gown or a disposable lab coat should be donned first and the gloves pulled over the sleeves. This technique will minimize exposure to the hands and arms. If the protective clothing becomes contaminated with blood or body fluids, it should be removed immediately and the exposed skin should be washed with soap and water.

Protective clothing worn during procedures should be removed before leaving the department or hospital building.

Equipment consideration. As awareness to the hazards of bloodborne pathogens increases, a variety of protective equipment and instruments is being made available for use in the cardiac catheterization laboratory.

Most companies that make manifolds offer closed drainage systems. This system incorporates a 1000-ml bag in the manifold system, which allows aspirated blood to be flushed directly into a sealed bag. This system reduces the potential exposure during the procedure and at the end of the procedure during cleanup.

Another product to reduce exposure improves on the conventional waste bowl frequently used on the sterile back table (the Backstop, Merit Medical). The closed bowl design allows bloody, fluid-filled syringes to be emptied into the receptacle and prevents backsplashing by incorporating a diaphragmed slot in which the syringe can be inserted and emptied.

Employer responsibility

HBV VACCINATION. The OSHA standard states that HBV vaccination must be made available to all employees with potential for occupational exposure as a prerequisite of employment. If the employee declines vaccination, it is mandatory that a HBV vaccine declination is signed.

RISK CATEGORY. The OSHA standard requires employers to inform employees of a job's risk category upon employment. Table 1-4 outlines the risk categories. Most, if not all, catheterization laboratory staff will fall into category I.

EMPLOYEE TRAINING. The employer must provide proper training to employees regarding bloodborne pathogens and the OSHA standards. Records must be kept documenting the dates, content, name of person conducting the training, and the names of the persons attending the session. These records must be maintained at least 3 years. The training should include the information in Table 1-1.

ELIMINATING CARELESS PRACTICES REDUCES RISKS. Often in the cardiac catheterization laboratory employees are exposed due to lack of attention to procedures and carelessness. All incidents of employee exposure should be properly documented. A periodic review should be conducted to determine ways to eliminate future exposure.

Careless practices that should be avoided in the catheterization laboratory include
- Careless disposal of blood in syringes into the back table waste bowl, resulting in excessive splashing
- Throwing of bloody gauze 4 × 4s into trash receptacles

1-4. Risk categories

Risk category I	Employment and procedures will require exposure to blood/body fluids
Risk category II	Employment and procedures may require exposure to blood/body fluids
Risk category III	Employment and procedures usually do not require exposure to blood/body fluids

- Improperly handled guidewires and catheters that may spring out of the saline bowl and cause splashing
- Needles that are not properly returned to a needle counter on the back table

Extra attention and care in such areas will prevent careless exposure of staff.

Summary. Personnel working in the cardiac catheterization laboratory should make every effort to reduce the risk of exposure to blood and body fluids. Department-specific exposure control plans will help minimize the chance of occupation exposure to contaminated agents.

Radiation Safety The catheterization laboratory environment should be made as safe as possible for the staff and patient. Because radiation cannot be seen, felt, or heard, it is easy to become lackadaisical about proper protective measures.

Standards for radiation protection in the cardiac catheterization laboratory have been published by the Society for Cardiac Angiography and Intervention. Four principles should be kept in mind when developing radiation exposure control procedures.

1. The less exposure, the less chance of absorbed energy biologic interaction.
2. No known level of ionizing radiation is a permissible dose or absolutely safe.
3. Radiation exposure is cumulative. There is no washout phenomenon.
4. All participants in the cardiac catheterization laboratory have voluntarily accepted some degree of radiation exposure, but they are obliged to minimize and reduce risks to other personnel and themselves.

The source of radiation in the cardiac catheterization laboratory is the primary x-ray beam emanating from the undertable x-ray tube upward through the patient and onto the image intensifier. Scatter of this beam exposes all subjects to radiation in a dose geometrically inverse to the distance from the source. Radiation scatter is increased when the angle of the tube is set obliquely. A high degree of angulation with large obliquities increases the amount of radiation scatter (see Fig. 4-43). Acrylic shields and table-mounted lead aprons should be used to reduce the amount of scatter.

Fluoroscopy generates approximately one-fifth the x-ray

exposure of cineangiography. The increased use of cineangiography for complex catheterization procedures has increased to total exposure to radiation and should be a consideration in procedures requiring extensive intracardiac manipulation, such as angioplasty or valvuloplasty.

Every cardiac catheterization laboratory should have a department-specific radiation safety policy. This policy should include:

1. Routine monitoring of personnel radiation exposure
2. Continuing education programs for personnel on radiation safety
3. Making personnel aware of the risks associated with radiation exposure
4. Requiring protective equipment be worn by all personnel
5. Procedures to check safety of all equipment (x-ray dose output, integrity of lead aprons, thyroid shields, etc.)

Lead eyeglasses. It has been known that a single x-ray exposure of 200 R can produce cataract formation in humans. Eyeglasses made of 0.5 to 0.75-mm lead-equivalent glass should be worn by personnel exposed to radiation on a daily basis (Fig. 1-7). Glasses containing 0.50 mm of lead offer four times the protection of regular eyeglasses. Glasses with

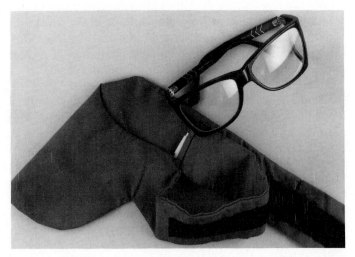

Fig. 1-7. Radiation safety glasses and thyroid shield should be worn by all personnel inside the catheterization suite.

photochromic lenses offer two times the protection of regular eyeglasses. Plastic lenses offer no eye protection from radiation.

It is important that radiation-protective glasses contain a wraparound side shield. Glasses with proper fitting side shields are good not only for radiation protection but also provide protection from blood products splashing into the eyes.

Radiation badges. All personnel should wear a radiation-monitoring badge when in the catheterization laboratory. To ensure accurate readings, badges should always remain on the person to whom it is assigned. Badges should never be left lying on a counter or attached to a lead apron in an area where there is potential radiation exposure. When badges are not being used, they should be stored in an area away from any potential radiation exposure.

At the end of each month, exposed badges are collected and sent for analysis. A monthly exposure report indicates each staff member's exposure for that month. This information should be posted in the laboratory so that each staff member can monitor his or her individual exposure. The report should be reviewed each month by the laboratory medical director as well as the institution's radiation safety officer.

Radiation dose limitation. Although no known threshold for radiation exposure exists to define specific risks, the NCRP (National Council on Radiation Protection and Measurements) has provided specific guidelines. No dose of greater than 3 rem should be allowed over a 3-month period.

Definitions of radiation units.

1. Roentgen (R) is the measure of ionization delivered to a specific point (exposure). One chest x-ray equals 3 to 5 mR.
2. Radiation absorbed dose (rad) is the amount of radiation energy deposited per unit mass of tissue. The amount of absorbed dose per given exposure is dependent upon tissue type. For example, for soft tissue, 1 R = 1 rad; for bone 1, R = 4 rad (i.e., greater absorption).
3. Radiation equivalent dose in man (rem) is used to express the biologic impact of a given exposure. For x-radiation, 1 rad = 1 rem.

Methods to limit exposure.

1. Wear leaded aprons (preferably wraparound): ≥0.5 mm thickness provides 80% protection.
2. Limit the fluoroscopic/cineangiographic time (cineangiographic time produces much greater exposure than fluoroscopic time).
3. Use collimators.
4. Reduce the distance between the x-ray source and patient.
5. Maximize the distance between the x-ray source and the operator and assitants.
6. Limit the milliamperes per kilovolts as much as possible for an adequate image.
7. Use slower panning, and provide good initial angiographic setup. Angled views almost double the radiation.
8. Keep the image magnification as low as possible.
9. Use extra shielding (leaded thyroid guards, lead glasses, and protective table shields).

Radiation exposure is greater during agioplasty than during diagnostic catheterization. If the protective shields are employed carefully, the radiation exposure for single- and double-vessel angioplasty as compared to diagnostic catheterization may be comparable. However, it should be understood that radiation exposures are generally higher for these procedures, especially when biplane angiography is performed.

Lead aprons. Lead aprons should contain 0.5-mm-thick lead lining. When properly cared for, an apron will provide years of service. However, the lead lining can crack or become torn. This is usually caused by careless handling or improper storage. Aprons should be placed in an appropriate hanger or storage rack after use. Repeatedly throwing an apron over a chair or stretcher may damage the lead lining (Fig. 1-8).

To assess the integrity of the lead, aprons should be fluoroscopied at least once a year. Documentation should be kept regarding the integrity of each apron. To do this, each apron should contain some sort of identification (number, color, name, etc.).

Due to the nature of work in the catheterization laboratory, personnel are not always able to maintain a frontal position to the x-ray beam. Therefore, wraparound lead

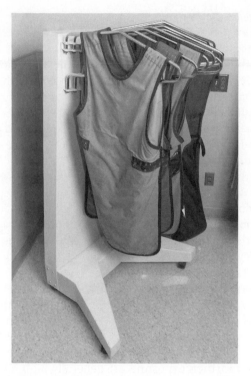

Fig. 1-8. One proper storage method to prevent lead aprons from developing cracks, which reduce radiation protection. All aprons should be hung up when not in use.

aprons should be considered. Aprons should be long enough to cover the long bones (femur) and should extend to the knee or just below the knee. Because proper fit is important, many companies will take measurements in order to ensure a proper fit.

Thyroid shields. Because the thyroid gland is particularly sensitive to ionizing radiation, a lead thyroid shield should be worn in the presence of ionizing radiation. Like aprons, thyroid shields should be properly stored and the lead periodically checked radiographically.

Responsibilities of laboratory management personnel

1. Budget and finance
2. Develop policies and procedures

3. Establish laboratory standards
4. Develop quality assurance programs
5. Recordkeeping
6. Develop training and continuing education programs

Physician Training Requirements in Cardiac Catheterization

Diagnostic catheterization in adults.   The following are the proposed physician requirements for certification in the performance of cardiac catheterization. The physician should spend a minimum of 12 months in the cardiac catheterization laboratory. The trainee will acquire a clear understanding of the indications, limitations, complications, and medical and surgical implications of the findings of cardiac catheterization and angiography. This background includes an understanding of the pathophysiology and the ability to interpret a wide variety of hemodynamic and angiographic data in adults. (Pediatric catheterization requires a special training track.) All trainees will receive basic instruction in radiation safety, use of fluoroscopy, and radiologic anatomy. The trainee will learn to perform right and left heart catheterization by the cutdown and/or percutaneous routes. Temporary right ventricular pacing, endo-myocardial biopsy, pericardiocentesis, and standard ventriculography and coronary angiography will be performed.

A working knowledge of catheterization laboratory equipment, including physiologic recorders, pressure transducers, blood gas analyzers, image intensifiers and other x-ray equipment, cineangiographic processing, and quality control of films, will be emphasized for those seeking advanced catheterization laboratory experience.

All trainees will be exposed to adult patients with valvular, congenital, cardiomyopathic, pericardial, and ischemic heart disease. Studies in acutely ill patients (cardiogenic shock, acute myocardial infarction, or unstable angina) are currently a routine part of invasive cardiology. Techniques of myocardial biopsy, transseptal catheterization, and intraaortic balloon counterpulsation require advanced, specialized training. At the end of the cardiac catheterization training period, a trainee should have performed at least 300 catheterization procedures; in 150 of them the trainee should have been the primary operator.

Interventional cardiology (PTCA, valvuloplasty). Because the potential for harm is greater with interventional techniques, only those individuals highly skilled and thoroughly trained in the fundamentals of diagnostic catheterization should undertake this course of specialized training. To meet the proposed training standards of the Society for Cardiac Angiography and of the Task Force of the American College of Cardiology for advanced cardiac catheterization procedures such as angioplasty, at least 1 year of additional training in the cardiac catheterization laboratory is recommended.

SUGGESTED READINGS

Abrams HL, editor: *Coronary arteriography: a practical approach*, Boston, 1983, Little, Brown.

Conti CR, Faxon DP, Gruentzig A, Gunnar RM, Lesch M, Reeves TJ: Task force III: training in cardiac catheterization, *J Am Coll Cardiol* 7:1205–1206, 1986.

Davidson CJ, Hlatky M, Morris KG, Pieper K, Skelton TN, Schwab SJ, Bashore TM: Cardiovascular and renal toxicity of a nonionic radiographic contrast agent after cardiac catheterization: a prospective trial, *Ann Intern Med* 110:119–124, 1989.

Douglas JS, Pepine CJ, Block PC, Brinker JA, Johnson WL Jr, Klinke WP, Levin DC, Mullins CE, Nissen SE, Topol EJ, Ellyot DJ, Vetrovec GW, Vogel JHK: Recommendations for development and maintenance of competence in coronary interventional procedures, *J Am Coll Cardiol* 22:629–631, 1993.

Friesinger GC, Adams DF, Bourassa MG, Carlsson E, Elliott LP, Gessner IH, Greenspan RH, Grossman W, Judkins MP, Kennedy JW, Sheldon WC: Optimal resources for examination of the heart and lungs: cardiac catheterization and radiographic facilities, *Circulation* 68:893A–930A, 1983.

Greenberger PA, Patterson R, Simon R, Lieberman P, Wallace W: Pretreatment of high-risk patients requiring radiographic contrast media studies, *J Allergy Clin Immunol* 67:185–187, 1981.

Grossman W, editor: *Cardiac catheterization and angiography*, ed 3, Philadelphia, 1986, Lea & Febiger.

Heiss HW: Werner Forssmann: a German problem with the Nobel prize. *Clin Cardiol* 15:547–549, 1992.

Johnson LW, Moore RJ, Balter S: Reviews of radiation safety in the cardiac catheterization laboratory, *Cardiac Cath and CV Diagn*, 25, 186–194, 1992.

Kelly JF, Patterson R, Lieberman P, Mathison DA, Stevenson DD: Radiographic contrast media studies in high-risk patients, *J Allergy Clin Immunol* 62:181–184, 1978.

Krone J and Morton MJ, editors: *Complications of cardiac catheterization and angiography: prevention and management*, Mount Kisco, NY, 1989, Futura Publishing.

Lasser EC, Berry CC, Talner LB, Santini LC, Lang EK, Gerger FH, Stolberg HO: Pretreatment with corticosteroids to alleviate reactions to intravenous contrast material, *N Engl J Med* 317:845–849, 1987.

Lieberman P, Siegle RL, Taylor WW: Anaphylactoid reactions to iodinated contrast material, *J Allergy Clin Immunol* 62:174–180, 1978.

Mudd JG: Should coronary angiograms be reviewed with patients? *Am J Cardiol* 57:501, 1986.

OSHA standards, Friday, Dec 6, 1991. 29 CER Part 1910.1030 Occupational exposure to bloodborne pathogens; final rule, *Federal Register*, 45(235):64175–64182.

Pepine CJ: *Diagnostic and therapeutic cardiac catheterization*, Baltimore, 1989, Williams & Wilkins.

Ryan TJ, Faxon DP, Gunnar RM, Kennedy JW, King SB III, Loop FD, Peterson KL, Reeves TJ, Williams DO, Winters WL Jr: Guidelines for percutaneous transluminal coronary angioplasty: a report of the American College of Cardiology/American Heart Association Task Force on Assessment of Diagnostic and Therapeutic Cardiovascular Procedures (subcommittee on percutaneous transluminal coronary angioplasty), *Circulation* 78:486–502, 1988.

Schwab SJ, Hlatky MA, Pieper KS, Davidson CJ, Morris KG, Skelton TN, Bashore TM: Contrast nephrotoxicity: a randomized controlled trial of a nonionic and an ionic radiographic contrast agent, *N Engl J Med* 320:149–153, 1989.

Shehadi WH, Toniolo G: Adverse reactions to contrast media: a report from the Committee on Safety of Contrast Media of the International Society of Radiology, 137:299–302, 1980.

Spittell JA Jr, Creager MA, Dorros G, Isner JM, Nanda NC, Ochsner JL, Wexler L, Young JR: Recommendations for peripheral transluminal angioplasty: training and facilities, *J Am Coll Cardiol* 21:546–548, 1993.

Spittell JA Jr, Creager MA, Dorros G, Isner JM, Nanda NC, Ochsner JL, Wexler L, Young JR: Recommendations for training in vascular medicine, *J Am Coll Cardiol* 22:626–628, 1993.

Stewart WJ, McSweeney SM, Kellett MA, Faxon DP, Ryan TJ: Increased risk of severe protamine reactions in NPH insulin-dependent diabetics undergoing cardiac catheterization, *Circulation* 70:788–792, 1984.

Weaver WF, Myler RK, Sheldon WC, Huston JT, Judkins MP, and the Laboratory Performance Standards Committee, Society for Cardiac Angiography and Interventions: Guidelines for free-standing cardiac catheterization laboratories, *Cathet Cardiovasc Diagn* 11:109–112, 1985.

Yang SS, Bentivoglio LG, Maranhao V, Goldberg H, editors: *Cardiac catheterization data to hemodynamic parameters*, ed 3, Philadelphia, 1978, FA Davis.

Zweiman B, Mishkin MM, Hildreth EA: An approach to the performance of contrast studies in contrast material-reactive persons, *Ann Intern Med* 83:159–162, 1975.

2

ARTERIAL AND VENOUS ACCESS

Ubeydullah Deligonul, Robert Roth, and Michael Flynn

The most common catheterization problem involves the initial access to the circulation. Although often relegated to the novice, this important step deserves full study. Because most aspects of cardiac catheterization are learned through apprentice-type experience, watching, reading, and doing under supervision are the keys to success.

This section of the handbook will not describe every detail but highlight the key points, some of which may not seem important to the uninitiated. Full and detailed descriptions of each technique are available elsewhere.

Entry into the circulation is generally the only painful part of the catheterization procedure. For best patient response, adequate local anesthesia should be provided using a gentle approach. Pain during entry into the vessel may cause vagal reaction or spasm, prolonging the procedure and potentially causing more significant complications.

The site and type of access (percutaneous or cutdown) are determined by the planned investigation and anticipated anatomic and pathologic conditions of the patient's cardiovascular system. A review of previous procedures and difficulties encountered should be obtained from old reports if possible. Assessment of all peripheral pulses is mandatory.

Indications for Alternative Routes to Femoral Arterial Catheterization

Claudication
Absent dorsalis pedis and posterior tibialis pulses
Absent popliteal pulses
Femoral bruits
Absent femoral pulses
Prior femoral artery graft surgery
Extensive inguinal scarring from radiation therapy, surgery, or
    prior catheterization
Excessively tortuous or diseased iliac arteries
Severe back pain, inability to lie flat
Patient request

PERCUTANEOUS FEMORAL APPROACH
Percutaneous Femoral Artery Puncture

Percutaneous femoral arterial catheterization is the most widely used technique. In patients with significant obstructive disease in the distal aorta, iliofemoral, or popliteotibial systems as indicated by a history of claudication, signs of chronic arterial insufficiency, diminished or absent pulses, or bruits over the iliofemoral area, alternate entry sites should be used rather than risking further impairment of the arterial circulation in the legs. The presence of arterial conduit grafts or previous balloon angioplasty of the iliofemoral system is not an absolute contraindication for femoral percutaneous technique. Graft puncture has been shown to be safe provided special care has been taken (although generally an alternative route should be selected).

In patients with diminished pedal pulses the femoral arterial approach using small-size (5 to 6 French*) sheaths and catheters is possible. However, even subtotal occlusions in the femoral artery site may cause a significant drop in distal perfusion pressure and blood supply to the already compromised foot. A small embolus in this patient may not be tolerated as in patients with patent distal vessels (see the box above).

The femoral percutaneous arterial entry is explained as

---

* The term *French size* converts the diameter in millimeters to standard numbered sizes: 1 French = 0.33 mm diameter (see Table 2-1).

follows. Usually the patient's right femoral artery is entered with the operator standing at the right side of the patient.

Locate the artery (Fig. 2-1).   The inguinal (groin) skin crease is located. The inguinal ligament, which lies directly beneath the inguinal skin crease from the iliac crest to pubis, is palpated. In obese patients the inguinal skin crease may be lower than the inguinal ligament, and there also may be several skin folds below and above the inguinal ligament. Therefore it is important to locate the inguinal ligament.

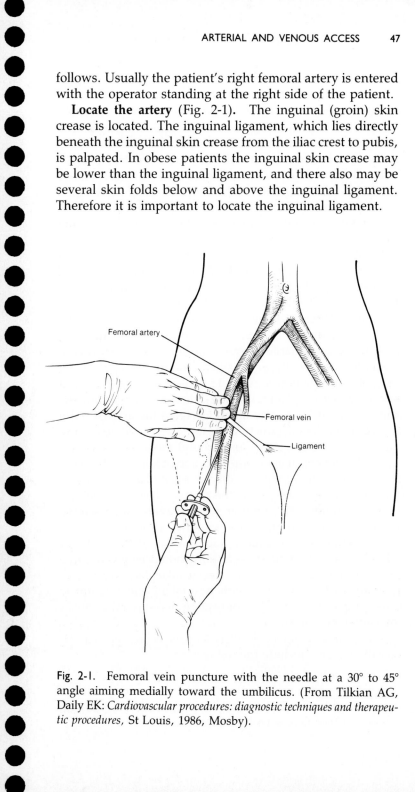

Fig. 2-1.   Femoral vein puncture with the needle at a 30° to 45° angle aiming medially toward the umbilicus. (From Tilkian AG, Daily EK: *Cardiovascular procedures: diagnostic techniques and therapeutic procedures,* St Louis, 1986, Mosby).

The femoral artery crosses the inguinal ligament at an imaginary point dividing the ligament into $\frac{1}{3}$ medial and $\frac{2}{3}$ lateral portions. The femoral artery is a tube approximately 1 cm in diameter running across the inguinal ligament. As in any tube the center line is the highest point with the edges of the tube lower on each side. The femoral artery pulse is located with middle and index fingers with the fingers placed parallel to the long axis of the femoral artery. The index finger palpates the artery 1 to 2 cm below the inguinal ligament where the site of actual arterial entry with the needle will be.

Local anesthesia.   With a 25-gauge needle the skin is infiltrated superficially with 2 to 3 ml 1% lidocaine 1 to 2 cm distal to where the index finger is placed as described above. This point will be the skin entry site. In obese patients with thick subcutaneous tissue, the entry site should be slightly lower to assure a ≤45° entry angle of the needle. In obese patients, because large amounts of lidocaine may obscure the pulse, repeatedly inject small amounts instead. Next, using a 22-gauge needle, 10 to 15 ml lidocaine is introduced into deep tissue planes. During lidocaine infiltration, left and middle index fingers should palpate the arterial pulse to avoid accidental puncture of the artery and to ensure infiltration of tissue above and around the artery.

Gentle aspiration before the injection of lidocaine is essential to make sure that the needle tip is not in a blood vessel. Inserting the needle first to the deepest level desired and then continuing infiltration at several layers may decrease the patient's discomfort. Local anesthesia should cover the whole depth of the expected skin-to-artery path. Sufficient lidocaine (about 20 ml 1% solution) should be given 2 to 3 minutes for the full anesthetic effect to take place. HINT: Give lidocaine early; while the anesthetic is taking effect, complete other preparations such as connecting pressure lines, flushing catheters, and the like.

Although rare, lidocaine allergies have been reported. Alternative agents include the following:*

---

* From Tilkian AG, Daily EK: *Cardiovascular procedures: diagnostic techniques and therapeutic procedures,* St Louis, 1986, Mosby.

Group I
Procaine (ester prototype)

Benoxinate
(Dorsacaine)
Benzocaine
Butacaine (Butyn)
Butethamine
(Monocaine)

Butylaminobenzoate
(Butesin)
Chloroprocaine
(Nesacaine)
Procaine (Novocain)
Tetracaine (Pontocaine)

Group II
Lidocaine (amide prototype)

Amydricaine (Alypin)
Bupivacaine (Marcaine)
Cyclomethycaine
(Surfacaine)
Dibucaine (Nupercaine)
Dimethisoquin (Quotane)
Diperodon (Diothane)
Dyclonine (Dyclone)
Etidocaine (Duranest)
Hexylcaine (Cyclaine)
Mepivacaine (Carbocaine)

Oxethazaine (Oxaine)
Phenacaine (Holocaine)
Piperocaine
(Metycaine)
Pramoxine
(Tronothane)
Prilocaine (Citanest)
Proparacaine
(Ophthaine)
Pyrrocaine (Endocaine)

Skin entry. With the left-hand fingers placed over the artery as described above, a skin incision of 2 to 4 mm length is made with a #11 scalpel blade, holding the blade perpendicular to the skin and penetrating 2 to 3 mm into the subcutaneous tissue 1 to 2 cm below the expected point of actual arterial entry.

Subcutaneous tunnel. A subcutaneous tunnel is made with blunt dissection using straight forceps. This channel makes the catheter/sheath entry easier and, more important, permits blood to drain to the outside of the leg after the catheters have been removed. While creating the channel, it is important to avoid extensive disruption of skin and subcutaneous tissue because these are the natural barriers to infection.

Arterial puncture (Fig. 2-2). Single anterior arterial wall entry technique is preferred. This is especially important in patients being treated with anticoagulants (e.g., heparin), antiplatelet agents, or thrombolytic agents. The original Seldinger double wall puncture technique will not be explained. Single wall technique begins with the left-hand fingers positioned over the femoral artery as described above. The arte-

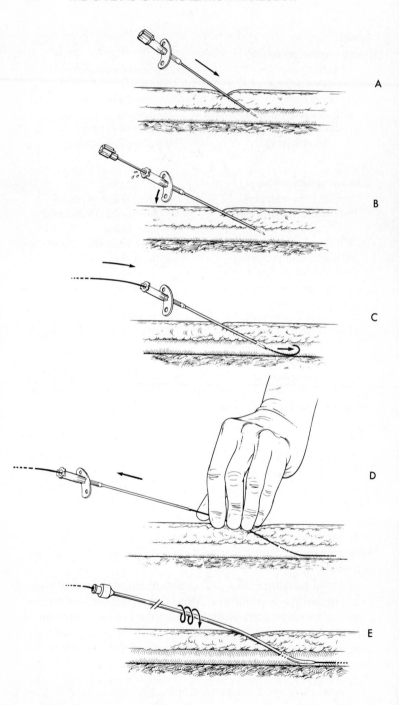

rial needle hub is held between the index and middle fingers of the right hand (like holding a pencil) with the needle tip bevel directed upward. The needle is introduced through the skin incision and advanced slowly toward the artery at a 30° to 45° angle with the horizontal plane. Too vertical an entry into the artery creates problems in advancing the guidewire and promotes sheath and catheter kinking. The pulsation may be felt when the needle contacts the arterial wall. A slight resistance to the needle can be felt as it passes through the arterial wall. At this point a jet of blood from the needle hub confirms arterial puncture. The immediate, strong spurt of pulsatile arterial blood should be maintained by holding the needle hub stable with the left-hand fingers. Resting the left wrist on the patient's thigh is helpful. The J-tipped guidewire is straightened and introduced into the needle with the right hand. The wire should be introduced only when good pulsatile blood flow is present.

Guidewire insertion. The guidewire is advanced gently into the artery. A soft J guidewire is the safest. Although straight-tipped guidewires have been used, the potential for subintimal dissection or tearing of the blood vessel wall is high. The wire should move without resistance. If resistance is encountered, the wire is pulled out and pulsatile blood return confirmed. Fluoroscopy should be used frequently to check wire movement. Repositioning of the needle may be necessary if the wire cannot be advanced freely. Sometimes the needle tip may partially penetrate the posterior wall. In this case there is good blood return, but the wire cannot be advanced because it is directed into the posterior wall rather than the arterial lumen. Withdrawing the needle 1 to 2 mm

---

Fig. 2-2. Basic procedure for the Seldinger technique. **A,** The vessel is punctured with the needle at a 30° to 40° angle. **B,** The stylet is removed and free blood flow is observed; the angle of the needle is then reduced. **C,** The flexible tip of the guidewire is passed through the needle into the vessel. **D,** The needle is removed over the wire while firm pressure is applied at the site. **E,** The tip of the catheter is passed over the wire and advanced into the vessel with a rotating motion. (From Tilkian AG, Dailey EK: *Cardiovascular procedures; diagnostic techniques and therapeutic procedures,* St Louis, 1986, Mosby.)

usually solves this problem. Care must be taken to puncture the artery close to the midline of the anterior wall. Puncturing the lateral arterial wall may create a problem in advancing the guidewire or, worse, controlling bleeding after the procedure.

If the tip of the arterial needle is not in the artery's long axis, the guidewire may be directed toward the wall rather than the lumen, impeding guidewire passage, despite excellent blood return. In this case the wire is withdrawn into the needle, and the needle hub is moved a few millimeters laterally or medially after which the guidewire is slowly readvanced. With this maneuver it is important not to move the needle hub excessively in either direction, slicing the arterial lumen. In the case of a too vertical (>45° angle) entry into the artery, as is sometimes encountered in obese patients, lowering the needle hub several millimeters may improve the artery/needle tip alignment and permit easier guidewire passage.

Another guidewire problem may be encountered if the puncture is made too low in the superficial femoral artery. In this case the needle is removed, and after obtaining adequate hemostasis, the puncture is attempted at a higher level.

If it is not possible to advance the wire or if the needle comes out of the artery during these manipulations, the needle is withdrawn and pressure applied over the puncture site for 3 to 5 minutes to ensure hemostasis. The procedure is then repeated using a slightly different angle or direction. If the artery is not encountered, the needle is again completely withdrawn and advanced in a different direction. Because of the sharp edge of the needle used for single wall entry, the direction of the needle generally should not be changed once the needle tip is in the subcutaneous tissue.

From guidewire to catheter insertion.   If there is no resistance, the guidewire is advanced several centimeters. The guidewire is advanced further into the abdominal aorta using fluoroscopy. Fluoroscopy during guidewire advancement through the iliac artery identifies large arterial plaques as well as excessive tortuosity that will complicate later catheter manipulation. As noted earlier, use of a J-tipped soft spring guidewire is recommended because a straight wire may pass under a plaque resulting in dissection. After the guidewire is well positioned in the aorta, the arterial needle can be removed. Apply firm pressure over the puncture site (to control bleeding) with the left-hand fingers while removing the needle from the skin and maintaining puncture site pressure. Grasp the guidewire firmly with the finger tips to avoid accidental removal of the wire from the artery. An assistant may help at this point to withdraw the needle over the wire and wipe the wire clean with a wet gauze.

Use of a sheath assembly (Fig. 2-3).   A catheter sheath is used in many laboratories. The advantages of a sheath include single arterial entry with increased patient comfort and limitation of the number of catheter exchanges through the artery. The sheath also maintains constant arterial access. An accidental removal of the guidewire by an enthusiastic assistant will not result in loss of arterial access. In addition, arterial access may be maintained for alternative procedures or later therapeutic interventions (e.g., PTCA). The alternative of leaving the catheter in without a sheath during decision making is acceptable. The incidence of complications and hematoma either with or without a sheath appears to be similar, although in the experience of many laboratories, the patient's comfort is greater with the sheath.

The sheath/dilator assembly has a valved end with a side arm. *Unvalved* sheaths *should not be used* because they leak and arterial pressure around a catheter cannot be measured through the side arm. A catheter one French size smaller than the sheath size is necessary for satisfactory side arm pressure recording. After guidewire insertion into the artery the assistant then advances the sheath/dilator assembly over the wire, holding the guidewire straight and stable. The operator introduces the sheath/dilator assembly into the artery by firmly holding it close to the tip, making clockwise and counterclockwise half rotations, and applying firm advancing pressure (see Fig. 2-3). The sheath should not be advanced if much resistance is encountered. The guidewire should be held straight and stable because otherwise it may kink at the site of the sheath tip. After the sheath is inserted completely, the sheath hub is held firmly in place and the dilator and guidewire are removed. Two to three milliliters of blood is aspirated from the side arm of the sheath, and the sheath is flushed with heparinized saline solution. The

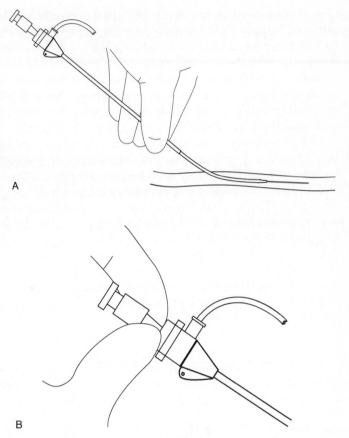

Fig. 2-3. Method of introducing valve sheath into artery. **A,** Valve sheath is advanced over a guidewire. **B, C,** Obturator is removed from the valve. **D,** Stylet can be inserted to plug valve after procedure. Arrows indicate position of sewing rings to attach valve to skin should prolonged insertion be required. (Courtesy of Cordis Corporation, Miami, FL.) *Continued on page 55.*

arterial pressure can be checked immediately by connecting a pressure manifold to the side arm of the sheath. After each catheter removal the sheath should be aspirated and flushed.

Patient's awareness note.   Three steps may be associated with pain and vagal reaction: (1) initial administration of lidocaine; (2) arterial needle insertion; (3) sheath assembly advancement. The operators should be listening to the heart

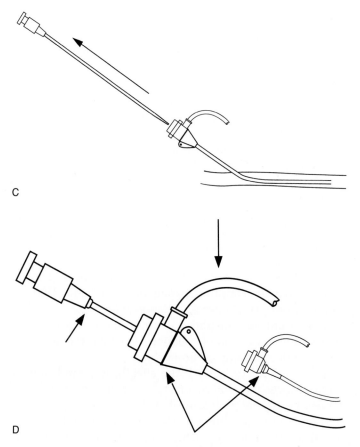

Fig. 2-3. *Continued*

rate monitor and feeling the strength of the arterial pulse to detect early vagal responses. Remember, vasovagal reaction can occur with no change in heart rate, most commonly in the elderly.

Ultrasound-facilitated arterial and venous access. Standard access may be difficult to obtain in patients who have altered anatomy or scarring secondary to prior surgical procedures (i.e., peripheral vascular surgery, multiple prior catheterization, or prior CPS systems). Arterial and venous access may be achieved with either ultrasonic direct visualization (SiteRite) or with Doppler-assisted differentiation of high or low-velocity flow (Smart Needle).

Hemostasis after sheath and catheter removal.   After the catheterization has been completed, blood pressure is observed, and the catheter is removed. The sheath is aspirated and flushed to clear the thrombi. The patient is transferred to the holding area on a stretcher. If heparin has been given during the procedure, reversal with protamine sulfate (25 to 50 mg) usually is given before sheath removal; administration of this dose should take no less than 5 minutes. Caution should be used in giving protamine to patients receiving NPH insulin (see Chapter 1). Protamine reactions include the following:

• Shaking
• Flushing
• Chills
• Back, chest, or flank pain
• Vasomotor collapse

Treatment for protamine reaction. Treatment for protamine reactions involves symptom management with 2 mg IV morphine or 25 mg IV Demerol, sedation with 25 to 50 mg IV Benadryl, fluid administration, and support of low blood pressure due to vasomotor collapse. Usually these reactions are self-limited, lasting <1 hour.

Sheath removal. To remove the sheath, left-hand fingers are placed over the femoral artery as described previously. Because the arterial puncture site is higher (more proximal) than the skin incision, the fingers should be placed over the femoral artery above the actual puncture site. While firm pressure is applied, the sheath is removed gently from the leg, taking care not to crush the sheath and "strip" clot into the distal artery. A small spurt of blood purges the arterial site of retained thrombi. Manual pressure is held firmly for 15 to 20 minutes (5 minutes of full pressure, 5 minutes of 75% pressure, 5 minutes of 50% pressure, and 5 minutes of 25% pressure). In patients receiving antiplatelet treatment (e.g., aspirin), 20 to 30 minutes of puncture site compression may be necessary. During pressure application, pedal pulses are checked every 2 to 3 minutes. A diminished pulse is acceptable during full pressure application, but the distal pulses should not be obliterated completely. If the pulse is absent during compression, the pressure over the artery should be slightly decreased periodically to allow distal circulation.

Some laboratories employ mechanical clamps to assist in puncture site hemostasis. The clamp is effective but must be applied carefully by a trained individual and must be monitored frequently for misalignment, bleeding, or excessive pressure with limb ischemia.

Recently, special collagen plugs that can be delivered directly over the arterial puncture site via a special sheath system have been shown to reduce the time to obtain hemostasis. This device may especially be helpful in anticoagulated patients (Fig. 2-4).

Hematoma monitoring. After 15 to 20 minutes of pressure, the hand is removed slowly and the area is inspected for 1 to 2 minutes for hematoma or bleeding. In obese, hypertensive, or elderly female patients and patients with aortic insufficiency, it may be difficult to obtain hemostasis. In some patients (e.g., those who are obese or who have large thighs), more than 500 ml of blood can be lost before the patient or nurse identifies the problem. For this same reason, a large opaque occlusive dressing over the puncture site is not recommended. Patients at high risk for groin hematoma and arterial complications who may need longer pressure application include the following:
- Obese patients
- Patients with hypertension
- Elderly
- Women
- Patients with aortic insufficiency
- Patients who have undergone prior puncture
- Patients with advanced peripheral atherosclerosis
- Patients who suffer from coagulopathy or those taking anticoagulants or antiplatelets

Firm three-finger pressure should be enough to control most femoral bleeding. Occasionally a rolled gauze pack may be placed over the artery to the groin and pressure applied by the palm of the hand. Standing on a short stool permits upper body weight to be used for pressure application.

In patients with low cardiac output, mitral stenosis, or cardiomyopathy with a small pulse pressure, the femoral artery can be obliterated easily. In these patients the distal pulses should be checked more frequently and less pressure applied to the groin.

After hemostasis is obtained the area is cleaned with an

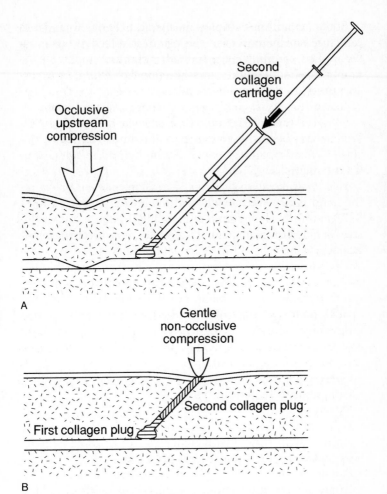

Fig. 2-4. **A,** Application of the second plug (100 mg collagen) through the applicator sheath, filling the space between the first plug and the skin. **B,** The applicator sheath is removed after both plugs are placed. Upstream compression of the artery can be stopped. (Courtesy of Datascope, Inc.)

antiseptic solution. A sterile tape or clear porous dressing is applied. Large pressure dressings or sandbags are not used routinely. A large occlusive dressing will obscure bleeding and possibly delay identification of a growing hematoma. While holding pressure, the clinical findings may be discussed (by the physician) and postcatheterization instructions reviewed.

If the femoral artery and vein are both used, ensure arterial hemostasis first and then remove the venous sheath to decrease the risk of arteriovenous fistula formation. Also, preservation of venous access for the first 15 minutes of arterial compression may provide a useful means of treating a vagal reaction should the peripheral IV inadvertently be lost.

Postcatheterization patient instructions. Depending on the catheter/sheath size, patients are kept at bed rest for 6 to 8 hours after femoral artery puncture. With small-diameter catheters (i.e., 5 French), shorter times (<4 hours) can be used. The patient is given the following instructions:

1. Keep head down.
2. Hold groin site when coughing.
3. Keep punctured leg straight.
4. Stay in bed.
5. Drink fluids.
6. Call nurse for assistance if there is bleeding or chest pain.

Percutaneous Femoral Vein Puncture

The femoral vein is located approximately 1 cm medial to the femoral artery; sometimes it is located partially behind the artery. The femoral arterial pulse is the landmark for the femoral vein. The procedure for femoral vein percutaneous entry involves the following steps.

Locate femoral vein.   The femoral artery pulse is located as described previously. If arterial and venous puncture is planned, the area infiltrated by lidocaine must be wide enough to provide adequate anesthesia to both puncture sites.

Skin entry.   The skin incision is made at the same level as the arterial skin entry site, but 0.5 to 1.0 cm medial and slightly distal to it. Because vein puncture may be successful only after several attempts, the skin incision may be made after the wire has been placed in the vein.

Vein puncture.   Because venous pressure is low, it may be difficult to see unassisted back bleeding from the needle on entry. A 10- or 20-ml syringe with 5 ml saline is attached to the Seldinger or Cook needle and gently aspirated during needle advancement. While the femoral artery pulse is palpated by the left-hand fingers, the needle is inserted through the skin at a 30° to 45° angle to the horizontal plane. The needle tip is introduced 0.5 to 1.0 cm medial to the artery.

(REMEMBER: N-A-V = nerve, artery, vein; i.e., outside in). If arterial pulsations are felt at the tip of the needle, the needle is withdrawn and redirected at a slightly more medial angle. A small amount of saline is injected to clear tissue or fat from the needle and a gentle suction is created with the syringe. If the vein has been entered, venous (nonpulsatile) dark blood will fill the syringe. Blood should come easily and without application of much negative pressure. If the vein has not been entered, the same gentle flush-aspiration cycle is repeated while withdrawing the needle a few millimeters at a time. If the attempt is unsuccessful, the needle is flushed and reintroduced in a slightly more lateral or medial direction. (Should the artery be entered and not used the needle is removed and firm manual pressure is applied over the artery for 3 to 5 minutes.) Another attempt can be made after bleeding has stopped. Several attempts may be needed to puncture the vein. Sometimes this may be necessary to direct the needle very close to the artery because the vein may be located partially under the artery.

A vein that has been entered mistakenly during a femoral artery puncture attempt should be used only if the needle tip did not puncture both walls of the artery and go into the vein behind it. Placing a sheath through the artery into the vein may create an arteriovenous fistula or cause uncontrolled bleeding from a large hole in the posterior wall of the femoral artery.

The remainder of the venous sheath placement is completed in the same fashion as described for the femoral arterial sheath insertion.

After the catheterization is completed, finger pressure is applied over the vein as described for femoral artery sheath removal. Five to ten minutes is usually enough time to obtain adequate hemostasis after percutaneous femoral vein puncture.

BRACHIAL APPROACH
Percutaneous Brachial Artery Puncture

In most cases percutaneous brachial artery puncture is a safe and effective alternative to brachial arterial cutdown. It can be performed more easily and often more quickly than brachial arteriotomy. Although very similar to femoral arterial puncture, there are several important differences. The brachial artery is smaller (3 to 5 mm in diameter) than the femoral artery. Because of the relatively loose subcutaneous tissues, the course of the brachial artery may change considerably. Spasm can occur very easily in the brachial artery with considerable decrease in pulse amplitude making the puncture more difficult. Care should be taken to puncture the artery successfully on the first attempt. Because of the smaller space in the arm, a hematoma formation can readily cause compression syndrome with ischemia of the forearm and hand. Remember the medial nerve lies immediately medial to the brachial artery. Accidental touching of the medial nerve causes a peculiar "electrical shock" sensation in the hand.

Before attempting brachial arterial puncture, check the brachial and radial pulses. They should be strong and equal on both arms. The patency of the ulnar artery and palmar arcus is checked by performing an Allen maneuver. The Allen maneuver is performed by compressing both radial and ulnar arteries at the wrist, and then releasing one to check patency by observing blood return to the hand. Check the arteries separately.

In cases where femoral access is not possible because of severe atherosclerosis, the same type of occlusive disease may exist in the subclavian arterial system. The subclavianaxillary artery system should be auscultated carefully for bruits above and below the clavicula.

Location of the brachial artery and anesthesia administration. The maximum point of brachial arterial pulse is located 1 to 2 cm above the elbow crease. With a 25-gauge needle, the skin and subcutaneous tissue are infiltrated with 2 to 3 ml lidocaine. At this point, injecting excessive amounts of local anesthetic may make palpation of the artery difficult or obscure the pulse completely.

Puncture of the artery and introduction of the guidewire. An 18-gauge needle with plastic cannula (Medicut or Angiocath) is used to puncture the brachial artery, entering the skin at a 45° angle. To facilitate the arterial puncture, the artery can be stabilized with the index and middle fingers placed below and above the puncture point. Arterial entry is confirmed by brisk bleeding from the needle. At this point, the needle is removed while the plastic outer sheath is advanced slowly into the artery. After removal of the needle, the sheath is held stable with the left-hand fingers and a 0.032-inch small-curve J guidewire is advanced into the artery and then into the aorta under fluoroscopic control.

Needle sheath removal.   Firm pressure is kept over the arterial puncture site and the wire is held firmly while the plastic sheath is removed over the wire. The wire is wiped clean with a wet gauze.

Skin preparation and entry.   The tip of a #11 scalpel blade is used to make a small skin incision at the entry point of the guidewire. Additional lidocaine can be given to the deeper tissue planes at this point.

Introduction of catheter sheath.   The sheath/dilator assembly is advanced over the wire and placed in the artery as described for femoral arterial puncture.

The sheath is aspirated and flushed after removal of the guidewire and dilator. The blood pressure is checked.

Sheath selection.   The brachial artery can accommodate up to size 8 French sheaths in large men. In smaller individuals and in women, smaller-size sheaths should be utilized. The new small-diameter (e.g., 5 to 6 French) equipment is very helpful in these patients.

Heparin administration.   Heparin (3000 to 5000 U) is given through the sheath or through a catheter advanced to the central aortic position. The patient must be warned about a temporary burning sensation in the hand caused by heparin (when injected into a vein at this location).

Catheter selection.   Multipurpose, Sones, or brachialtype (Castillo) catheters are easier to manipulate from the right arm. However, performed Judkins-type catheters can be used from the left arm and may work as well.

Hemostasis after brachial percutaneous catheterization. The radial pulse is checked before sheath removal. If pulse is weak or absent, 0.2 to 0.4 mg nitroglycerin can be delivered into the artery through the sheath. Administration of IV protamine, as for femoral artery hemostasis, is optional.

A board can be placed behind the elbow to facilitate pressure application.

The sheath is removed with firm finger pressure applied over the puncture site. A small amount of bleeding is allowed to purge possible clots. Do not "strip" the sheath, pushing thrombus out into the artery. The radial pulse is palpated continuously by the right hand while the amount of pressure applied over the artery by the left hand is adjusted to stop bleeding without completely obliterating the radial pulse.

After 15 to 20 minutes the pressure is released slowly. The pulse is checked and recorded. The arm circumference at the site of puncture is measured to facilitate the detection of hematoma formation. The patient is instructed to keep the arm in a relaxed but straight position for 4 to 6 hours. Sitting up in bed is permitted, but ambulation is restricted until after the hemostasis period (4 to 6 hours).

Percutaneous Brachial Vein Puncture

Because the antecubital vein anatomy varies greatly among patients, a successful vein puncture depends on visual identification of an adequately sized medial antecubital vein. The veins located on the lateral antecubital area should not be used because of their course through the cephalic venous system over the deltoid muscles, making it difficult to advance a catheter through the relatively sharp turns in the shoulder area. Application of a tourniquet several centimeters above the elbow may facilitate the identification of a suitable vein. The entry into the vein and placement of a sheath is accomplished through the same steps as described for brachial arterial entry. Heparin injection is not necessary. Because of the low flow in the vein only very gentle aspiration should be applied to the sheath prior to flushing.

Brachial Artery Cutdown Technique (Fig. 2-5)

The brachial artery and superficial antecubital or brachial veins can be accessed by direct cutdown technique as described below.

Arterial localization.   The brachial arterial pulse is located as described previously.

Using 5 to 10 ml 1% lidocaine, the skin and subcutaneous tissue are infiltrated deeply and widely enough to make an incision 1 to 2 cm wide.

Skin entry.   A 1-cm skin incision perpendicular to the long axis of the artery is performed. The length of the incision depends on the thickness of the subcutaneous tissue; thus a smaller incision may be enough in a thin patient.

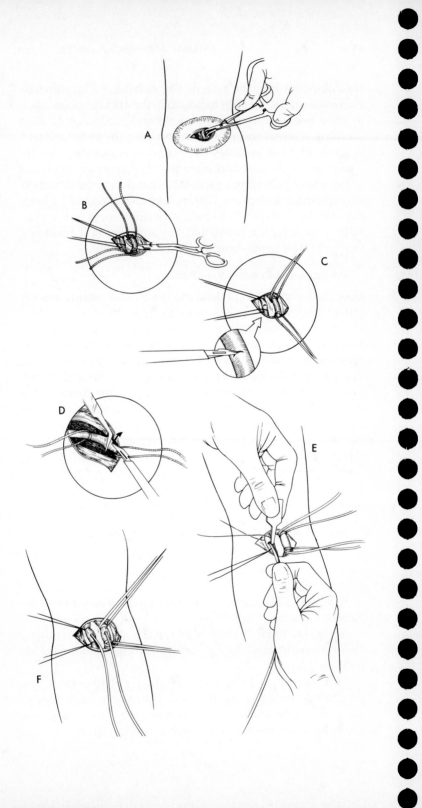

Blunt dissection.   The subcutaneous tissue is dissected carefully using blunt technique with a curved hemostat. The hemostat is held firmly and dissection is performed parallel to the long axis of the artery. A retractor or second hemostat is helpful to hold aside the tissue planes above the artery. There may be one or more superficial veins in the way; most are pushed aside. One should be selected with an encircling 4-0 silk tie in case urgent venous access is needed. The brachial artery lies in the superficial muscle plane under the bicipital tendon surrounded by adventitial fat, the brachial vein branches, and, medially, the median nerve.

Control of artery.   With careful blunt dissection a 1- to 2-cm length of the brachial artery is freed from surrounding tissue and adventitia. Silastic tapes are placed proximally and distally.

Arteriotomy.   While an assistant gently pulls the proximal and distal tapes to control bleeding, a small arteriotomy is performed using a pair of fine-point eye scissors or #11 scalpel blade. Do not perforate the posterior wall of the artery. The arteriotomy should only be wide enough to introduce the tip of the Sones catheter into the artery. A large arteriotomy may cause significant bleeding around the catheter. Such bleeding can be controlled by placing a rubber band around the artery.

Before the arteriotomy, the Sones or multipurpose catheter is flushed and connected to the pressure manifold in preparation for arterial insertion. Catheter introduction is facilitated by opening the arteriotomy site with a fine-curved eye forceps or a small vessel introducer. Once the Sones or multipurpose catheter is advanced 3 to 5 cm into the brachial

←

Fig. 2-5.   Arterial and venous cutdown technique. **A,** Through a transverse skin incision, the subcutaneous tissues are longitudinally dissected. **B,** The selected vessel is brought to the surface with use of a forceps and the proximal and distal segments of the vessel are tagged. A small incision is made into the vein (**C**) or into the artery (**D**) with the sharp point of a #11 scalpel. **E,** Venous catheter insertion is facilitated with use of a small vein dilator. **F,** Arterial and venous catheter insertion. (From Tilkian AG, Daily EK: *Cardiovascular procedures: diagnostic techniques and therapeutic procedures,* St Louis, 1986, Mosby.)

artery and an undamped arterial pressure wave form is observed on the monitor (excluding the possibility of subintimal introduction of the catheter), the catheter is held firmly in place to avoid accidental ejection from the artery by blood pressure. The proximal and distal tapes are released and the catheter is advanced to the subclavian artery at this point. Heparin (3000 to 5000 U) is administered through the catheter. The patient should be warned about a peculiar temporary burning sensation in the hand related to heparin. (The alternative method for injecting heparin into the distal artery is to use a 25-gauge needle, which is inserted into the artery at the planned arteriotomy site and directed distally.) The catheter is then advanced slowly under fluoroscopic control. A short sheath with a hemostatic valve can be placed in the artery if vigorous catheter manipulation or exchanges are anticipated.

Closure of brachial arteriotomy. After the catheterization, while gentle traction is applied on the proximal and distal tapes by an assistant, the catheter is removed by the operator. Keeping traction on the distal tape, the proximal tape is released slowly for a moment to eject clots and confirm pulsatile blood flow. Then the proximal tape is held tightly again, and the distal flow is checked in the same fashion. Distal bleeding should be brisk, although it may not be spurting as strongly as the proximal. After ensuring arterial patency in this fashion, the arteriotomy is closed with a running or pursestring suture using 6-0 Prolene. If the arteriotomy is too large or if the artery is too small, the pursestring technique can cause considerable obliteration of lumen. A running, continuous suture or interrupted suture technique is required. With this technique, lumen obliteration is minimal; however, the technique is more time-consuming. Heparinized saline solution often is instilled into the artery proximal and distal to the arteriotomy site. Vascular (bulldog) clamps are placed above and below the arteriotomy site. After the last suture has been placed, air is purged from the artery by first releasing the distal (furthest from the heart) tape or clamp and then reapplying it. Then the proximal tape or clamp is released and removed. Moderate pressure applied over the sutured artery by a fingertip for 5 to 10 minutes will control minimal bleeding. A full radial artery pulse should return immediately. If the pulse is not satisfactory, the arteriotomy site is inspected for obliterating sutures that must be corrected. In case of distal thrombotic occlusion, Fogarty embolectomy—often done in the catheterization laboratory—is required. If the operator is not experienced in this technique, a vascular surgery consultation should be obtained.

Sometimes local vasospasm may be responsible for a decreased radial pulse that responds to topical application of nitroglycerin. Sublingual nitroglycerin or nifedipine may be useful. Occasionally, pulse loss is caused by dissection at the arteriotomy site. In this case the arteriotomy should be reopened and inspected thoroughly. If flaps are seen, these can be removed. The artery is closed again in the same fashion. For dissected arteries, a vascular surgeon should be contacted for consultation. A corrective procedure can be performed by the surgeon in the catheterization laboratory or the skin can be closed temporarily and the patient transferred to the operating room for arterial repair.

Venous Cutdown (Fig. 2-5)

If brachial arteriotomy also is planned, the procedure should be performed as described in the section on brachial artery cutdown technique. In this case a deeper vein also can be utilized.

A superficial antecubital vein can be entered using a cutdown technique as follows:

1. Find a superficial medial antecubital vein at or below the elbow crease before the procedure.
2. After local anesthesia with 2 to 3 ml 1% lidocaine, a 5-mm skin incision is made over the vein as described in the arterial cutdown section. The subcutaneous tissue is dissected gently using a curved hemostat. The antecubital vein lies in the superficial plane. Once the vein is located the surrounding tissue and adventitia are separated using a curved mosquito hemostat passed under the vein several times. A 4-0 silk tie is placed at the distal end and (if the vein is not large) tied down. Another 4-0 silk tie is placed proximally.
3. A small venotomy incision is made using a blade or a fine pair of scissors. While the distal tie is pulled gently, the

vein is held using a mosquito hemostat or a curved forceps. Then the proximal tie is released, and while gentle traction is kept on the distal tie, the catheter is introduced gently into the vein and advanced slowy. Catheter insertion may be facilitated by opening the venotomy using a curved eye forceps or a small vessel introducer. Spasm in the antecubital veins is not uncommon. In this case the catheter is removed completely. Injection of 0.5 to 1 ml 1% lidocaine in the vein may relieve the spasm. The catheter can be reintroduced in a few minutes.

Possible Vascular Access Routes

ARTERIAL

Axillary
Brachial
Femoral
Radial—rarely used for cardiac catheterization
Subclavian—*not* used for cardiac catheterization
Translumbar—*not* used for cardiac catheterization

VENOUS

Brachial
Femoral
Internal jugular
Subclavian

---

4. To obtain hemostasis after venous cutdown, small veins simply are tied distally and proximally using 4-0 silk. Large veins are closed using the pursestring technique as described for arteriotomy. Thrombotic occlusion develops in most repaired veins.

Other vascular access (see the box above).   Access to the circulation is not limited to the above-mentioned techniques. However, techniques that are used rarely in the catheterization laboratory such as axillary artery puncture only should be attempted by experienced operators. Percutaneous subclavian and jugular vein puncture and techniques will not be explained here because they are used infrequently for routine cardiac catheterization.

Vascular access through synthetic graft conduits.   Access through synthetic peripheral vascular grafts should be avoided if possible. A limited experience indicates complications were <2% when grafts were at least 6 months old using 5 to 9 French sheaths for diagnostic but not interventional procedures.

USE OF HEPARIN DURING CARDIAC CATHETERIZATION

Heparin has been used in cardiac catheterization since the development of a suitable preparation for humans. Use of heparin for standard femoral approach and left-sided heart catheterization with coronary arteriography does not reduce or increase procedural complications. The appropriate doses of heparin and measurement of satisfactory anticoagulation are controversial. An intravenous (5000 U) bolus can achieve therapeutic anticoagulation status in 94% of patients. Heparin doses of 3000 U will provide measurable anticoagulant effect for most patients undergoing standard catheterization of short duration with low likelihood of prolonged anticoagulant effect requiring therapeutic reversal. Heparin routinely is recommended for patients in whom a prolonged (>20 minutes arterial time) catheterization procedure is anticipated or in whom prior clinical indications for use of heparin exist (e.g., thrombotic tendency, known severe peripheral vascular disease, embolic phenomenon on previous study). In most centers, heparin can be omitted for routine left heart catheterization when the procedure is performed in a timely and accurate manner.

Heparin reversal with protamine sulfate should be selected for patients in whom fish allergy or previous use of NPH insulin is not a concomitant factor (see Chapter 1).

PROBLEMS OF VASCULAR ACCESS

"Save time: do it right the first time" is an old catheterization laboratory saying. A thoughtful and systematic approach to the catheterization procedure decreases problems of access. The order of arterial or venous access is often a matter of personal preference. For novice operators whose stereotactic "view" through their fingers needs refinement, attempts at femoral venous entry before arterial sheath insertion are recommended for the following reason. If the arterial sheath is inserted first, firm palpation to establish the landmarks for venous entry may crimp the arterial sheath with formation of a generous hematoma. This rapidly forming hematoma makes venous location very difficult. Obviously, if the artery is punctured inadvertently while attempting venous access, the arterial sheath can be inserted so long as the precautions described in the section on the percutaneous femoral approach are observed. Once the arterial entry is established, difficulties next may be encountered at the thoracic or ascending aorta or in selectively cannulating the coronary arteries, vein grafts, or left ventricle. If the reader is unfamiliar with catheterization tools, a review of the guidewires and catheters to be used is provided in this chapter on p. 74. A special needle equipped with a disposable Doppler transducer (Smart Needle, Peripherial Systems Group, Mountain View, CA) may be helpful in case of difficulty locating the artery or vein.

Vessel Tortuosity

The most frequently encountered difficulty in advancing the guidewires or catheters into the aorta is tortuosity of the iliac or subclavian vessels, a condition often found in elderly patients. The steerable 0.035-inch Wholey guidewire has excellent characteristics for negotiating a tortuous vessel. Its flexible, relatively atraumatic curved tip is steerable and increases safety. In cases of extreme tortuosity it might be necessary to advance a catheter close to the guidewire tip (within several centimeters) to increase torque control and pushability of the guidewire. A right Judkins coronary catheter can be used to change the direction of the guidewire tip.

Equipment for tortuous vessels.   In patients with tortuous iliac vessels, a long (20-cm) sheath may be used, recognizing the trade-off of multiple friction points for some straightening of the vessel. Catheter exchanges over a long (300-cm) exchange guidewire may be required to avoid undue procedure prolongation by repeated attempts to advance catheters across tortuous atherosclerotic segments.

In patients with extreme tortuosity in the iliac or subclavian system, the torque control of the catheter is markedly decreased; use of a preshaped catheter is preferred in these cases because it often requires only minimal manipulation to engage the coronary arteries. In addition, advancing a pigtail catheter into the left ventricle of these patients may also be very difficult, involving loss of catheter length and

control in the tortuous segments. This problem may be overcome partially by inserting a 0.038-inch J-tipped guidewire
into the catheter and advancing and manipulating the catheter with the wire in place.

REMEMBER: Wire contact with blood will form thrombi
despite anticoagulation. Limit wire-loaded catheter manipulations to 2 to 3 minutes and use meticulous flush technique.

Complications of arterial access. The most common
complication from femoral cardiac catheterization is hemorrhage and local hematoma formation, increasing in frequency with the increasing size of the sheath, the amount
of anticoagulation, and obesity of the patient. Other common
complications (in order of decreasing frequency) include
pseudoaneurysm, arterio-venous (AV) fistula formation, arterial thrombosis secondary to intimal dissection, stroke,
sepsis with or without abcess formation, cholesterol embolization, and retroperitoneal hematoma. The frequency of
these complications is increased in procedures in high-risk
critically ill elderly patients with extensive atheromatous disease; the use of anticoagulation, antiplatelet, and fibrinolytic
therapies; and concomitant interventional procedures. The
brachial rather than femoral approach is also known to have
a higher risk of vascular complications.

Infections are more frequent in patients undergoing repeat
ipsilateral femoral punctures or prolonged duration (1 to 5
days) of femoral sheath maintenance. Cholesterol embolism
may be a subclinical finding in up to 30% of high-risk patients. Manifestations include abdominal pain or headache
(from mesenteric or central nervous system [CNS] ischemia),
skin mottling, renal insufficiency, and lung hemorrhage.

A retroperitoneal hematoma should be suspected in patients with a rapidly falling hematocrit postcatheterization,
lower abdominal or back pain, or neurological changes in
the leg with the puncture. This complication is associated
with high femoral arterial puncture and full anticoagulation.
Pseudoaneurysm is a complication associated with low femoral arterial puncture (usually below the head of the femur).

In the past, all femoral pseudoaneurysms were routinely
repaired by the vascular surgeon to avoid further neurovas-
cular complication or rupture. With ultrasound imaging techniques, these false channels can be easily identified to predict

which will require surgical repair or spontaneously thrombose. Nonsurgical closure by manual compression of the expansile groin mass guided by Doppler ultrasound has become a documented therapy for femoral pseudoaneurysm (Fig. 2-6) even in patients fully anticoagulated.

Common Problems in Accessing and Cannulating Coronary Arteries and Grafts

Left coronary artery

Short left main, separate ostia for left anterior descending and circumflex arteries. In these cases it may be necessary to cannulate the left anterior descending (LAD) and circumflex (CX) arteries separately. Slightly advancing the left Judkins

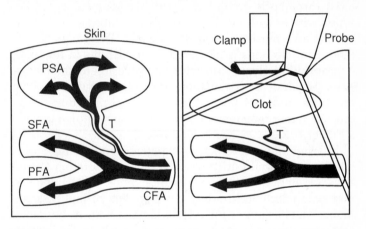

Fig. 2-6. Noninvasive technique for closure of a femoral artery pseudoaneurysm (*PSA*) by external compression. Arrows represent the course and direction of blood flow. *Left panel,* Blood is shown flowing from the common femoral artery (*CFA*) into a large pseudoaneurysm (*PSA*) through a large tract (*T*). *Right panel,* External application of pressure using a vascular clamp guided by Doppler ultrasound color flow probe (P) results in obliteration of the tract and clot formation in the pseudoaneurysm. *PFA,* Profunda femoris artery; *SFA,* superficial femoral artery. (Redrawn from Agrawal SK, Pinheiro L, Roubin GS, Hearu JA, Cannon AD, MacAnder PJ, Barnes JL, Dean LS, Nanda NC: Nonsurgical closure of femoral pseudoaneurysms complicating cardiac catheterization and percutaneous transluminal coronary angioplasty. *J Am Coll Cardiol* 20:610–615, 1992.)

catheter or using a left Judkins catheter that is one size smaller (i.e., 3.5 cm from 4.0 cm size) permits cannulation of the LAD artery. Slight withdrawal and clockwise rotation of the catheter or use of a left Judkins catheter that is one size larger permit cannulation of the CX artery. An Amplatz-type catheter is especially useful to cannulate the CX artery separately but must be used with care to avoid dissection of arteries.

High left coronary artery takeoff. An unusually high origin of the left main coronary artery from the aorta usually can be cannulated using a multipurpose catheter or an Amplatz-type catheter. In some cases, a brachial Castillo-type catheter (100-cm length) introduced through the femoral artery also gives excellent results. To cannulate the high-origin left main trunk through the brachial approach a long tapered tip Sones catheter may be utilized.

Wide aortic root. In patients with a relatively horizontal and wide aortic root with upward takeoff of the left main coronary artery, a large-curve left Judkins (5 or 6 cm), an Amplatz-type left coronary catheter, or a multipurpose catheter may be required.

Right coronary artery.   The origin of the right coronary artery shows more variation than the left coronary artery. A powerful hand injection into the low right coronary cusp will show the origin of the right coronary artery and will help in directing the catheter. If the right coronary is not seen with this injection, it may be totally occluded or may originate anteriorly or from the left sinus of Valsalva. In this case the orifice usually is located above the sinotubular ridge. A left Amplatz catheter or a left bypass graft catheter can be utilized successfully to engage right coronary artery orifice located anteriorly or in the left cusp. Minimal anterior displacement of the right coronary artery from the right coronary sinus is more common. In this case the right Judkins catheter tip may not be directed towards the right, but rather looks foreshortened in the familiar left anterior oblique (LAO) view. Directing the catheter tip to the right in the usual fashion using the lateral view permits easy cannulation of the anteriorly directed right coronary orifice.

Wide aortic root. In a patient with horizontal and wide aortic root, cannulation of the right coronary orifice and right coronary cusp may require manipulation of an Amplatz or multipurpose catheter.

High right coronary artery takeoff. A relatively high origin of the right coronary artery may require a left or right (modified) Amplatz-type catheter.

The most common coronary anomaly (see below) is the circumflex artery originating from the right coronary artery or right coronary cusp and coursing posteriorly and downward. This location may be cannulated easily using a right Amplatz catheter.

Bypass grafts (Figs. 2-7 and 2-8).   In patients with previous coronary bypass surgery, the operative and prior catheterization records with previous angiograms must be reviewed for helpful remarks. The number, type of grafts (i.e., sequential or Y grafts), and the presence of mammary artery grafts should be known before the procedure. Special care must be taken to visualize all grafts and native vessels. An aortic root injection may be necessary to document the occlusion of aortic anastomosis of a vein graft. Metallic markers placed during the operation are thought to be helpful in locating the aortic anastomosis site but do not always pinpoint the graft ostia.

Vein bypass grafts are anastomosed to the anterior wall of the ascending aorta. The right coronary artery graft usually is anastomosed to the anterior wall of the aorta a few centimeters above and anterior to the right coronary orifice. Left anterior descending and diagonal grafts usually are anastomosed somewhat higher and slightly to the left. Obtuse marginal grafts are usually the highest and furthest left.

Right coronary bypass vein graft catheterization (Fig. 2-8).   The right coronary vein graft usually can be entered using a 4-cm right Judkins-type catheter. In some cases simple pullback of the catheter from the right coronary orifice, after right coronary angiogram has been completed, will be enough to engage the right coronary vein graft ostium. In other cases the right coronary catheter is placed in the ascending aorta at a level that is slightly higher than the expected level of the right coronary vein graft orifice and the catheter is rotated clockwise for 45° to 90°. This will cause the catheter tip to move along the left border of the ascending aortic silhouette in the LAO position. Advancement or withdrawal while ro-

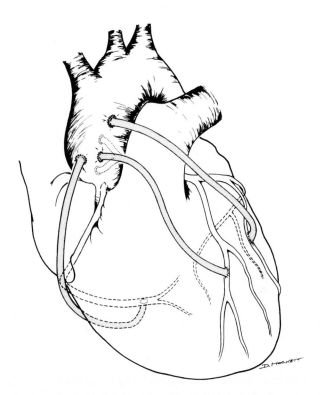

Fig. 2-7. Usual insertion sites of vein grafts to coronary arteries. The proximal (aortic) anastomosis site of the graft to the right coronary artery is most anterior and usually the lowest. Grafts to the branches of the left coronary artery are usually inserted in a progressively higher and more posterolateral position. Variations frequently occur. (From Tilkian AG, Daily EK: *Cardiovascular procedures: diagnostic techniques and therapeutic procedures*, St Louis, 1986, Mosby.)

tating the catheter tip might be necessary for graft engagement. In case of right vein graft vertical takeoff, the right coronary Judkins catheter tip may be directed toward the wall rather than into the lumen making adequate opacification of the vein graft difficult. In these cases a right coronary bypass vein graft catheter should be used. Because of the wider primary curve, the right vein graft catheter tip usually points downward and more parallel to the axis of the graft. Sometimes this catheter may have a tendency to move deeply

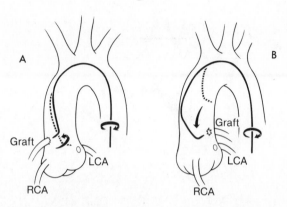

Fig. 2-8. Use of the Judkins right and left vein bypass catheters. **A,** For right coronary artery *(RCA)* grafts, the catheter is rotated clockwise in the left anterior oblique projection until the tip is superior to the graft orifice. It is then advanced down the aortic wall to the orifice of the graft. **B,** For left coronary artery *(LCA)* grafts, clockwise rotation is applied in the left or right anterior oblique projection. (From Tilkian AG, Daily EK: *Cardiovascular procedures: diagnostic techniques and therapeutic procedures,* St Louis, 1986, Mosby.)

into the right coronary vein graft. A right modified Amplatz catheter can also be used for horizontal or vertical takeoff vein grafts.

LAD vein graft catheterization. Often a LAD vein graft can be entered easily by simply pulling back the right Judkins catheter after right coronary vein graft injection has been completed. Alternatively the right Judkins catheter is placed at a level slightly higher than the expected level of the LAD vein graft orifice and 30° to 45° clockwise rotation is applied. The catheter tip will appear foreshortened in the LAO view and will be pointing toward the right border of the ascending aorta silhouette in the right anterior oblique (RAO) view. In some patients it may be necessary to use a left coronary vein graft catheter or left Amplatz catheter. A slight clockwise rotation of the catheter at the level of expected aortic anastomosis site of the LAD graft will engage the catheter into the ostium.

Circumflex vein graft catheterization. This graft usually is located above the LAD vein graft site. Therefore it can be engaged by simply withdrawing the right Judkins catheter from the LAD graft orifice or by repeating the same maneuver described for LAD vein graft cannulation using right Judkins or left vein graft catheters.

There are many alternative catheters for vein grafts. In some cases it may be necessary to search the whole anterior ascending aortic wall in the LAO and RAO projections systematically by injecting small amounts of contrast. In a patient with a large ectatic ascending aorta, it may be necessary to use a curved multipurpose catheter, a left Amplatz catheter, or a Castillo catheter.

Avoid unnecessary manipulation of catheters in vein grafts, especially in old grafts that may contain friable atherosclerotic material with potential risk of embolization.

If a coronary vein graft orifice cannot be entered an aortic root injection should be performed to document the patency of the graft and assist in further cannulation attempts.

Internal mammary artery graft cannulation (Figs. 2-9 and 2-10). The left internal mammary artery originates anteriorly from the caudal wall of the subclavian artery distal to the vertebral artery origin. The left subclavian artery can be entered using a right Judkins catheter. The right Judkins catheter is advanced into the aortic arch up to the level of the right brachiocephalic truncus with the tip directed caudally. Subsequently the catheter is withdrawn slowly and rotated counterclockwise. The catheter tip is deflected cranially, usually engaging the left subclavian artery at the top of the aortic knob in the anteroposterior projection. There are many variations in the shape of the aortic arch and origin and direction of the subclavian artery. More than one attempt is often necessary to engage into the subclavian artery. Once the subclavian artery is engaged the catheter is advanced slightly over a guidewire beyond the internal mammary orifice. We recommend a J-tipped guidewire or a Wholey wire to guide the catheter into the subclavian artery. In some patients the proximal portion of the subclavian artery can be straightened and the angle between the aortic arch and the subclavian artery can be improved by removing the pillows under the patient's head and hyperextending the neck to the right. Once the catheter has been advanced beyond the internal mammary artery takeoff, it is withdrawn slowly and

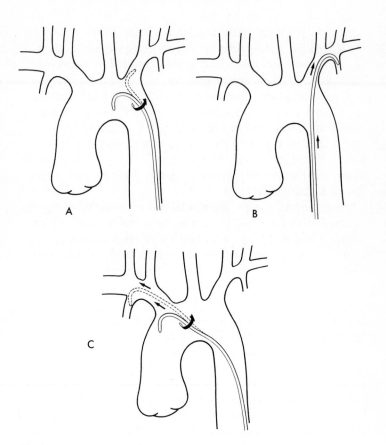

Fig. 2-9. Catheterization of the internal mammary arteries. **A,** To catheterize the left internal mammary artery, the catheter is located in the aortic arch in a neutral position, with its tip pointing downward. The catheter is then rotated counterclockwise until it falls into the left subclavian artery. **B,** The catheter is then advanced with a slight anterior rotation until it engages the origin of the left internal mammary artery. **C,** The right internal mammary artery is entered by counterclockwise rotation of the catheter at the origin of the right innominate artery and advanced until the origin of the internal mammary artery is engaged. (From Tilkian AG, Daily EK: *Cardiovascular procedures: diagnostic techniques and therapeutic procedures,* St Louis, 1986, Mosby.)

small contrast injections are given to visualize the internal mammary artery orifice. The catheter tip should be directed caudally. At the level of the internal mammary orifice a slight

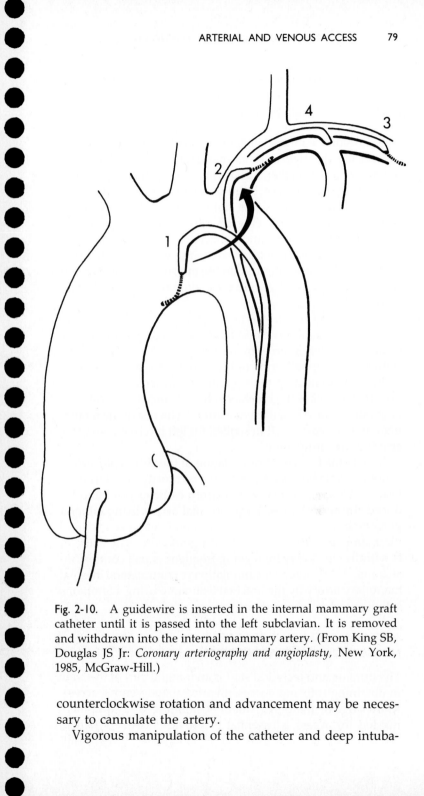

Fig. 2-10. A guidewire is inserted in the internal mammary graft catheter until it is passed into the left subclavian. It is removed and withdrawn into the internal mammary artery. (From King SB, Douglas JS Jr: *Coronary arteriography and angioplasty,* New York, 1985, McGraw-Hill.)

counterclockwise rotation and advancement may be necessary to cannulate the artery.

Vigorous manipulation of the catheter and deep intubation of the internal mammary artery should be avoided because of the hazard of dissection. During internal mammary artery injections, the patient should be warned about a painful, burning sensation in the shoulder and anterior chest wall (nonionic contrast media is less painful). In cases with a vertically directed internal mammary artery, an internal mammary artery catheter and a more acute tip angle can be used. This catheter can be introduced into the subclavian artery (as described for the right Judkins catheter) or the subclavian artery can be entered using a right Judkins catheter (as described above) and replaced with an internal mammary artery catheter over an exchange guidewire. Because of the peculiar tip configuration the internal mammary curve catheter usually engages into the ostium without much difficulty.

Right internal mammary artery graft catheterization. Right internal mammary artery cannulation is less common and more difficult than left internal mammary artery cannulation. The right brachiocephalic truncus is entered using a right Judkins catheter by deflecting the tip with a counterclockwise rotation at the level of the brachiocephalic truncus. The catheter is advanced into the subclavian artery. The rest of the manipulation is similar to that described for left internal mammary artery graft cannulation.

In patients for whom cannulation of the subclavian artery is not possible because of excessive tortuosity or obstructive lesions, an internal mammary artery catheter can be introduced through the ipsilateral brachial artery using either a percutaneous or cutdown approach and is advanced beyond the mammary artery orifice over a guidewire. The catheter is withdrawn slowly by making frequent, small contrast injections. A technique for cannulation of contralateral internal mammary artery by the brachial technique using a Simmons catheter also has been described.

ARTERIAL AND VENOUS ACCESS: NURSE/TECHNICIAN VIEWPOINT

The nursing and technical staff is an integral part of the team in obtaining safe and successful arterial and venous access. Knowledge of anatomy, patient positioning, and equipment needed for access is essential to provide adequate patient care and technical support during the access phase of the procedure.

Precatheterization Assessment

Because vessel trauma is inflicted while obtaining access, vascular compromise may occur as a result of the procedure. Upon the patient's arrival in the cardiac catheterization laboratory, the nursing and technical staff must (1) assess the patient's baseline peripheral vascular status; (2) properly position the patient on the procedure table for either femoral or brachial approach; and (3) prepare the access site in a manner that will facilitate vascular access by the physician. Pulses should be palpated or when necessary Doppler assessment should be performed. Information concerning the presence and stability of the pulse must be conveyed to the physician.

Baseline Vascular Assessment

The patient's preprocedure peripheral vascular status (i.e., pulse quality) should be assessed and documented on the catheterization chart before the start of the procedure. In some laboratories this will be the responsibility of the nurse whereas in other labs all personnel will share this duty. It is a good idea for the person responsible for postcatheterization care to do the initial assessment so that any changes in vascular status will be recognized easily. Many laboratories are set up in such a fashion that the entry/preparation area and recovery area are managed by the same staff members. This setup is ideal, as the staff member responsible for precatheterization and postcatheterization care can easily assess any change in the patient's baseline status.

If the femoral approach is used, the femoral artery, dorsalis pedis (top of the foot just below the ankle), and posterior tibial (inside behind ankle) artery pulses should be assessed, graded, and recorded on a scale of 0 to 4+ (4 being maximal or a bounding pulse). It is also helpful to use a marking pen to indicate the location and grade of the pulse on the patient's foot to facilitate postcatheterization assessment.

If the brachial approach is used a precatheterization assessment of the brachial and radial pulses must be performed. Again, the location should be marked and the grade documented on the chart.

Before the procedure the staff member should warn the patient as to what sensations may be experienced while the physician is obtaining access.

Patient Positioning

Femoral approach.   Proper positioning of the patient on the catheterization table by laboratory personnel is important to facilitate arterial and venous access. For the femoral approach the patient should be in the supine position. The x-ray table being used may dictate placement of the patient's arms. In some laboratories the patient's arms are placed behind the head. This ensures that the hands and arms are away from the sterile field and will not be in the way of the C-arm of the x-ray unit. The problem with placement of the arms above the head is that the patient will become very uncomfortable (and fatigued) during a long procedure. Positioning the arms at the patient's side is probably the most common method. Patients should be instructed to keep their arms as close to their body as possible and under the sterile drape at all times. Instructing patients to *tuck their hands under their hips* may help remind them to keep their arms at their side and aid in maintaining a comfortable position during the procedure. Positioning of patients' arms at their sides will cause the arms to appear in the x-ray field and compromise angiography performed in the lateral projections. For lateral projections the arms should be raised and placed behind the head. Positioning aids are available that facilitate arm positioning on the x-ray table.

Patients should be instructed to spread their legs slightly such that their knees are 8 to 12 inches apart. This position facilitates access to the groin by pulling the skin folds apart at the inguinal crease, a landmark for access.

The patient should be positioned as far toward the head of the catheterization table as possible. This allows travel of the C-arm of the x-ray unit to cover the inguinal area. If access is difficult because of vessel obstruction or tortuosity, it is necessary to use the fluoroscope over the insertion site. If the patient is positioned too far toward the foot of the x-ray table, fluoroscopic visualization of this area will be impossible because most C-arms will not reach the insertion site.

Special problems positioning the obese patient: femoral approach. Obese patients present a challenge to the staff in terms of positioning and site preparation. The first problem encountered is that most catheterization tables are narrow, which leaves no room for comfortable positioning of the patients' arms. A plexiglass arm retainer gives some support and helps keep the patients' arms at their sides. For short procedures the arms-above-the-head position is recommended for obese patients.

The second challenge is that of groin preparation. The protruding abdomen and panniculus of the obese patient usually extend and rest over the groin area, presenting an obstacle for access. The abdomen can be retracted toward the chest and retained in this position by using 3- to 4-inch wide tape. The tape can be criss-crossed over the retracted abdomen and secured to the sides of the catheterization table. Once the abdomen folds are retracted, the groin can be prepared in the usual fashion. Because excessive skin folds in the obese patient may result in higher than normal counts of skin bacteria, extra care should be taken in regard to skin cleansing and application of antiseptic solutions.

Positioning for brachial approach. Brachial artery access is obtained either by cutdown technique or percutaneous entry. Proper positioning of the arms is important in order to orient the brachial artery for easy access. The arm should be positioned on an arm board that stabilizes the position of the arm. Proper orientation will occur if the arm is placed on the arm board with the hand secured in the palm up position. This position forces rotation of the antecubital fossa into the correct position. Most x-ray tables have accessory arm boards that mount on the side of the x-ray table.

The arm should be placed at a 45° to 60° angle to the body. Less than 45° or greater than 60° may hinder catheter movement at the entrance to the subclavian artery. The arm board must not be secured to the table but be allowed to move freely should the physician need to redirect arm position to aid in catheter manipulation.

EQUIPMENT AND INSTRUMENTS USED FOR ACCESS
(Figs. 2-11 and 2-12)

A variety of needles, guidewires, vessel dilators, and introducer sheaths are available for use in obtaining access. Be-

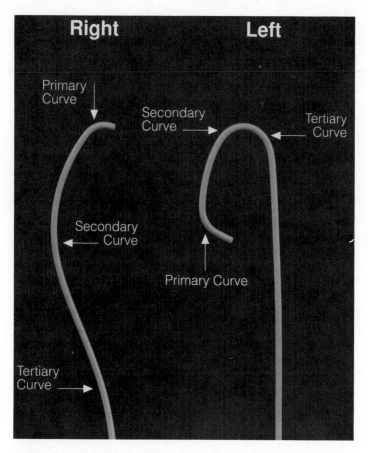

Fig. 2-11. Right and left Judkins catheters identifying primary, secondary, and tertiary curves of each catheter. These curves are designed to facilitate entry into the ostia of each coronary artery, respectively. (Courtesy of Cordis, Corporation, Miami, FL.)

cause components necessary for access come in many different sizes, the staff member must be knowledgeable regarding compatibility of the different components. For example, certain needles will accept only certain sized guidewires. The same is true for compatibility between wires, catheters, and introducer sheaths. Package inserts contain information regarding size and component compatibility.

The catheterization team members should understand the anatomy of the vasculature system for access and catheter

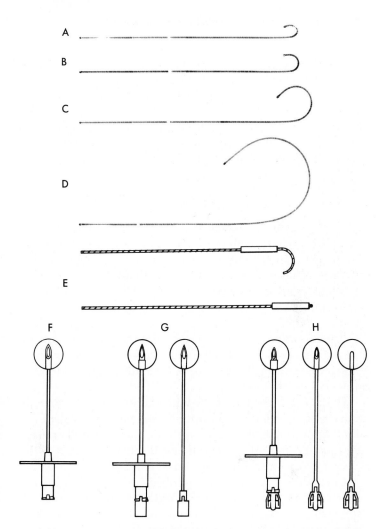

Fig. 2-12. Various-size curves of the J-curve guidewire. **A,** Small (1.5-mm) curve. **B,** 3-mm curve. **C,** 6-mm curve. **D,** Large (15-mm) curve. **E,** The curve of the J-curve guidewire is straightened out before vascular entry by sliding the accompanying plastic sleeve over the distal wire tip. **F** through **H,** Three types of percutaneous vascular entry needles. **F,** One-part needle. **G,** Two-part needle consisting of an inner beveled stylet and an outer cannula of metal or plastic. **H,** Three-part needle consisting of an inner beveled stylet, outer cannula, and rounded obturator (note the two cutting edges of the needle tip). (From Tilkian AG, Daily EK: *Cardiovascular procedures: diagnostic techniques and therapeutic procedures,* St Louis, 1986, Mosby.)

placement. Femoral, brachial, and axillary arterial entry give access to the aorta and left side of the heart, while femoral, brachial, subclavian, or internal jugular venous entry give access to the right side of the heart. Depending on the clinical presentation the patient may be scheduled for a right heart catheterization, left heart catheterization, or combined right and left heart catheterization (see Hemodynamic Data, Chapter 3).

Guidewires (Fig. 2-12)

Spring guide.   A guidewire is commonly called a *spring guide*. Other names often used are *wire guide, leader, wire,* or *guide*. They all refer to the same basic instrument, which consists of some type of core wire with another wire coiled tightly around it. Viewed from the outside, it looks like a thin, tightly coiled spring and usually is made of stainless steel.

Proximal tip.   The end of the wire that extends outside the patient's body is called the *proximal tip*. The doctor manipulates this end of the wire. It is the end that is nearest, or proximal, to the doctor.

Distal tip.   The end of the wire that makes percutaneous entry into the patient and through the vessels is called the *distal tip*. It is farthest away, or distal, from the doctor. This tip must be especially smooth and flexible because it is the "leading" or "working" end of the wire.

Core wire.   As already described, most guidewires are constructed with an inner wire or rod surrounded by a coiled, springlike wire. The inner wire is called the *core wire*. Both wires usually are made of stainless steel. The core wire also may be called a *mandrel*. Its purpose is to give the wire body some stiffness so that it can be manipulated, but the wire must also be flexible; different core wire designs allow different degrees of flexibility.

Safety ribbon.   As mentioned above a fixed core usually is attached to the proximal end of a guidewire, but not to the distal end. The distal end of the guidewire is just a flexible spring. If this spring were somehow to break off, it could be lost in the patient's bloodstream. To prevent this, a safety ribbon or safety wire is built into almost all guidewires. This safety ribbon is a flat, round, or braided wire strand that is attached to the distal tip of the guidewire on one end. In a fixed-core guidewire the other end of the safety ribbon may attach to the end of the fixed core or it may run all the way to the proximal end of the guidewire. In a movable-core guidewire, the safety ribbon must run all through the wire and attach at both ends because the core is attached only to the movable handle section.

Spring wire.   The outer part of the guidewire formed by a piece of stainless-steel wire tightly coiled around the inner core is called a *spring wire* or a *spiral wire.* The rounded wire does not have sharp cutting edges when bent and its coils have maximum contact with each other to prevent the spreading of coils that might trap blood and encourage clotting.

Fixed core guide.   A fixed core guide is a type of guidewire that has a rigid core that is fixed at the proximal end of the wire but usually is unattached at the distal end. The fixed core runs almost the full length of the guidewire. It stops about 3 to 5 cm from the distal tip, leaving an end that is just a spring without a core. Naturally, this end is more flexible than the part of the wire that has a core.

Moveable core guide.   A movable core guide is a type of a guidewire that has a rigid core, that is not fixed at either end of the wire. Instead the core can be attached to a handle at the proximal end of the wire. The handle is a similar but separate segment of spring bonded to the proximal end. By manipulating the handle, the doctor can extend the core closer to the distal tip of the wire or pull it farther away from the distal tip. This adjusts the length of the flexible spring at the distal tip to suit the doctor's needs.

Tapered core wire.   A regular core wire ends abruptly within the lumen of the spring guide, but a tapered core wire gradually diminishes in diameter as it approaches the distal tip of the guide. This allows a smoother transition between the flexible tip and the more rigid section of the wire containing the core. The smoother transition makes the wire itself a bit easier to control and it gives the wire greater flexibility. If the wire is utilized to place the catheter in a small, tortuous vessel, the more smoothly the catheter moves, and the less chance there is of the guidewire jolting or flipping its distal portion out of the desired vessel. Stainless-steel and Teflon-jacketed guides have tapered cores.

Long tapered core wire.   Most tapered ends of the core are about 3 cm long, but long tapered core wires have tapers that are 10, 15, or 20 cm in length. These extra-long tapers are designed specifically to minimize the problem of the guidewire flipping or jolting out of the vessel entrance.

Dagger effect.   In some wires there is a possibility that with severe kinking the core (whether fixed or movable) can separate the coils of the spring wire and poke through them. This is called a *dagger effect* and could result in damage to the vessel.

J-Tip spring guides.   Guidewires that have a curve in the distal tip, usually with a radius of 3, 6, or 15 mm, are called *J-tip spring guides* (Fig. 2-12). They are used for especially tortuous vessels that often are found in older people. These vessels are therefore more likely to have plaques in them. A straight guidewire might not follow the twisting path of a tortuous vessel easily. In addition, it might even dislodge plaques. The leading end of a J-tip wire, however, is more curved. The shoulder of the J-tip wire negotiates curves and glides over rough spots and plaques more easily than a straight guidewire. The J-tip wire is gaining popularity because of its great versatility.

Catheters (Table 2-1)

Femoral arterial technique.   The Judkins femoral arterial catheterization technique permits selection of various preformed or preshaped catheters in contrast to the Sones technique where the operator must form loops to position the catheter. The catheters can be manipulated through the skin directly or through an introducer sheath.

Improvements in catheter manufacturing technology have made large lumen preshaped coronary catheters (6 French or smaller) preferred in many laboratories. These catheters may allow early patient ambulation after the procedure because of the smaller arterial puncture hole. However, 5 French (or smaller) catheters may need to be replaced with larger French-size catheters occasionally when coronary ar-

TABLE 2-1. Catheter size specifications

Inches	mm	cm	French	Inches	mm	cm	French	Inches	mm	cm	French
0.004	0.10	0.01	0.3	0.038	0.96	0.10	2.9	0.072	1.83	0.18	5.4
0.005	0.13	0.01	0.4	0.039	1.00	0.10	3.0	0.073	1.85	0.19	5.5
0.006	0.15	0.02	0.5	0.041	1.04	0.10	3.1	0.074	1.88	0.19	5.6
0.008	0.20	0.02	0.6	0.042	1.07	0.11	3.2	0.076	1.93	0.19	5.7
0.009	0.23	0.02	0.7	0.044	1.12	0.11	3.3	0.077	1.95	0.20	5.8
0.010	0.25	0.03	0.8	0.045	1.14	0.11	3.4	0.078	1.98	0.20	5.9
0.012	0.30	0.03	0.9	0.046	1.17	0.12	3.5	0.079	2.00	0.20	6.0
0.013	0.33	0.03	1.0	0.048	1.22	0.12	3.6	0.081	2.06	0.21	6.1
0.014	0.36	0.04	1.1	0.049	1.24	0.12	3.7	0.082	2.08	0.21	6.2
0.016	0.41	0.04	1.2	0.050	1.27	0.13	3.8	0.084	2.13	0.21	6.3
0.017	0.43	0.04	1.3	0.052	1.32	0.13	3.9	0.085	2.16	0.22	6.4
0.018	0.46	0.05	1.4	0.053	1.33	0.13	4.0	0.086	2.18	0.22	6.5
0.020	0.51	0.05	1.5	0.054	1.37	0.14	4.1	0.088	2.23	0.22	6.6
0.021	0.53	0.05	1.6	0.056	1.42	0.14	4.2	0.089	2.26	0.23	6.7
0.022	0.56	0.06	1.7	0.057	1.45	0.14	4.3	0.091	2.31	0.23	6.8
0.024	0.61	0.06	1.8	0.059	1.50	0.15	4.4	0.092	2.33	0.23	7.0
0.025	0.63	0.06	1.9	0.060	1.52	0.15	4.5	0.100	2.54	0.25	7.5
0.026	0.67	0.07	2.0	0.061	1.55	0.15	4.6	0.105	2.67	0.27	8.0
0.028	0.71	0.07	2.1	0.063	1.60	0.16	4.7	0.113	2.87	0.29	8.5
0.029	0.74	0.07	2.2	0.064	1.62	0.16	4.8	0.118	3.00	0.30	9.0
0.030	0.76	0.08	2.3	0.065	1.65	0.16	4.9	0.126	3.20	0.32	9.5
0.032	0.81	0.08	2.4	0.066	1.67	0.17	5.0	0.131	3.33	0.34	10.0
0.033	0.84	0.08	2.5	0.068	1.73	0.17	5.1	0.139	3.53	0.35	10.5
0.035	0.89	0.09	2.6	0.069	1.75	0.18	5.2	0.144	3.67	0.37	11.0
0.036	0.91	0.09	2.7	0.071	1.80	0.18	5.3	0.153	3.88	0.39	11.5
0.037	0.94	0.09	2.8					0.158	4.00	0.40	12.0

tery opacification is poor because of dislodgment of the catheter during contrast injection.

All femoral catheters are inserted with a J-tipped guidewire. The J-tipped guidewire is advanced into the ascending thoracic aorta under fluoroscopic guidance and is followed by the catheter. Once the catheter tip has reached the desired location in the aorta, the guidewire is removed, the catheter is aspirated (2 to 3 ml of blood), flushed, and connected to the pressure manifold.

Except in cases involving known severe atherosclerotic disease or the presence of thrombi in the aortoiliac system the catheters can be removed without a guidewire.

The guidewire or catheter tip should be visible on the fluoroscopy screen whenever the catheter or guidewire is manipulated.

Coronary angiographic catheters (Figs. 2-13 and 2-14)

Judkins-type coronary catheters. Coronary angiography can be completed using Judkins catheters from the femoral approach in more than 90% of patients. The Judkins catheters have special preshaped curves and tapered end-hole tips. The Judkins left coronary catheter has a double curve. The length of the segment between the primary and secondary curve determines the size of the catheter (i.e., 3.5, 4.0, 5.0, or 6.0 cm). The proper size of left Judkins catheter is selected depending on the length and width of the ascending aorta. In a small person with a small aorta, a 3.5-cm catheter is appropriate, while in a large person or in those with an enlarged or dilated ascending aorta (e.g., as a result of aortic stenosis, regurgitation, or Marfan's syndrome) a 5.0- or 6.0-cm catheter may be required (Figs. 2-15 and 2-16).

The ingenious design of the left Judkins catheter permits cannulation of the left coronary artery without any major catheter manipulation except the slow advance of the catheter under fluoroscopic control. The catheter tip follows the ascending aortic border and falls into the left main coronary ostium, often with an abrupt jump. In the words of its inventor "the (Judkins) catheter knows where to go if not thwarted by the operator."

A left 4-cm Judkins catheter fits in most adult patients. When catheter size is adequate, the catheter tip is aligned with the long axis of the left main coronary trunk. A smaller

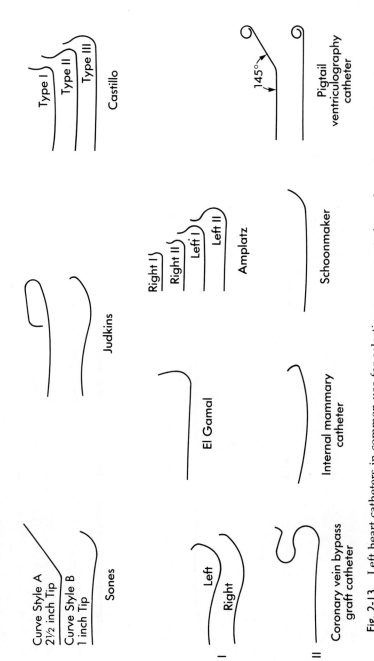

Fig. 2-13. Left heart catheters in common use for selective coronary arteriography and ventriculography.

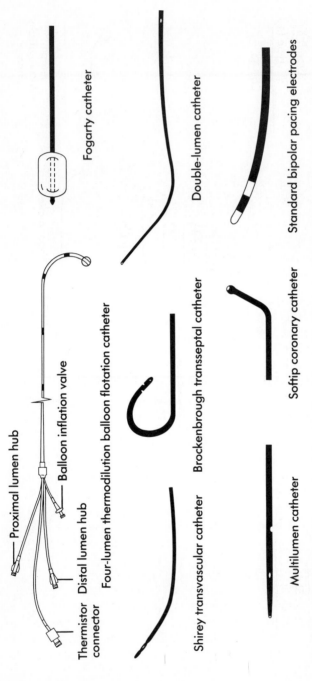

Proximal lumen hub

Balloon inflation valve

Distal lumen hub

Thermistor connector

Four-lumen thermodilution balloon flotation catheter

Fogarty catheter

Shirey transvascular catheter

Brockenbrough transseptal catheter

Double-lumen catheter

Multilumen catheter

Softip coronary catheter

Standard bipolar pacing electrodes

Fig. 2-14. Various special purpose catheters for right and left heart catheterization. Fogarty catheter is used to remove arterial thrombus. The Softip catheter has an atraumatic flared tip for coronary angiography. (Modified from Tilkian AG, Daily EK: *Cardiovascular procedures: diagnostic techniques and therapeutic procedures*, St Louis, 1986, Mosby.)

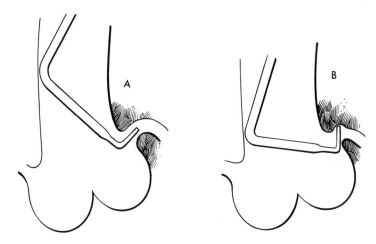

Fig. 2-15. Left Judkins coronary catheter position. **A,** Correct alignment. **B,** Incorrect position and overinsertion. (From King SB, Douglas JS Jr: *Coronary arteriography and angioplasty,* New York, 1985, McGraw-Hill.)

(3.5-cm) catheter in the same patient will tip upward and a larger (5.0-cm) catheter will tip downward into the coronary cusp. When the coronary orifice is not cannulated appropriately, the catheter should be replaced with a better-fitting catheter rather than manipulated into the coronary artery (see Fig. 2-15). Sometimes a slight counterclockwise rotation of the catheter may be necessary to improve alignment of the catheter tip with the left main trunk.

The Judkins right coronary catheter is sized by the length of the secondary curve and comes in 3.5, 4.0, and 5.0-cm sizes. The 4.0-cm catheter is adequate in the majority of cases.

The right Judkins catheter is advanced into the ascending aorta (usually with LAO projection) with the tip directed caudally (see Fig. 2-16).

The right coronary artery can be entered in most cases by one of two maneuvers:

1. The catheter is advanced into the right coronary cusp. The catheter is rotated 45° to 90° clockwise while the tip is pulled back 2 to 3 cm at the same time. Rotation of the tip toward the right cusp and downward motion of the catheter are seen while engaging the right coronary orifice.

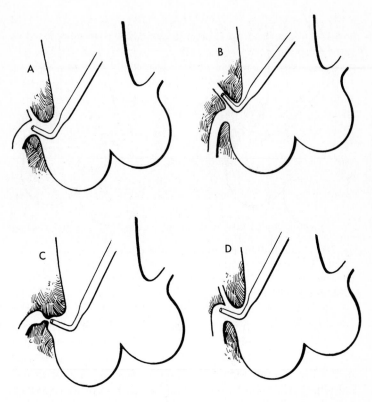

Fig. 2-16. Right Judkins coronary catheter position. A, Correct alignment. B, Tip subselectively in conus artery. C, Tip wedged in proximal stenosis. D, Tip impinging on lateral vessel wall. (From King SB, Douglas JS Jr: *Coronary arteriography and angioplasty*, New York, 1985, McGraw-Hill.)

2. The catheter tip is advanced to 2 to 4 cm above the valve. When the catheter is rotated clockwise for 45° to 90°, the tip will rotate toward the right cusp and descend approximately 1 to 2 cm engaging the right coronary ostium from above.

If the coronary ostium is not engaged, the maneuvers are repeated starting at a slightly different level each time. A brief contrast injection into the right coronary cusp may show the right coronary artery orifice and help in directing the catheter. A slight but firm push and pull on the catheter is necessary to translate rotational motion at the hub down to the tip. If stored rotational energy is not released by a small counterrotation after seating, the catheter may spring out of the right coronary ostium when the patient takes a deep breath.

Amplatz-type catheters (Fig. 2-17). The left Amplatz-type catheter is a preshaped half circle with the tapered tip extending perpendicular to the curve. Amplatz catheter sizes (left 1, 2, and 3 and right 1 and 2) indicate the diameter of the tip curve. In most normal-sized adults, #2 left and #1 right (modified) Amplatz catheters give satisfactory results. In the LAO projection, the tip is advanced into the left aortic cusp. Further advancement of the catheter causes the tip to move upward into the left main trunk. It is necessary to push the Amplatz catheters slightly to disengage by backing the catheter tip upward and out of the left main ostium. If the catheter is pulled instead of first being advanced, the tip moves downward and into the left main or CX artery. Unwanted deep cannulation of the CX might tear this branch or the left main trunk. Amplatz catheters have higher incidence of coronary dissection than Judkins-style catheters.

The right Amplatz (modified) catheter has a smaller but similar hook-shaped curve. The catheter is advanced into the right coronary cusp. As with Judkins right catheters the catheter is rotated clockwise for 45° to 90°. The same maneuver is repeated at different levels until the right coronary artery is entered. After coronary injections the catheter may be pulled, advanced, or rotated out of the coronary artery.

Multipurpose catheters. Multipurpose catheters usually are straight catheters with an end hole and two side holes placed close to the tip. Preshaped, mildly angled configurations are also available. The multipurpose catheter can be used for both left and right coronary injections and left ventriculography. (For a description of manipulation, see the section on Sones catheterization on p. 104.)

Special purpose femoral angiography catheters. The right coronary vein graft catheter is similar to a right Judkins catheter with a wider, more open primary curve allowing cannulation of vertically oriented coronary artery vein graft.

The left vein graft catheter is similar to the right Judkins catheter with a smaller and sharper secondary curve allowing easy cannulation of LAD and left CX vein grafts, which are usually placed higher and more anterior than the right

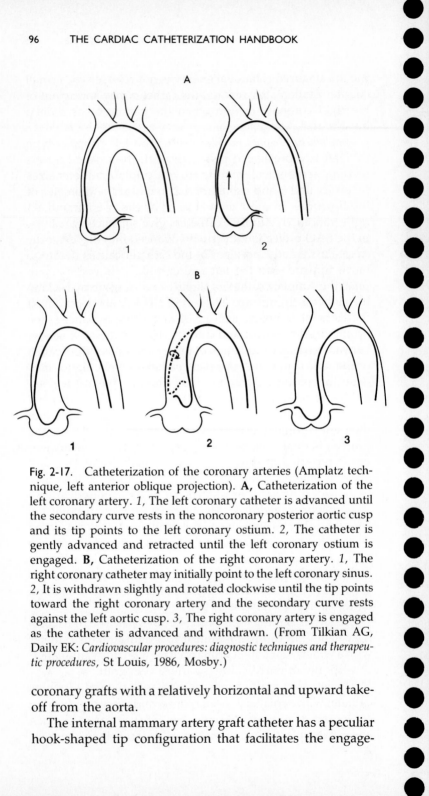

Fig. 2-17. Catheterization of the coronary arteries (Amplatz technique, left anterior oblique projection). **A,** Catheterization of the left coronary artery. *1,* The left coronary catheter is advanced until the secondary curve rests in the noncoronary posterior aortic cusp and its tip points to the left coronary ostium. *2,* The catheter is gently advanced and retracted until the left coronary ostium is engaged. **B,** Catheterization of the right coronary artery. *1,* The right coronary catheter may initially point to the left coronary sinus. *2,* It is withdrawn slightly and rotated clockwise until the tip points toward the right coronary artery and the secondary curve rests against the left aortic cusp. *3,* The right coronary artery is engaged as the catheter is advanced and withdrawn. (From Tilkian AG, Daily EK: *Cardiovascular procedures: diagnostic techniques and therapeutic procedures,* St Louis, 1986, Mosby.)

coronary grafts with a relatively horizontal and upward take-off from the aorta.

The internal mammary artery graft catheter has a peculiar hook-shaped tip configuration that facilitates the engagement of internal mammary artery grafts, especially in patients with very vertical origin of the internal mammary artery.

Femoral ventriculography catheters. For the femoral approach, two catheters generally are used:

1. *The pigtail catheter* has a tapered tip, preshaped to make a full circle 1 cm in diameter. Five to twelve side holes are located on the straight portion of the catheter above the curve. To enter the left ventricle, the pigtail catheter is advanced to the aortic valve. The loop is positioned to the left in the RAO projection and the catheter is pushed against the valve to make a U shape that facilitates the entry into the ventricle during deep inspiration. The catheter is placed in front of the mitral valve with the loop directed away from the valve (in the RAO position). A slight rotation, advancement, or withdrawal may be necessary to find a "quiet" position (one that does not cause frequent premature ventricular contractions) in the ventricle (Fig. 2-18). For this purpose an angled (145°) pigtail catheter may be helpful, especially for horizontally ori-

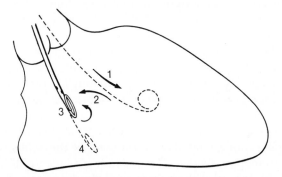

Fig. 2-18. Judkins method of left ventricular catheterization. *1,* Having crossed the aortic valve, the pigtail catheter will be in position. *2,* The catheter is withdrawn 2 to 3 cm and rotated 70° to 90° counterclockwise. *3,* The coiled loop will be in the inflow tract of the mitral valve. *4,* If the catheter moves excessively in this position, it should be advanced until it is stable. (From Judkins MP, Judkins E: Coronary arteriography and left ventriculography: Judkins technique. In King SB III, Douglas JS Jr: *Coronary arteriography and angioplasty,* New York, 1985, McGraw-Hill, p 201. Reproduced with permission.)

ented hearts. A novel 5 French catheter with a helical tip with inward-directed side holes (Halo catheter, Angiodynamics) appears to produce equivalent left ventriculograms with minimal ectopy.

2. *The multipurpose catheter* is also used for femoral ventriculography. It is advanced across the aortic valve directly or, after making an upward loop with slight rotation, falls into the ventricle. This catheter should be positioned freely in the left ventricular chamber so that the high-pressure contrast jet does not produce ventricular tachycardia or contrast injection in the myocardial tissue (contrast staining). See p. 107.

The pigtail catheter produces less ectopy than the multipurpose catheter, and it rarely causes myocardial contrast staining.

Catheters for the brachial technique. The Sones catheter is a straight woven Dacron catheter with a gradually tapered tip with two side holes and a single end hole. It comes in different tapered tip lengths and in straight or preformed tip angle shapes.

SONES CATHETER INTRODUCTION. The Sones catheter is introduced through a right brachial arteriotomy or percutaneous sheath and usually is advanced over a guidewire into the subclavian artery under fluoroscopic guidance. There may be a sharp caudal turn near the origin of the carotid artery that usually requires a J-tipped guidewire for passage. An inexperienced operator manipulating the catheter in this area may dissect or perforate the subclavian artery. To decrease the kinking and tortuosity of brachiocephalic vessels, the patient is instructed to turn his or her head to the left, with the chin extended (as if trying to see the ceiling corner), and to inspire deeply. The operator also may pull the arm straight and raise the arm toward the head at a 90° angle with the chest wall.

SONES CORONARY CANNULATION (FIG. 2-19). Cannulation of the *left coronary artery* using a Sones catheter is performed in the LAO projection. The catheter tip is advanced against the aortic valve and pushed to form a U-shaped loop with upward movement of the tip toward the left main trunk. The tip position is verified with small contrast injections. Once the catheter tip is near the left main coronary artery

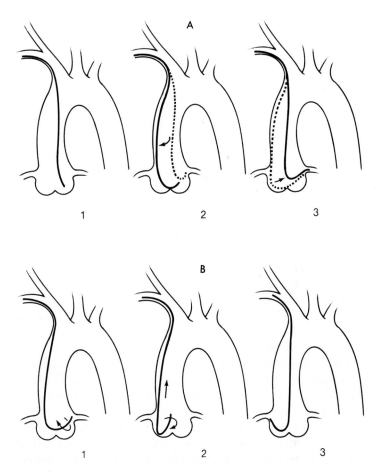

Fig. 2-19. Catheterization of the left (**A**) and right (**B**) coronary arteries in the left anterior oblique projection using the Sones technique. (From Tilkian AG, Daily EK: *Cardiovascular procedures: diagnostic techniques and therapeutic procedures,* St Louis, 1986, Mosby.)

orifice, a slight counterclockwise rotation of the catheter brings the tip into the left main. Slightly withdrawing the catheter causes the tip to seat in the left main, achieving a more stable angiographic position. Because the catheter moves considerably with breathing, stability is assured by advancing or withdrawing the catheter slightly as needed.

Cannulation of the right coronary artery is also performed in the LAO projection. A smaller U-shaped curve can be formed in the right cusp with the tip directed to the left coronary orifice. Rotate the catheter clockwise into the right cusp keeping the shortened U-shaped loop. Once the tip is engaged the catheter has a tendency to go very deeply into the right coronary artery, which requires catheter adjustments during respiratory cycles. In patients with a vertically originating right coronary artery, the Sones catheter may go directly into the right coronary artery when it is first advanced through the right arm.

Preshaped coronary catheters for brachial use. Judkins left and right coronary catheters can be used through the left arm with satisfactory results. Compared to the femoral technique, a left Judkins catheter of smaller curve may be necessary with the left brachial technique. The preshaped catheter should be introduced and advanced over the J-tipped guidewire. A preshaped brachial (Castillo, Fig. 2-20) catheter (size 1, 2, or 3) with a curved tip configuration similar to the Amplatz catheter is used effectively from the right or left arm. This catheter is manipulated in a fashion similar to that described for the Amplatz catheter. Although the preshaped coronary catheters can be removed without a guidewire, a pigtail ventriculography catheter should be removed over a guidewire to straighten the pigtail loop and prevent it from kinking or lodging in the subclavian or axillary artery.

Brachial ventriculography catheters

The Sones catheter. Entering into the left ventricle with a Sones catheter is usually easy. A U loop can be formed by pushing the catheter against the aortic valve. Keeping tension on the catheter during deep inspiration will cause the catheter to drop into the left ventricle. The catheter should be placed in front of the mitral valve in the RAO position with the tip directed toward the apex. The catheter should be free in the ventricle. It is important to avoid direct contact with the myocardium because the injection of contrast may result in myocardial contrast penetration or perforation (Fig. 2-21).

The Sones catheter can perform all the functions of the Judkins catheters. However, ventriculography with the Sones catheter is more difficult and carries a higher risk of injury than use of closed-end catheters or the multiple side hole (pigtail) catheters. Complications of Sones ventriculography include contrast injection into the myocardium with

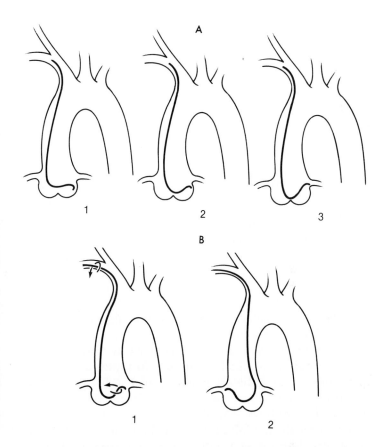

Fig. 2-20. Castillo modification of the Amplatz technique. **A,** Catheterization of the left coronary artery. *1,* The Castillo catheter is advanced until the secondary curve rests in the noncoronary posterior aortic cusp and its tip points to the left coronary ostium. *2* and *3,* The catheter is gently advanced and retracted until the left coronary ostium is engaged. **B,** Catheterization of the right coronary artery. *1,* Initially the catheter points to the left coronary sinus. *2,* It is withdrawn slightly and rotated until the tip points toward the right coronary artery. The right coronary ostium is engaged as the catheter is advanced and withdrawn. (From Tilkian AG, Daily EK: *Cardiovascular procedures: diagnostic techniques and therapeutic procedures,* St Louis, 1986, Mosby.)

staining of the myocardium, perforation of the myocardium, ejection out of the ventricle with dissection of the aorta during high-pressure jet injection into the wall of the aorta, and

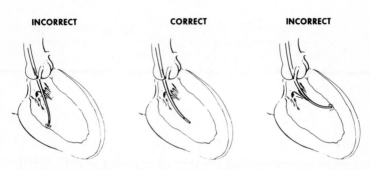

Fig. 2-21. Catheterization of the left ventricle in the 35° right anterior oblique projection. When positioned correctly *(center)*, the catheter tip should be near the tip of the papillary muscles, aiming toward the apex. If it is touching the inferior or inferolateral wall *(left)* it should be rotated clockwise. If it is touching the anteroseptal wall *(right),* it should be rotated counterclockwise. (From King SB, Douglas JS Jr: *Coronary anteriography and angioplasty,* New York, 1985, McGraw-Hill.)

excessive ventricular ectopy making ventriculograms suboptimal for interpretation.

Alternative catheters. For ventriculography through the brachial approach, pigtail, National Institutes of Health (NIH), or Lehman catheters are also available. The NIH catheter has a closed tip with six side holes. It is a relatively stiff but large-bore catheter that allows injection of large amounts of contrast with minimal ectopy. The Lehman catheter is also a closed-tip catheter with side holes placed before the tapered distal end. Both NIH and Lehman catheters are placed into the ventricle as described for the Sones catheter. The Lehman catheter must be advanced deeply into the ventricle because the side holes are some distance from the tip.

The multipurpose catheter can be used via the brachial or femoral artery route and is manipulated in the same fashion as described for the Sones catheter. It carries the same risk for complications as the Sones catheter.

Catheters for right heart catheterization

HEMODYNAMIC MEASUREMENTS. A balloon-tipped flotation catheter (Fig. 2-22)—originally designed by Drs. H.J.C. Swan and W. Ganz—is the most widely used catheter for right heart hemodynamics. The balloon tip allows the catheter to float through the right side of the heart safely and easily in a majority of cases. The pulmonary capillary wedge

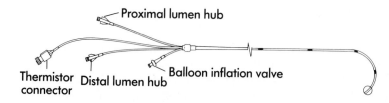

Fig. 2-22. Multilumen balloon-tipped pulmonary artery catheter for right heart hemodynamic measurements. (From Tilkian AG, Daily EK: *Cardiovascular procedures: diagnostic techniques and therapeutic procedures,* St Louis, 1986, Mosby.)

pressure (reflecting left ventricular filling pressures) can be obtained easily. Thermodilution cardiac output measurements are routine and exclusive to this catheter. The balloon-tipped catheter can be introduced through any venous access route. The balloon is inflated with room air. Carbon dioxide is used if passage to the arterial circulation is anticipated.

BALLOON CATHETER TECHNIQUE FOR THE RIGHT HEART. From the femoral approach, two techniques can be used to traverse the right heart:

1. The catheter is directed toward the lateral wall of the right atrium. A loop is made with the tip directed in a circle and under and across to the tricuspid valve. As it is advanced, the catheter floats across the tricuspid valve and up through the right ventricle and into the pulmonary artery.

Conditions of Patients in Whom Superior Vena Caval Approach for
Right Heart Catheterization Is Preferred

Pulmonary hypertension
Right ventricular hypertension
Tricuspid regurgitation/stenosis
Massive right atrial dilation
Massive right ventricular dilation
Anomalous inferior vena cava
Inferior vena cava filter (for pulmonary embolism)
Suspected femoral/iliac vein thrombus (may precipitate pulmonary
    embolus)
Renal vein thrombosis

2. The catheter tip is passed directly (medially) across the tricuspid valve and allowed to float just beyond the tricuspid valve in the right ventricle. The catheter is then pulled back slightly and a clockwise rotation is applied. When the balloon tip is deflected upward toward the right ventricular outflow tract, the catheter is advanced quickly into the pulmonary artery well beyond the pulmonary valve.

The balloon-tipped catheters do not provide good torque control, making catheterization of the pulmonary artery in patients with right atrial or ventricular enlargement, pulmonary hypertension, or tricuspid regurgitation difficult. This difficulty is especially prominent when the femoral technique is used. In cases where a guidewire (0.025 inch) does not add control to catheter manipulations, the catheter can be introduced through the antecubital, jugular, or subclavian vein (see the box above). A Mullins-type long sheath may also be helpful to direct the catheter tip toward the lateral right atrial wall and into the tricuspid valve by forming a large loop. Once the catheter is in the pulmonary artery the tip (with the inflated balloon) is advanced to obtain a pulmonary artery wedge pressure.* (See Chapter 3.)

Complications of Pulmonary Artery Catheterization

Complications of vascular access
Pulmonary infarction
Pulmonary artery rupture
Injury to chordae in right ventricle
Tricuspid regurgitation
Right bundle branch block
Dislodgement of pacemaker leads

Pulmonary capillary wedge pressure can be identified from adequate pressure waveforms and should be confirmed with oximetry, especially in cases where a critical measure

---

* For an excellent review of problems with balloon-tipped catheters, see Matthay MA, Chatterjee K: Bedside catheterization of the pulmonary artery: risks compared with benefits, *Ann Intern Med* 109:826–834, 1988.

of mitral valvular function is required. Often it is impossible to obtain adequate saturation with the balloon inflated. Advancement of the catheter tip with the balloon deflated into the deep wedge position may yield a satisfactory and confirmatory oxygen saturation. The best location of the pulmonary wedge pressure has been questioned, but for practical purposes any of the four locations (left or right upper lobes or left or right lower lobes) within the pulmonary tree are generally acceptable. The right lower lobe is the most common location for positioning of the pulmonary artery balloon-tipped catheter. In patients with high pulmonary artery pressures (>50 mm Hg) an inflated balloon should not be left in place for more than 10 minutes. In other patients the balloon can be inflated for longer periods, but excessive prolongation of balloon inflation may cause pulmonary infarction or damage to the pulmonary artery. In addition, care should be taken not to inflate a balloon vigorously in distal portions of the lung where the balloon may tear a small pulmonary vessel. Complications of pulmonary artery catheter are described in the box above.

Several other types of catheters provide high-quality right heart pressure measurement and permit rapid aspiration of blood samples for oxygen saturation measurements, but do not have thermodilution cardiac output capability. End hole (Cournand) catheters can be introduced through the femoral or brachial veins and manipulated in a fashion similar to the balloon-tipped method described here. The end hole design allows wedge pressure measurement when the catheter is advanced deeply into the pulmonary artery. A deep inspiration and simultaneous catheter advancement with a cough facilitate a wedge placement with these catheters. The Goodale-Lubin, a similar catheter with two closely located side holes, also allows easier pressure measurement and blood sampling.

CATHETERS FOR RIGHT HEART ANGIOGRAPHY. The NIH catheter is relatively stiff with a closed blunt tip that should always be manipulated gently through the right heart. The Berman catheter is a balloon-tipped angiographic catheter without an end hole; it has side holes placed proximally to the balloon. It is introduced easily into the right heart and can be used to measure pulmonary artery pressures. Keeping the balloon inflated increases the catheter stability during angiography. This catheter allows flow rates as high as a pigtail catheter. A regular pigtail catheter or one with a special obtuse angle (Grollman) also can be utilized for right ventriculography.

A comprehensive discussion of all available catheter types and techniques is beyond the limits of this handbook. The new operator should concentrate on mastering a few types of catheters and gain extensive experience in using them effectively.

SUGGESTED READINGS

Adams DF, Abrams LH: Complications of coronary arteriography: a follow-up report, *Cardiovasc Radiol* 2:89–96, 1979.

Barry WH, Levin DC, Green LH, Bettman MA, Mudge GH Jr, Phillips D: Left heart catheterization and angiography via the percutaneous femoral approach using an arterial sheath, *Cathet Cardiovasc Diagn* 5:401–409, 1979.

Davis K, Kennedy JW, Kemp HG, Judkins MP, Gosselin AJ, Killip T: Complications of coronary arteriography from the collaborative study of coronary artery surgery (CASS), *Circulation* 59:1105–1111, 1979.

Ernst SPMG, Tjonjoegin M, Schrader R, Kaltenbach M, Sigwart U, Sanborn TA, Plokker HWT: Immediate sealing of arterial puncture sites after cardiac catheterization and coronary angioplasty using a biodegradable collagen plug: results of an international registry, *J Am Coll Cardiol* 21:851–855, 1993.

Kern MJ, Cohen M, Talley JD, Litvack F, Serota H, Aguirre F, Deligonul U: Early ambulation after 5F diagnostic catheterization: results of a multicenter trial, *J Am Coll Cardiol* 15:1475–1483, 1990.

Kim D, Orron DE, Skillman JJ, Kent KC, Porter DH, Schlam BW, Carrozza J, Reis GJ, Baim DS: Role of superficial femoral artery puncture in the development of pseudoaneusyrm and arteriovenous fistula complicating percutaneous transfemoral cardiac catheterization, *Cathet Cardiovasc Diagn* 25:91–97, 1992.

Lesnefsky EJ, Carrea FP, Groves BM: Safety of cardiac catheterization via peripheral vascular grafts, *Cathet Cardiovasc Diagn* 29:113–116, 1993.

Llia R, Kimbiris D, Hakki A, Edlin D, Iskandrian AS, Bemis DE, Mintz GS, Segal BL: Percutaneous left heart catheterization and coronary arteriography with and without an arterial sheath in patients without peripheral vascular disease, *Cathet Cardiovasc Diagn* 11:463–466, 1985.

Maouad J, Hebert JL, Fernandez F, Gay J: Percutaneous brachial approach using the femoral artery sheath for left heart catheterization and selective coronary angiography, *Cathet Cardiovasc Diagn* 1:539–546, 1985.

Matthay MA, Chatterjee K: Bedside catheterization of the pulmonary artery: risks compared with benefits, *Ann Intern Med* 109:826–834, 1988.

Rich JM, Cobb TC, Leighton RF: Percutaneous transfemoral coronary arteriography without systemic anticoagulation: a review of 648 consecutive procedures, *Cathet Cardiovasc Diagn* 1:275–281, 1975.

Tilkian AG, Daily EK: *Cardiovascular procedures: diagnostic techniques and therapeutic procedures,* St Louis, 1986, Mosby.

Vacek JL, Bellinger RL, Phelix J: Heparin bolus therapy during cardiac catheterization, *Am J Cardiol* 62:1314–1317, 1988.

3

HEMODYNAMIC DATA

Morton J. Kern, Ubeydullah Deligonul, Thomas Donohue, Eugene Caracciolo, and Ted Feldman

SECTION I: HEMODYNAMIC DATA

Cardiac catheterization (Fig. 3-1) provides anatomic information through cineangiograms and equally important physiologic information through the recording of hemodynamic data, including pressure measurements, cardiac output (CO) determinations, and blood oximetry.

PRESSURE WAVES IN THE HEART

Blood within the heart or vessels exerts pressure. A pressure wave is created by cardiac muscular contraction and is transmitted along a closed, fluid-filled column (catheter) to a pressure transducer, converting the mechanical pressure to an electrical signal that is displayed on a video monitor. Cardiac pressure waveforms are cyclical, repeating the pressure change from the onset of one cardiac contraction (systole) to the onset of the subsequent contraction. The physiology of heart function is beyond the scope of this text, but an examination of the diagram of the cardiac cycle and corresponding pressures (Figs. 3-2 and 3-3) will provide the essentials for the understanding of basic hemodynamics in the cardiac catheterization laboratory.

The collection of hemodynamic data for cardiac catheterization is an integral part of every protocol. Even complex

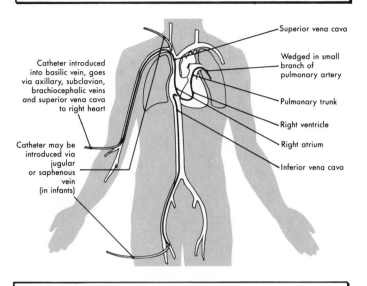

Catheter introduced into basilic vein, goes via axillary, subclavian, brachiocephalic veins and superior vena cava to right heart

Catheter may be introduced via jugular or saphenous vein (in infants)

Superior vena cava

Wedged in small branch of pulmonary artery

Pulmonary trunk

Right ventricle

Right atrium

Inferior vena cava

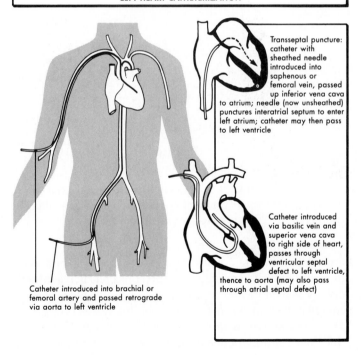

LEFT HEART CATHETERIZATION

Transseptal puncture: catheter with sheathed needle introduced into saphenous or femoral vein, passed up inferior vena cava to atrium; needle (now unsheathed) punctures interatrial septum to enter left atrium; catheter may then pass to left ventricle

Catheter introduced via basilic vein and superior vena cava to right side of heart, passes through ventricular septal defect to left ventricle, thence to aorta (may also pass through atrial septal defect)

Catheter introduced into brachial or femoral artery and passed retrograde via aorta to left ventricle

Fig. 3-1. Right and left heart catheterization from the brachial and femoral approaches.

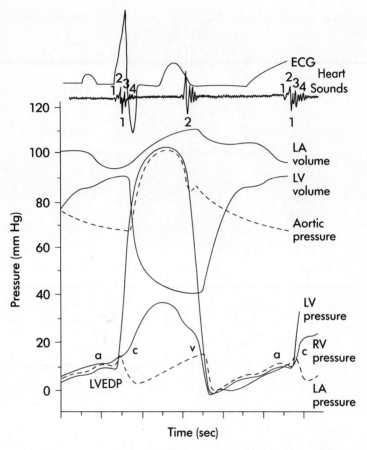

Fig. 3-2. Normal hemodynamics. *LA,* left atrial; *LV,* left ventricle; *RA,* right atrial; *RV,* right ventricle; *a,* atrial contraction
wave; *c,* ventricular contraction wave; *v,* ventricular filling
wave; *LVEDP,* left ventricular end-diastolic pressure.

hemodynamic data recording can be accomplished accurately and rapidly if an efficient and consistently used methodology is established in the laboratory. The measurement
sequence used in our laboratory (see the boxes on pp. 112,
113, 115, and 116) is one example of such a methodology.
It facilitates simultaneous pressure measurements across the
heart, concentrating on the aortic and mitral valves, those
which are affected most commonly by disease. Ninety per-

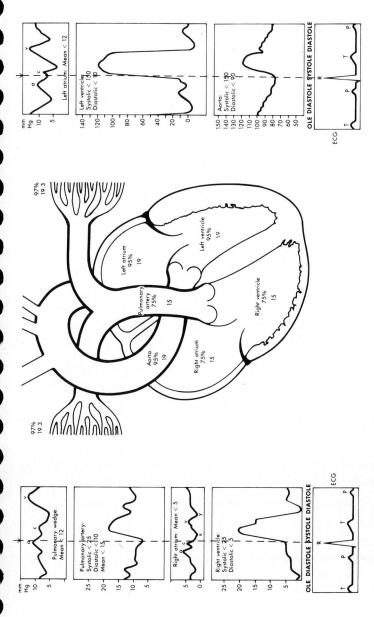

Fig. 3-3. Normal oxygen saturation, oxygen volume percentage, and pressure ranges in heart chambers and great vessels with pressure tracings in relation to ECG.

cent of all hemodynamic questions can be answered by examining the data collected in this way. As with most brief formulas, this technique is not all inclusive. Different hemodynamic measurements for specific clinical situations are necessary. Specific examples are included in the case studies.

The routine collection of right and left heart hemodynamic data with appropriate sampling for blood oxygen saturations and cardiac output measurements can be accomplished rapidly and safely in less than 30 minutes. Cardiac output by thermodilution technique is routine. Fick (oxygen consumption method) cardiac output is used for valvular lesions (green dye curves are reserved for suspected cardiac shunt studies). Arterial, right atrial (RA), and pulmonary artery (PA) oxygen saturations are collected routinely. Multiple oxygen saturation samples are obtained throughout the right (and left) heart for intracardiac shunt identification.

PROTOCOLS FOR RIGHT AND LEFT HEART CATHETERIZATION

The protocol used during right heart catheterization is summarized in the box on p. 113. Right heart catheterization is not required for all left heart studies.

Indications

Right heart catheterization is indicated in patients with a history of dyspnea, valvular heart disease, or intracardiac shunts. Patients with a history of pulmonary edema occurring on a previous hospital admission often have only dyspnea with no objective evidence of left ventricular (LV) dysfunction (e.g., chest x-ray, echocardiography). Dyspnea caused by lung disease cannot be differentiated from that caused by pulmonary hypertension or LV dysfunction.

Complications of Right Heart Catheterization (Table 3-1)

The most common problem during right heart catheterization is stimulation of the right ventricular (RV) outflow tract, which may result in ventricular arrhythmias, advanced atrioventricular block, or, rarely, right bundle branch block. Significant but transient ventricular arrhythmias occur in 30% to 60% of patients undergoing right heart catheterization and are self-limited, not requiring treatment. The arrhythmia is terminated when the catheter is readjusted. Sustained

Right Heart Catheterization Protocol

RIGHT ATRIUM (RA)

1. Advance catheter to RA.
2. Obtain oxygen saturation sample (1- to 3-ml heparinized*
   syringe).
3. Turn recorder on (40 mm Hg scale); zero pressure.
4. Record phasic pressure (25 mm/sec paper speed).
5. Check mean pressure (10 mm/sec paper speed), inspiration
   maneuver, phasic pressure; zero check pressure.
6. Turn recorder off.

RIGHT VENTRICLE (RV)

1. Advance catheter to RV.
2. Turn recorder on; record phasic pressure (25 mm/sec paper
   speed).
3. Zero check pressure.
4. Turn recorder off.

PULMONARY CAPILLARY WEDGE (PCW)

1. Advance catheter to PCW.
2. Turn recorder on.
3. Record phasic/mean/phasic pressure (25-10-25 mm/sec paper
   speed).

PULMONARY ARTERY (PA)

1. From PCW let balloon down, pull catheter back for PA
   pressure.
2. Record phasic/mean/phasic pressure (25-10-25 mm/sec paper
   speed).
3. Zero check pressure.
4. Turn recorder off.
5. Obtain oxygen saturation samples.

* 1- to 3-ml heparinized syringes should only have 1 to 2 drops of
heparin aspirated and flushed out.

ventricular arrhythmias have been reported, especially in
unstable patients or those with electrolyte imbalance, acidosis, or concurrent myocardial ischemia. The prophylactic use
of lidocaine is not necessary. However, many high-risk patients entering the catheterization laboratory may be already
receiving this medication.

In patients with left bundle branch block, a temporary

TABLE 3-1.   Complications of right heart (pulmonary artery) catheterization

| | Complications | |
	Major	Minor
Access	Pneumothorax	Hematoma
	Hemothorax	Thrombosis
	Tracheal perforation (subclavian route)	
	Sepsis	Cellulitis
Intracardiac	Right ventricular perforation	Ventricular arrhythmia
	Heart block (right bundle branch block)	
	Pulmonary rupture	
	Pulmonary infarction	

pacemaker may be needed if right bundle branch block occurs.

Use of the Pulmonary Wedge Pressure

The pulmonary capillary wedge (PCW) pressure closely approximates left atrial (LA) pressure. PCW pressure overestimates LA pressure in patients with acute respiratory failure, chronic obstructive lung disease with pulmonary hypertension, pulmonary venoconstriction, or LV failure with volume overload. Reported discrepancies between LA and PCW may be due, in part, to different types of catheters: balloon-tipped flotation catheters are soft with small lumens; LA pressure catheters (e.g., Brockenbrough or Mullins-type sheath) are stiff with large lumens. In most patients the PCW is sufficient to assess LV filling pressure. However, in patients with mitral valvular disease or mitral valve prostheses a significant error may be introduced by using a balloon-tipped flotation catheter for pulmonary wedge pressure. Transseptal LA catheterization should be considered in these cases.

Rules for obtaining an accurate PCW pressure that agrees with LA pressures are as follows:

1. Obtain correct position and verify through waveform, oximetry (oxygen saturation >95%), and fluoroscopy.
   a. Confirm position of catheters (end-hole wedge) by oxygen saturation sample >95% (obtaining this saturation not contaminated by low saturation pulmonary artery blood is difficult when the balloon is inflated).

b. Confirm that waveform of PCW pressure with precise a and v waves is not damped pulmonary artery pressure with waveform timing against ECG or LV pressure.

c. During fluoroscopy, 2 to 5 ml of contrast is injected into the catheter; a lack of contrast washout 15 seconds after injection indicates proper catheter position. Fluoroscopic method has been confirmed correct in 95% of attempts. A "fern" pattern of contrast seen on the fluoroscope may help when the hemodynamic tracing is in question in patients on mechanically assisted ventilation or in those patients with rapid deep inspiratory efforts.

2. Use a stiff, large-bore end-hold catheter.
3. Use stiff, short pressure tubing to connect the catheter to the pressure manifold.
4. Flush system thoroughly before accepting wedge pressure.
5. For mitral valve area determinations, correct for the time delay (phase shift PCW pressure v wave to match the LV downstroke). Also see p. 127.

Left Heart Catheterization

The protocol for left heart catheterization is summarized in the box on pp. 115–116. Indications for left heart catheterization are summarized in Chapter 1 (see box on p. 3). A combined right and left heart protocol is the most precise and complete method of addressing the vast majority of hemodynamic problems encountered in the catheterization laboratory (see the box on pp. 116–117).

Left Heart Catheterization Protocol*

MATCHING PERIPHERAL TO CENTRAL AORTIC PRESSURE

1. Pigtail catheter inserted through arterial sheath (sheath should be one French size larger than catheter.)
2. Administer heparin (3000 to 5000 U per lab routine).
3. Advance catheter to aortic valve.
4. Zero check pigtail pressure (200 mm Hg scale).
5. Zero check sheath pressure (200 mm Hg scale).
6. Turn recorder on; record femoral artery (sheath) and central

aortic pressure (phasic/mean/phasic 25-10-25 mm/sec paper speed).
7. Zero check both pressures.
8. Turn recorder off.

AORTIC VALVE ASSESSMENT

1. Advance pigtail to LV chamber.
2. Zero check pressures; turn recorder on.
3. Turn recorder on; record LV and femoral artery (FA) pressures (25 mm/sec speed, 200 scale) phasic/mean FA/phasic pressure.[†]
4. Turn recorder off.

* Right heart studies often precede left heart hemodynamic studies. Simultaneous left and right heart pressures will provide the most precise and accurate information.
† 100 mm/sec paper speed if aortic valve gradient present.

COMPUTATIONS FOR HEMODYNAMIC MEASUREMENTS

Once the hemodynamic data have been obtained, computations are made to clarify and enhance quantitation of cardiac function. In this section only the most common computations and standard formulas are provided. Computations most often used involve assessment of cardiac work, calculation of flow resistance, computation of valve areas, and shunt calculations. Specific derivations and applications of these formulas can be found elsewhere.

Combined (Left and Right Heart) Hemodynamic Measurements

Begin studies after right heart catheterization completed with PCW tracing ready and LV protocol completed with pigtail catheter in LV before LV pullback.

AORTIC VALVE ASSESSMENT

Follow left heart protocol (see the box on pp. 115–116).

MITRAL VALVE ASSESSMENT

1. Zero check PCW, femoral artery, and LV pressures.
2. Turn recorder on; record LV vs PCW (50 mm/sec speed, 40 mm Hg scale) phasic/mean phasic PCW pressure.
3. Zero check LV pressure.
4. Let down balloon or pull back PCW to PA (25 mm/sec speed, 40 mm Hg scale) and record phasic/mean/phasic PA pressure.
5. Turn recorder off.

NOTE: 100 mm/sec paper if mitral valve gradient present.

CARDIAC OUTPUT

1. Perform Fick oxygen collection (Waters oximetry hood or Douglas bag).
2. Measure thermodilution outputs × 3.
3. Obtain arterial and PA oxygen saturation samples (in duplicate).

RIGHT HEART PULLBACK

1. Zero check all pressures.
2. Turn recorder on (25 mm/sec paper speed; 40 mm Hg scale).
3. Record PCW to PA phasic/mean/phasic pressure.
4. Record PA to RV.
5. Continue recording RV and add LV pressure (to establish presence of constrictive/restrictive physiology) (100 mm/sec paper speed, 40 mm Hg scale).
6. Zero check LV pressure.
7. Record RV to RA (phasic/mean/phasic 25-10-25 mm paper speed; 40 mm Hg scale zero check).
8. Turn recorder off.

NOTE: Left ventriculography usually performed at this point.

POSTVENTRICULOGRAPHY HEMODYNAMICS

1. Zero check LV, aortic pressures.
2. Turn recorder on.
3. Record post ventriculography LV end diastolic pressure (50 mm/sec paper speed, 40 mm Hg scale).
4. Perform LV pullback to aorta with femoral artery pressures displayed (25 mm/sec paper speed; 200 mm Hg scale).
5. Check mean aortic pressures.
6. Zero check pressures.
7. Turn recorder off.

Cardiac output by Fick (O_2 consumption) method

$$\frac{O_2 \text{ consumption (ml/min)}}{AVo_2 \text{ difference (ml } O_2/100 \text{ ml blood)} \times 10}$$

O_2 consumption is measured from metabolic "hood" or Douglas bag; it can also be estimated as 3 ml O_2/kg or 125 ml/min/m^2. AVo_2 (arteriovenous oxygen) difference calculated from arterial − mixed venous (pulmonary artery) O_2 content, where O_2 content = saturation × 1.36 × hemoglobin.

For example, if the arterial saturation is 95%, then the O_2

content = $0.95 \times 1.36 \times 13.0\,g = 16.7\,ml$, pulmonary artery saturation is 65%, and O_2 consumption is 210 ml/min (70 kg $\times$ 3 ml/kg) or measured value, then cardiac output would be determined as follows:

$$\frac{210}{(0.95 - 0.65) \times 1.36 \times 13.0 \times 10^*} = \frac{210}{53} = 3.96\,L/min$$

Cardiac index (CI, L/min/m²)

$$CI = \frac{CO\,(L/min)}{BSA\,(m^2)}$$

where CO is cardiac output and BSA is body surface area.

Stroke volume (SV, ml/beat)

$$SV = \frac{CO\,(ml/min)}{HR\,(bpm)}$$

where HR is heart rate.

Stroke index (SI, ml/beat/m²)

$$SI = \frac{SV\,(ml/beat)}{BSA\,(m^2)}$$

Stroke work (SW, g·m)

SW = (mean LV systolic pressure − mean LV diastolic pressure) × stroke volume × 0.0144[†]

Pulmonary arteriolar resistance (PAR, units)

$$PAR = \frac{\text{mean pulmonary arterial pressure } - \text{ mean LA pressure (or PCW)}}{CO}$$

Total pulmonary resistance (TPR, units)

$$TPR = \frac{\text{mean pulmonary arterial pressure}}{CO}$$

Systemic vascular resistance (SVR, WOOD units)

$$SVR = \frac{\text{mean systemic arterial pressure } - \text{ mean right atrial pressure}}{CO}$$

Converting to Resistance in Metric Units (dynes·sec·cm⁻⁵)

SVR, PAR, TPR units × 80

---

[*] Correction factor when using O_2 content in the Fick formula.
[†] 0.0136 = conversion factor for mm Hg to cm H_2O.

COMPUTATIONS OF VALVE AREAS FROM PRESSURE GRADIENTS AND CARDIAC OUTPUT

A pressure gradient is defined as the pressure difference across an area of obstruction, such as a stenosis or an occlusion (Fig. 3-4).

Anatomic and Artifactual Variables That Affect Pressure Gradients

Physiologic variables
1. Velocity of blood flow
2. Cardiac output
3. Resistance to flow after obstruction
4. Proximal chamber pressure

Anatomic variables
1. Tortuosities of the vessels (for arterial stenosis)
2. Multiple lesions (for both cardiac valves and arterial stenosis)

Artifactual variables
1. Miscalibrated pressure transducers
2. Pressure leaks on catheter manifold or connecting tubing
3. Pressure tubing type, length, and connectors
4. Air in system
5. Catheter sizes (especially small diameters)
6. Position of catheter side holes (aortic stenosis with pigtail catheter, see Fig. 3-64)

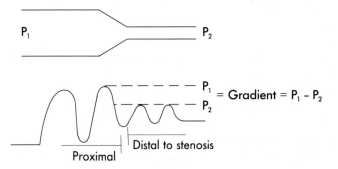

Fig. 3-4. Diagram of pressure gradient across a stenosis or occlusion. The pressure gradient is the difference between P_1 and P_2. P_1, Pressure before the narrowing; P_2, pressure after the narrowing.

Valve Area Calculation

$$\text{Area (cm}^2) = \frac{\text{valve flow (ml/sec)}}{K \times C \times \sqrt{\text{MVG}}}$$

where MVG is mean valvular gradient (mm Hg), K (44.3) is a derived constant by Gorlin and Gorlin,[*] C is an empirical constant that is 1 for semilunar valves and tricuspid valve and 0.85 for mitral valve, and valve flow is measured in milliliters per second during the diastolic or systolic flow period.

Mitral valve flow

$$\frac{\text{CO (ml/min)}}{\text{diastolic filling period (sec/min)}}$$

where diastolic filling period (sec/min) = diastolic period (sec/beat) × HR.

Aortic valve flow

$$\frac{\text{CO (ml/min)}}{\text{systolic ejection period (sec/min)}}$$

where systolic ejection period (sec/min) = systolic period (sec/beat) × HR.

———— Examples of Aortic and Mitral Valve Area Calculations: ————

NOTES FOR DATA USED IN THE FOLLOWING CALCULATIONS: A scale factor is calculated as millimeters of mercury per centimeter of paper deflection. However, 200 mm Hg full scale may not be exactly 10 cm on the recording paper. When using cardiac output, convert to milliliters per minute, not liters per minute. When computing flow, the ejection period and filling period are converted to fractions of the period in seconds by measuring the paper distance and converting that to time (i.e., 4.1 cm for systolic ejection period = 4.1 cm × 1 sec/10 cm = 0.41 second).

Data obtained at catheterization for aortic stenosis (Fig. 3-5)
1. CO = 4.0 L/min = 4000 ml/min
2. HR = 60 bpm

[*] Gorlin R, Gorlin SG: Hydraulic formula for calculation of stenotic mitral valve, other cardiac valves, and central circulatory shunts, *Am Heart J* 41:1-29, 1951.

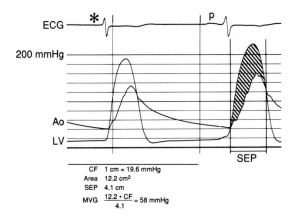

CF 1 cm = 19.6 mmHg
Area 12.2 cm²
SEP 4.1 cm
MVG $\dfrac{12.2 \cdot CF}{4.1}$ = 58 mmHg

Fig. 3-5. Aortic valve area as determined from the planimetered area of the aortic valve gradient. The aortic valve gradient area (*shaded area*) is bounded by the systolic ejection period (*SEP*). *Ao,* Aortic pressure; *LV,* left ventricular pressure (scale 0 to 200 mm Hg); *CF,* correction factor or scale factor; *SEP,* systolic ejection period; *MVG,* mean value gradient. See text for details.

3. Scale factor to convert recording deflection to pressure = 1 cm = 19.6 mm Hg (directly measured paper deflection of 200 mm Hg)
4. Tracing of LV-AO (aortic) pressures at 100 cm/sec paper speed (if using femoral artery pressure, shift upstroke to match LV upstroke)

Step 1:   Planimeter 5 aortic-LV gradients and average (if atrial fibrillation, planimeter 10 beats).

$$\text{Area} = 12.20 \text{ cm}^2$$

Step 2:   Measure systolic ejection periods (SEP) and average.

$$
\begin{aligned}
\text{SEP} &= 4.1 \text{ cm (next convert to time)} \\
&= 4.1 \text{ cm} \times 1 \text{ sec}/10 \text{ cm} = 0.41 \text{ second}
\end{aligned}
$$

Step 3:   Convert planimeter area to mean systolic pressure gradient.

Mean valve gradient (MVG) = (area × scale factor)/SEP

$$12.2 \text{ cm}^2 \times \frac{19.6 \text{ mm Hg}/1 \text{ cm}}{4.1 \text{ cm}} = \frac{239}{4.1} = 58 \text{ mm Hg}$$

Step 4:   Compute aortic valve flow.

$$\frac{CO}{SEP \times HR} = \frac{4000}{0.41 \text{ sec/beat} \times 60 \text{ bpm}} = \frac{4000}{24.6} = 162.6$$

Step 5:   Compute aortic valve area.

$$\frac{\text{Aortic valve flow}}{1.0 \times 44.3 \sqrt{\text{gradient}}} = \frac{162.6}{44.3 \times \sqrt{58}} = \frac{162.6}{44.3 \times 7.6}$$

$$= \frac{162.6}{336.6} = 0.48 \text{ cm}^2$$

NOTES ON THE AORTIC VALVE GRADIENT: The mean pressure gradient is measured by planimetry of the superimposed aortic and LV pressure tracings. Peak-to-peak pressure gradients are easily seen and often used as an estimate of the severity of stenosis. The peak-to-peak gradient is not equivalent to mean gradient for mild and moderate stenosis but is often close to mean gradient for severe stenosis. The delay in pressure transmission and pressure wave reflection from the proximal aorta to the femoral artery artificially increases the mean gradient. Femoral pressure overshoot (amplification) reduces the true gradient. If the femoral arterial pressure is used, phase shifting of the femoral arterial pressure to the left ventricle upstroke is important. In patients with gradients <35 mm Hg, more accurate valve areas were obtained with unadjusted LV-Ao pressure tracings.[*] Optimally a second catheter can be positioned directly above the aortic valve to reduce transmission delay and femoral pressure amplification. Transseptal cardiac catheterization can also be performed to obtain direct pressure (Fig. 3-5).

Simplified formulas provide quick in-lab determinations of aortic valve area. Aortic valve area can be estimated closely as cardiac output divided by the square root of the LV-AO peak-to-peak pressure difference.

$$\text{Peak-to-peak gradient} = 65 \text{ mm HG}$$
$$CO = 5 \text{ L/min}$$

[*] Brogan WC 3d, Lange RA, Hillis LD: Accuracy of various methods of measuring the transvalvular pressure gradient in aortic stenosis. *Am Heart J* 123:948–953, 1992.

$$\text{Quick valve area} = \frac{5 \, \text{L/min}}{\sqrt{65}}$$
$$= \frac{5 \, \text{L/min}}{8}$$
$$= 0.63 \, \text{cm}^2$$

NOTE: The quick formulas for valve area differ from the Gorlin formula by $18 \pm 13\%$ in patients with bradycardia (<65 bpm) or tachycardia (>100 bpm).*

The Gorlin equation at low flow states overestimates the severity of valve stenosis. In low flow states (CO <2.5 L/min), the Gorlin formula should be modified to employ the mean transvalvular gradient with new empirically derived constants.†

USE OF VALVE RESISTANCE FOR AORTIC STENOSIS

Valve resistance, a measure of valve obstruction, has recently been shown to have clinical utility. This index was first proposed for valve stenosis around the same time that the Gorlin valve area formula was initially reported. Valve resistance did not find favor when initially proposed because the relatively obscure unit of dynes per second per centimeter to the fifth power was not well understood.

Despite obvious strengths, valve area measurements have both practical and theoretical limitations. Area is a planar measurement without consideration of the funnellike nature of the mitral inflow or the more tubelike configuration of the aortic outlet. Valve area is based on laminar flow of a nonviscous fluid. Turbulence and blood viscosity are not considered. The constant in the denominator of the Gorlin formula is the square root of 2gH, or gravity, and assumes that blood flow is gravity driven rather than pulsatile as in the arterial system.

Valve areas under 0.7 cm^2 are almost always associated with an important clinical syndrome and areas greater than

* Hillis LD, Winniford MD: The simplified formula for the calculation of aortic valve area: potential inaccuracies in patients with bradycardia or tachycardia. *Cathet Cardiovasc Diagn* 13:301–303, 1987.
† See Cannon SR, Richards KL, Crawford M: Hydraulic estimation of stenotic orifice area: a correction of the Gorlin formula, *Circulation* 71:1170–1178, 1985.

1.1 cm^2 are usually not associated with significant symptoms, but the areas in between remain in a gray zone. One of the most common clinical situations is found in the patient with a valve area of 0.9 to 1.0 cm^2, a low transvalve pressure gradient and low cardiac output and poor LV function. There is uncertainty regarding the outcome following valve replacement with a high mortality if ventricular function does not improve following surgery.

Valve resistance provides an alternative method to assess valve obstruction. It is calculated using the same variables used for valve area measurement. In contrast to valve area, the mean pressure gradient is considered to be a linear variable rather than taken as a square root term (Fig. 3-6). Thus, the contribution of pressure gradient to the magnitude of valve resistance is greater. Resistance has also been shown to be more constant under conditions of changing cardiac output than valve area.

Resistance thus necessarily has a close relationship to valve area. Fig. 3-7 shows resistance and area calculated in a group of patients before and after balloon aortic valve dilatation. Resistance rises sharply above a valve area of 0.7 cm^2. The shoulder of this curve is between 0.7 and 1.1 cm^2, which is the common area of indeterminate significance of Gorlin aortic valve area. Some patients in this gray zone tend to have higher valve resistance than others. It has been shown in this setting that the patients with resis-

VALVE RESISTANCE
dynes.sec.cm^{-5}

$$\left[\frac{\text{Mean Gradient}}{\left(\dfrac{\text{C.O.(L/min)}}{\text{SEP(sec/min)}} \right) \times 60} \right] \times 80$$

Fig. 3-6. Formula for valve resistance. *CO*, cardiac output; *SEP*, systolic ejection period.

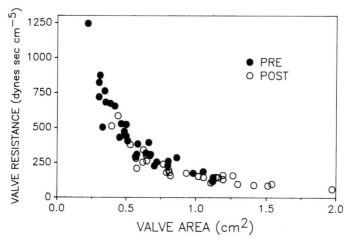

Fig. 3-7. Comparison of valve area by Gorlin formula versus valve resistance before (*pre*) and after (*post*) aortic valvuloplasty. Valve resistance <200 dynes · sec · cm^{-5} is associated with minimal obstruction, >250 dynes · sec · cm^{-5} with significant obstruction. This measure compliments and refines valve area decision making. (From Feldman T, Ford L, Chiu YC, Carroll J: Changes in valvular resistance power dissipation and myocardial reserve with aortic valvuloplasty, *J Heart Valve Dis* 1:55–64, 1992.)

tance >250 dynes·sec·cm^{-5} are more likely to have significant obstruction while those with resistance below 200 dynes·sec·cm^{-5} are less so. There remains a gray zone using this index as well. In addition, some patients may have a resistance below 250 despite a planar valve area of 0.7 to 0.8 cm^2.

Resistance represents a complimentary index. It is not a replacement for valve area. Valve resistance is not expected to remain consistent. Some of the changes in valve area observed in a single patient under different conditions or at different times might be more acceptable when considered as changes in valve resistance than planar area. As with peripheral resistance, valve resistance is interpreted in the context of the clinical conditions under which it is measured. A peripheral resistance of 1000 dynes·sec·cm^{-5} has a greatly different significance in a patient with presumed sepsis than it does in a patient with LV failure. Similarly, we can expect valve resistance to vary as cardiac output changes.

Catheter Selection for Aortic Stenosis

Initial catheter selection is a matter of operator choice based on previous experience. The pigtail ventriculography catheter is a good initial choice in most cases. The aortic valve is crossed with a 0.038-inch straight-tipped safety guidewire, extending the wire straightening the pigtail with a slight angled bend. The wire should be directed into the area of highest turbulence as detected by jet impaction on the wire noting the movement as visualized on the fluoroscopy monitor. Manipulating the wire and catheter allows positioning the wire in various directions needed to cross the valve. Advancing the pigtail over the wire and, in most cases, rapidly positioning the catheter for ventriculography and hemodynamic studies is a simple operation. When this method is successful, it is a one-step procedure, and for this reason the pigtail catheter is a logical first choice. Other choices for crossing the aortic valve include the left and, occasionally, right Amplatz catheter, right Judkins, multipurpose catheter, and specially designed catheters that have been reported in the technical literature. Crossing the aortic valve should not require more than 15 to 20 minutes, and if great difficulty is encountered, a transseptal approach should be considered early.

Points to remember for crossing the aortic valve with guidewires

1. Adequate heparinization (5000-U bolus) should be maintained and frequent flushing performed.
2. A maximal time of 3 minutes per crossing attempt is required before wire withdrawal, wiping, and flushing of the catheter.
3. A 0.035-inch guidewire may be insufficiently stiff to support the catheter on crossing severely deformed, calcific aortic valves, and a 0.038-inch guidewire should be substituted. Use large catheters that accept this size of wire.
4. Avoid guidewire configurations leading to the coronary ostia to prevent dissection of the coronary arteries that would complicate this otherwise benign maneuver.

5. Manipulation of the wire should be gentle to avoid damaging the valve or causing a perforation of the cusps or aortic root.

Data from catheterization laboratory for calculation of mitral valve area (Fig. 3-8)

1. Cardiac output = 3.5 L/min = 3500 ml/min
2. Heart rate = 80 bpm
3. Scale factor = 1 cm = 3.9 mm Hg (40 mm Hg full scale)
4. Tracing of LV-PCW at 100 mm/sec paper speed = (10 cm/sec paper speed) (align PCW v wave with downstroke of LV pressure)

Step 1:   Planimeter 5 LV-PCW areas (10 if in atrial fibrillation).

$$\text{Area} = 9.46 \ cm^2$$

Step 2:   Measure diastolic filling period (DFP).

$$DFP = 3.4 \ cm \ (\text{then convert to time})$$

$$3.4 \ cm \times 1 \ sec/10 \ cm = 0.34 \ second$$

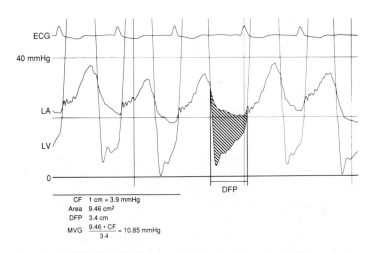

Fig. 3-8.   Hemodynamic tracing used to calculate mitral valve area. The shaded area is the diastolic mitral valve gradient surrounded by the diastolic filling period (*DFP*). *CF*, Correction factor or scale factor; *LA*, left atrial pressure; *LV*, left ventricular pressure (scale 0 to 40 mm Hg); *DFP*, diastolic filling period; *MVG*, mean value gradient. See text for details.

Step 3: Convert planimetered area to mean diastolic pressure gradient.

$$MVG = \frac{area \times scale\ factor}{DFP}$$
$$= \frac{9.46\ cm^2 \times 3.9\ mm\ Hg/1\ cm}{3.4\ cm}$$
$$= \frac{36.9}{3.4}$$
$$= 10.85\ mm\ Hg$$

Step 4: Compute mitral valve flow.

$$\frac{CO\ (ml/min)}{DFP \times HR} = \frac{3500\ ml/min}{3.4\ cm \times (1\ sec/10\ cm) \times 80\ bpm}$$
$$= \frac{3500}{0.34 \times 80}$$
$$= \frac{3500}{27.2}$$
$$= 128.7$$

Step 5: Compute mitral valve area.

$$\frac{Mitral\ valve\ flow}{0.85^* \times 44.3\ \sqrt{10.85}} = \frac{128.7}{0.85 \times 44.3 \times 3.3} = \frac{128.7}{124.3} = 1.0\ cm^2$$

NOTES ON MITRAL VALVE GRADIENT: Obtaining an accurate PCW pressure (discussed earlier in this chapter and in Chapter 2) is critical. PCW pressure overestimates LA pressure (transseptal catheterization) in patients with prosthetic mitral valves. Overestimation is due, in part, to large v waves increasing the phase delay, making correction and alignment of pressure tracings difficult.

Using direct LA pressure with transseptal measurement is the most accurate method. Transseptal catheterization should be performed to confirm large pressure gradients, especially for suspected prosthetic mitral stenosis. However, if the wedge pressure/LV pressure tracings show no significant gradients, transseptal catheterization is unnecessary.

A worksheet for valve area calculation is shown in Fig. 3-9.

---

* 0.85 is Gorlin factor for mitral valve area.

Determination of mitral valve gradient and area

Cardiac output (CO)   ml/min
Diastolic filling period per beat (dfp true)   sec/beat
Heart rate   beats/min
Diastolic filling period per minute (DFP) = HR × dfp   sec/min
Empiric constant (with true dfp)   0.85
Mitral diastolic mean gradient (by planimetry)   mm Hg

$$\text{Mitral valve flow} = \frac{CO}{DFP} = \boxed{} \text{ ml/sec}$$

$$\text{Mitral valve area} = \frac{\text{Mitral valve flow}}{0.85 \times 44.3 \times \sqrt{\text{mitral valve diastolic gradient}}} = \boxed{} = \boxed{} \text{ cm}^2$$

Determination of aortic valve gradient and area

Cardiac output (CO)   ml/min
Systolic ejection period per beat (sep)   sec/beat
Heart rate   beats/min
Systolic ejection period per minute (SEP) = HR × sep   sec/min
Empiric constant   1
Aortic systolic mean gradient (by planimetry)   mm Hg

$$\text{Aortic valve flow} = \frac{CO}{SEP} = \boxed{} \text{ ml/sec}$$

$$\text{Aortic valve area} = \frac{\text{Aortic valve flow}}{1 \times 44.3 \times \sqrt{\text{aortic valve systolic gradient}}} = \boxed{} = \boxed{} \text{ cm}^2$$

Fig. 3-9. Worksheet for determination of valve areas. (Adapted from Grossman W: *Cardiac catheterization and angiography*, ed 3, Philadelphia, 1986, Lea & Febiger.)

Tricuspid valve gradients (see Fig. 3-27 on p. 165). Because small gradients (5 mm Hg) across the tricuspid valve may lead to significant clinical symptoms, precise measurement of hemodynamics through two large lumen catheters is required. Pressures through two catheters should be matched before placement in the RA and RV to avoid technical error. Use the valve area formula for mitral stenosis. Validation of the Gorlin constant has not been established.

Pulmonic valve stenosis (Fig. 3-10). A pulmonary valvular stenosis gradient is obtained by catheter "pullback," continuously measuring pressure during catheter withdrawal across the stenotic valve. However, two catheters or multiple lumen balloon-tipped catheters or double-lumen Cournand catheters are more precise and can record simultaneous PA and RV pressures in the manner used for aortic valve stenosis. There is no formula for pulmonary valve area. In fact, prognostic data are based on RV pressure.

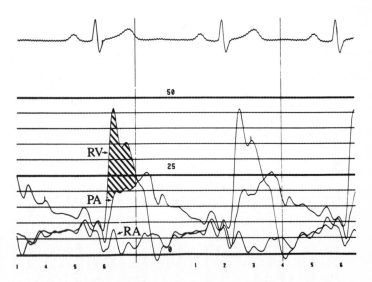

Fig. 3-10. Hemodynamic tracings from a patient with pulmonary stenosis. The shaded area is pulmonary stenosis gradient (scale 0 to 50 mm Hg, time lines are 1 second). *PA*, pulmonary artery pressure; *RV*, right ventricular pressure; *RA*, right atrial pressure.

SECTION II: TECHNIQUES FOR MEASUREMENT OF CARDIAC OUTPUT
OXYGEN CONSUMPTION MEASUREMENT (FICK METHOD)

In the cardiac catheterization laboratory, cardiac output is determined by one of two techniques:
1. Measurement of oxygen consumption (Fick technique)
2. Indicator dilution technique (thermodilution using a pulmonary artery catheter or indocyanine green dye curve)

Fick Principle for Measurement of Cardiac Output

The Fick principle states that uptake or release of a substance by any organ is the product of the arteriovenous concentration difference of the substance and the blood flow to that organ. Therefore, pulmonary blood flow (which is equal to systemic blood flow in the absence of an intracardiac shunt) is determined by measuring the arteriovenous difference of oxygen across the lungs and the uptake of oxygen from room air by the lungs. Cardiac output is then calculated as oxygen consumption divided by the arteriovenous oxygen concentration difference. The arteriovenous oxygen consumption difference is calculated (in ml oxygen) from the difference in LV oxygen content ($1.36 \times$ Hgb $\times$ LV O_2 saturation $\times$ 10) minus the pulmonary artery (mixed venous) oxygen content ($1.36 \times$ Hgb $\times$ PA O_2 saturation $\times$ 10).

Two methods are utilized in the cardiac catheterization laboratory for measuring oxygen consumption: (1) the polarographic cell method and (2) the Douglas bag method.

Polaragraphic Method (Metabolic Hood)

This method utilizes a polaragraphic oxygen sensor cell to measure the oxygen content of expired air. The MRM-2* is one example of a polaragraphic system (Fig. 3-11). Room air is withdrawn at a constant rate through a plastic hood that is placed over the patient's head while the patient is in a supine position. The unit measures the contents of the hood (room air/expired air) through a flexible tubing to the polaragraphic oxygen sensing cell. The metabolic rate meter gives a readout of oxygen consumption in liters per minute.

---

* Waters Instruments, Rochester, Minn.

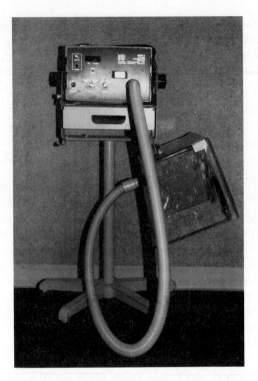

Fig. 3-11. Metabolic (Waters) Hood for determination of oxygen consumption. See text for details.

The following are important considerations when using a polaragraphic method for determining oxygen consumption:

1. Allow the unit to warm up for 30 minutes before use.
2. Check the cell voltage by turning the select knob to "cell." This reading should not be less than 30% of the reference cell voltage. The reference cell voltage is set at the time of cell installation and can be read by switching the select knob to "calibrate." If the cell voltage is less than 30% the reference voltage, it is time to replace the cell.
3. Remove any supplemental oxygen that the patient may be receiving; allow 10 to 15 minutes after discontinuation of the oxygen prior to using the hood.
4. Explain to the patient that the hood will not restrict his

flow of air, and instruct him to breathe in a normal fashion and to be still.

5. Make sure that there is a good seal around the base of the hood. A flat surface such as a board should be placed under the patient's head and shoulders before positioning the hood.

6. The air entrance holes of the hood should not be restricted.

7. The flexible tubing should be in good working condition and without holes or cuts. It is important that the flexible hose is the exact length specified by the manufacturer.

8. Zero the unit before initiating sampling.

9. Allow the patient to breathe normally for 3 to 5 minutes before recording data. Once the rate meter has stabilized, a steady hemodynamic state is present. Record data from the rate meter at this time. It is important to record data every 20 to 30 seconds for 2 to 3 minutes. It is also important to note the patient's heart rate during this period. Accurate oxygen consumption can only be recorded at steady-state conditions.

A calibration check of the polaragraphic unit should be done at routine intervals. A simple method involves filling the hood with a known flow rate of 100% nitrogen. The metabolic rate meter will give specific values for specific flow rates of nitrogen. If these values are inaccurate, the unit should be sent for further calibration by qualified personnel.

Douglas Bag Method

With this method the patient is asked to breathe into a large, sealed, air-tight bag (usually 60-L capacity*) for a specific period of time. The mouthpiece is connected to the bag by a two-way valve. This allows the patient to inspire room air, while the expired air is directed to the Douglas bag. The nose is clipped so that all expired air is forced into the collection bag.

After the specified interval, the bag is sealed and its contents analyzed. This requires analysis of room air as well as the contents of the Douglas bag. An oxygen analyzer is necessary for the analysis of the room air. A Tissot spirometer

---

* Sixty-liter Douglas bag, Warron Collins, Inc., Boston, Mass.

or gas meter is needed to measure the volume of expired air in the Douglas bag.

Points of importance:

1. Explain to the patient the importance of forming a good seal around the mouthpiece in order to direct all expired air into the bag.
2. Make sure the nose clip is placed securely to prevent expired air from exiting through the nose (ask about ear drum perforation as a cause of air leakage).
3. Do not allow the contents of the bag to escape from the time the sample is collected to when it is measured by a spirometer or gas meter. The integrity of the valve system must remain intact during this time.

Once the contents of the bag have been analyzed, the calculations can be made to determine oxygen consumption.

THE FICK OXYGEN CONSUMPTION METHOD

Determination of cardiac output by the Fick technique is the most accurate method of assessing cardiac output, particularly in patients with low cardiac output. Simultaneous reliable measurements of the arteriovenous oxygen content difference and oxygen consumption are critical for accurate cardiac output determination. Use of the polarographic (metabolic hood) and Douglas bag methods for determination of oxygen consumption require that patients breathe comfortably at steady state. If a steady state is not achieved due to anxiety, dyspnea, or any condition where measurement of oxygen is spuriously elevated, an abnormally high cardiac output will be calculated. Conversely, shallow breathing (alveolar hypoventilation), commonly seen with oversedation, results in a falsely low oxygen consumption and, therefore, low cardiac output determination.

Supplemental oxygen is often administered to a patient during diagnostic cardiac catheterization. Mixing the supplemental oxygen with room air makes determination of the oxygen content of the inspired air difficult (if not impossible) to calculate. Therefore, supplemental oxygen therapy should be discontinued at least 10 to 15 minutes before determination of the cardiac output by the Fick technique. If oxygen cannot safely be discontinued, an alternative to the Fick technique should be used.

INDICATOR DILUTION CARDIAC OUTPUT PRINCIPLE

The indicator dilution technique is based on the principle that a single injection of a known amount of an indicator (e.g., cold saline for the thermodilution technique or indocyanine green dye) injected into the central circulation mixes completely with blood and changes concentration as it flows to a more distal location. The change in the indicator concentration (or temperature) is plotted over time; the area under the curve is planimetered to calculate cardiac output.

The most common indicator dilution technique utilized in the cardiac catheterization laboratory is the thermodilution method. Primarily for technical considerations, the indocyanine method is used mainly for shunt studies today.

Thermodilution Indicator Method

The thermodilution indicator method requires a pulmonary artery balloon flotation catheter (Swan-Ganz) with a thermistor at the tip. The thermodilution method used iced or room temperature saline as the indicator substance. Iced (4°C) or room temperature (20°C) saline is cold relative to blood at normal body temperature (37°C). The basic Swan-Ganz catheter is a triple-lumen design: the proximal port, located 30 cm from the tip, is used for RA pressure measurement and for rapid infusion of the saline during cardiac output determination; the distal end hole is used for pressure measurement; and the lumen is used to inflate the balloon. A thermistor at the distal tip measures the blood temperature.

The balloon serves two purposes: (1) it is a positioning aid, and (2) it facilitates measurement of the PCW pressure. The inflated balloon helps to direct the catheter into the PA by "floating" with the flow of blood through the right heart chambers. Once positioned in the PA, the catheter can be advanced to the distal pulmonary vasculature, "wedging" in a small branch. The balloon forms a seal that isolates the tip from PA flow. This separation ensures that the pressure measured beyond the balloon is the pulmonary capillary pressure, which is generally equal to the LA pressure.

An additional feature of this catheter is a small thermistor near the end of the catheter. The thermistor is positioned in the PA when the proximal injectate port is in the right atrium.

Measuring Cardiac Output

Cardiac output is determined by rapidly injecting 10 ml saline (iced or at room temperature) through the proximal port of the PA catheter. An external thermistor measures the temperature of the injectate. Complete mixing of the injectate with blood causes a decrease in the blood temperature, which is sensed by the distal thermistor. The cardiac output computer calculates the change in the indicator concentration (temperature over time) to determine the cardiac output in liters per minute.

For saline injections, coiled tubing systems that are immersed in an ice water bath are commercially available to facilitate cooling of the injectate. With this system, the injectate is withdrawn from a room temperature bag of IV fluid, through the coil, and into the injectate syringe. Special syringes are available that isolate the operator's hand from the injectate syringe. This prevents warming of the injectate by the operator's hand.

Notes on Thermodilution Technique

In order to obtain consistent, reliable results, both the physician and the members of the technical staff must employ good technique. The following steps will contribute to thermodilution cardiac output accuracy.

1. The catheter must be properly positioned in the PA. Excessive coiling of the catheter in the RA or RV can result in poor positioning of the dual thermistor in relation to the injectate port. This problem is sometimes encountered with a large, dilated right heart. In these instances, a 0.025-inch guidewire should be used to give additional stiffness to the catheter.

2. Most thermodilution systems require that a computation constant (on the output computer) is used. Set the computer to the proper computation constant depending on the system being used. Some computers provide a table that gives a constant corresponding to the injectate volume, the injectate temperature, and size and type of catheter being used.

3. Inject the precise amount of injectate. In adults, 10 ml is the commonly used volume, while 5 ml is typical for pediatric procedures. In adults where fluid restriction is

important, a smaller bolus of injectate may be desired. If so, remember to change the computation constant on the output computer to reflect the change in injectate volume.

4. Avoid warming the barrel of the injectate syringe in the palm of the hand. This will introduce error into the output calculation. Special syringe holders are available to alleviate this problem.

5. Coordinate the start button. The technician must press the start button on the computer simultaneously with the delivery of the injectate. Injection before the release of the start button by the technician is a common error. When this happens the computer will not recognize the full bolus of injectate being delivered.

6. The bolus should be delivered rapidly at a consistent flow rate.

7. Connect the catheter to the computer securely. If the interface cable from the cardiac output computer is non-sterile, care should be taken that the sterile field is not violated (special cable drapes are available; see Fig. 6-17).

8. If room-temperature saline is used, there should be at least a 10°C difference between the injectate and body temperature. Most computers have built-in sensors that enable the technician to check these parameters before the start of the procedure.

9. Three to five outputs should be obtained. Any erroneous values should be recorded, but ignored in the final result.

10. The thermodilution technique is inaccurate with tricuspid regurgitation or low cardiac output. Both conditions interfere with the normal flow of injectate past the sensing thermistor (see Fig. 3-12).

ANGIOGRAPHIC CARDIAC OUTPUT

Cardiac output determined angiographically is computed as the end diastolic volume minus the end systolic volume (the stroke volume) times the heart rate. Angiographic cardiac output determination provides the best estimate of cardiac output through a stenotic valve when any degree of regurgitation is present. Errors in volumetric stroke volume computation are increased with enlarged ventricles, especially

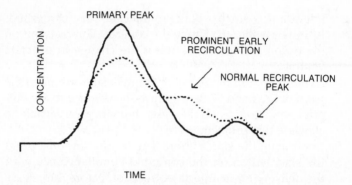

Fig. 3-12. Indocyanine green curves obtained by sampling its concentration in systemic arterial blood after injection into pulmonary artery. *Solid line,* Normal curve; *dotted line,* curve from patient with intracardiac left-to-right shunting. (Adapted from Boehrer JD, Lange RA, Willard JE, Grayburn PA, Hillis LD: Advantages and limitations of methods to detect, localize, and quantitate intracardiac left-to-right shunting, *Am Heart J* 124:448–455, 1992.

when single-plane cineangiography is employed. Angiographic cardiac output is not determined simultaneously with a transvalvular gradient and, therefore additional error may be introduced by delay in simultaneous measurements. (See Chapter 5 for calculation of angiographic output.)

DIFFERENCES AMONG CARDIAC OUTPUT TECHNIQUES

Discrepancies exist between Fick, thermodilution, and indocyanine green dye determinations of cardiac output in patients with low cardiac output or in those with aortic or mitral regurgitation. In low flow states or in valvular regurgitation, recirculation of the green dye may appear on the curve downslope before extrapolation to baseline. Failure to extrapolate to baseline will result in inaccurate cardiac output determinations. Hillis and others* have shown that, in patients with mitral and aortic valve regurgitation, and in patients with

---

* Hillis LD, Firth BG, Winniford MD: Analysis of factors affecting the variability of Fick versus indicator dilution measurements of cardiac output. *Am J Cardiol* 56:764–768, 1985.

low cardiac output, the dye dilution method varied by more than 20% from the Fick method in a significant number of patients. Thermodilution is inaccurate in low cardiac output states. Tricuspid regurgitation or intracardiac shunts further reduce the accuracy of thermodilution. Hillis and others* compared Fick and thermodilution methods and Fick and green dye methods in patients with low cardiac output and found the Fick/thermodilution percentage difference averaged 10 ± 10%, whereas Fick/green dye percent difference averaged 15 ± 12% (significantly higher). In patients with aortic or mitral regurgitation, the Fick/thermodilution percentage difference was 7 ± 7%, whereas the Fick/green dye percentage difference was 17 ± 15%, again statistically significant. Thermodilution is preferable to green dye because right-sided injection and right-sided sampling (of the cold indicator) yields a curve that is less subject to recirculation-induced distortion than right-sided injection and left-sided sampling of green dye.

INTRACARDIAC SHUNTS

A shunt is an abnormal communication between the left and right heart chambers. The direction of blood flowing through the shunt is left to right, right to left, or sometimes bidirectional. In the absence of shunting, the pulmonary blood flow (right heart) is equal to the systemic blood flow. Table 3-2 lists intracardiac shunt locations. A left-to-right shunt increases the amount of blood to the right heart and increases pulmonary blood flow. Therefore pulmonary blood flow is the sum of the systemic blood flow plus shunt flow. With a right-to-left shunt, the amount of blood shunted from the right side to the left is added to that normally ejected into the systemic circulation. Systemic blood flow is then greater than pulmonary blood flow by the amount of the shunt (Fig. 3-13).

Intracardiac shunts can be evaluated by four methods:
1. Oximetry
2. Indocyanin green dye dilution curves (Figs. 3-12 and 3-14)

* Hillis LD, Firth BG, Winniford MD: Comparison of thermodilution and indocyanine green dye, in low cardiac output or left-sided regurgitation. *Am J Cardiol* 57:1201–1202, 1986.

TABLE 3-2.   Cardiac shunt locations

Locations	Earliest step-up location (for left-to-right shunts)
Partial anomalous pulmonary venous return (pulmonary veins entering right atrium)	RA
Atrial septal defects	
Primum (low)	RA, RV
Secundum (mid)	RA
Sinus venosus (high)	RA
Ventricular septal defects	
Membranous (high)	RV
Muscular (mid)	RV
Apical (low)	RV
Aorticopulmonary window (connection of aorta to pulmonary artery)	PA
Patent ductus arteriosus (normally closed Ao-PA connection at birth)	PA

Ao, aortic; PA, pulmonary artery; RA, right atrium; RV, right ventricle.

3. Angiography
4. Radioactive tracers
Also, see Table 3-3 on shunt detection.

Sample Sites for Oxygen Saturations during Diagnostic Saturation Run

RIGHT HEART

LPA (left pulmonary artery)
RPA (right pulmonary artery)
MPA (main pulmonary artery)
PA_{PV} (above pulmonary valve)
RV_{PV} (right ventricle, below pulmonary valve)
RV (mid)
RV (apex)
RV_{TV} (tricuspid valve)
RA_{TV} (right atrium at tricuspid valve)
RA (mid)
SVC, high (superior vena cava)
SVC (low)
RA (high)
RA (low)
IVC, high (inferior vena cava, just beneath heart, above hepatic vein)

IVC (low, above renal vein, but below hepatic vein)

LEFT HEART

Arterial saturation, aortic
(If possible cross atrial septal defect, pulmonary vein saturation)
Patent foramen ovale (PFO) or LA (left atrium)

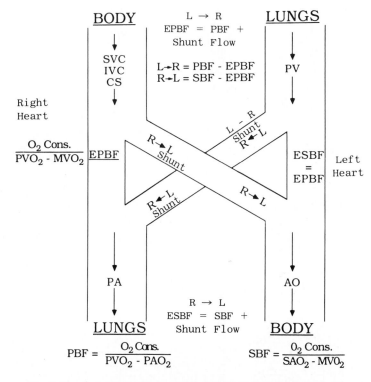

Fig. 3-13. Schematic diagram for right to left and left to right shunting across the heart. *L*, Left; *R*, right; *PBF*, pulmonary blood flow; *EPBF*, effective pulmonary blood flow; *SBF*, systemic blood flow; *ESBF*, effective systemic blood flow; O_2 *Cons.*, oxygen consumption; PAO_2, pulmonary artery oxygen saturation or content; PVO_2, pulmonary venous oxygen saturation or content; MVO_2, mixed venous oxygen saturation or content; SAO_2, systemic arterial oxygen saturation or content; *SVC*, superior vena cava; *IVC*, inferior vena cava; *CS*, coronary sinus; *AO*, aorta; *PA*, pulmonary artery.

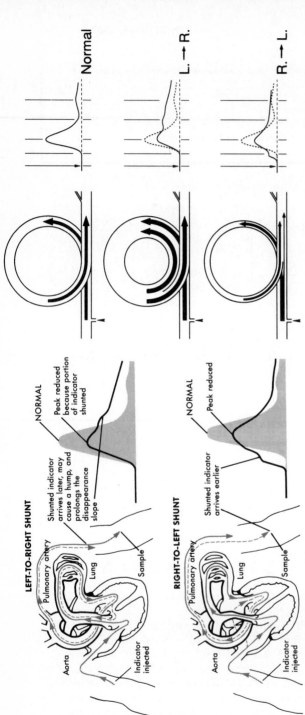

Fig. 3-14. *Left-to-right shunt (increased pulmonic flow).* Indicator is not cleared rapidly but recirculates through central circulation via defect. Based on magnitude of shunt, a constant fraction leaves the central pool with each circulation. Maximal deflection is reduced and the disappearance is prolonged as a result of slow clearance. *Right-to-left shunt (decreased pulmonic flow).* A portion of the indicator passes directly to the arterial circulation via the defect without passing through the lungs and arrives at the arterial sampling site before the portion that did traverse the pulmonary circulation.

TABLE 3-3. Comparison of methods to detect, localize, and quantitate intracardiac left-to-right shunting

Method	Able to localize?	Able to quantitate?	Minimal Qp/Qs reliably detected
Oximetry	Yes	Yes	1.5-1.9 Atrium
			1.3-1.5 Ventricle
			1.3 Great vessels
Indocyanine green			
Carter et al.*	No	Yes	1.35
Gamma variate	No	Yes	1.15
Hydrogen	No	No	1.01
Angiography	Yes	No	Unknown
Radionuclide	No	Yes	1.15
Echocardiography	Yes	Yes	Unknown

*Boehrer JD, Lange RA, Willard JE, Grayburn PA, Hillis LD: Advantages and limitations of methods to detect, localize, and quantitate intracardiac left-to-right shunting. *Am Heart J* 124:448–455, 1992.

Oximetry Procedure: The Diagnostic Saturation ("sat") Run

Oximetry is the most commonly used method. A diagnostic "saturation run" uses heparinized 1- to 3-ml syringes to obtain blood from the PAs and regions of the RV, RA, and superior (SVC) and inferior vena cavae (IVC) in a rapid, organized manner. A large-bore end-hole or side-hole catheter (NIH, Goodale-Lubin, or Cournand) is preferred for rapid sampling. Samples also can be obtained from a standard balloon-tipped Swan-Ganz–type catheter. Saturation syringes should be heparinized with less than 0.5 ml. The labels and list of sample sites also should be prepared in advance (see the box above).

The saturation run begins after diagnostic hemodynamic data and cardiac output have been obtained, and before right heart pullback. With the catheter positioned in the right or left PA, oxygen consumption (Fick method) is measured. After the oxygen consumption measurement is completed, one operator manipulates the catheter under fluoroscopic and pressure control while the assistant aspirates the blood samples at each location along the run. Each new sample is obtained after withdrawing and discarding several milliliters of blood within the catheter left from the previous site. If a sample cannot be obtained from a specific site because of ventricular ectopy, it may be necessary to reposition the catheter or skip the sample site until the rest of the run has been completed. The entire diagnostic run should take approximately 5 to 7 minutes.

Oxygen step-up.   A left-to-right shunt is suggested at a chamber or vessel when a step-up, or increase, of oxygen content in that chamber or vessel exceeds that of a proximal compartment (beyond a normal variation in the oxygen content between the right heart chambers). Thus a step-up in oxygen saturation at the PA by more than 7% (above the RA saturation) is indicative of a left-to-right shunt at the atrial level (Table 3-4). Similarly the desaturation of arterialized blood samples from the left heart chambers and aorta suggests a right-to-left shunt. In determining the site of the right-to-left shunt, sequential sampling can be made from the left atrium, left ventricle, and aorta.

Mixed venous blood is assumed to be fully mixed PA blood. If there is a left-to-right shunt, mixed venous blood is measured one chamber proximal to the step-up. In the case of an atrial septal defect, the mixed venous oxygen content is computed as the sum of three times the superior vena cava plus one inferior vena cava oxygen content and divided by four.

When pulmonary venous blood is not collected, PVo_2 (pulmonary vein) percentage saturation is assumed to be 95%.

Shunt calculation (see Fig. 3-13).   The Fick or left-sided indicator dilution methods of cardiac output determination

TABLE 3-4.   Oxygen saturation values for shunt detection

Level of shunt	Significant step-up difference* O_2 % saturation
Atrial (SVC/IVC to right atria)	≥7
Ventricular	≥5
Great vessel	≥5

SVC, superior vena cava; IVC, inferior vena cava; PA, pulmonary artery pressure.
*Difference distal-proximal chamber. For example for ASD:

$$PA - \frac{3\,SVC + 1\,IVC}{4} \text{ (should be ≥7\% normally.)}$$

are employed to measure systemic flow. Using the Fick method the following formulas apply:

Systemic flow (L/min)*

$$= \frac{O_2 \text{ consumption (ml/min)}}{10 \times \text{arterial} - \text{mixed venous } O_2 \text{ difference (vol \%)}}$$

Pulmonary flow (L/min)

$$= \frac{O_2 \text{ consumption (ml/min)}}{10 \times \text{pulmonary vein} - \text{pulmonary artery } O_2 \text{ difference (vol \%)}}$$

Normally, the effective pulmonary blood flow is equal to the systemic blood flow.

In a left-to-right shunt (see Fig. 3-14) the effective pulmonary blood flow is increased (by the amount of the shunt) as follows:

Effective pulmonary flow = systemic flow + shunt flow
(left-to-right)   (1)

However, in a right-to-left shunt the effective pulmonary blood flow is decreased (by the amount of the shunt):

Effective pulmonary flow = systemic flow − shunt flow
(right-to-left)   (2)

The shunt volume is determined using Equations (1) and (2).

The ratio of pulmonary to systemic flow (called Qp/Qs, where Q is flow, p is pulmonary, s is systemic) for a left-to-right shunt is called the shunt fraction. Flow ratios, Qp/Qs >1.5 often require closure.

_____ Example for Left-to-Right Shunt Atrial Septal _____
Defect (ASD) Calculation:

Data obtained at catheterization:

$$Hgb = 13.0 \text{ g}$$

$$O_2 \text{ consumption} = 210 \text{ ml/min}$$

Location	Saturation (%)
Arterial	92
SVC	70
Mid RA	85
Low RA	68

* See cardiac output calculation, p. 118.

Location	Saturation (%)
PA	83
Pulmonary vein	95
IVC	68

Step 1: Compute O_2 content.*

$$\text{Arterial } O_2 \text{ content} = 0.92 \times 1.36 \times 13.0 \times 10 = 163$$

$$\text{Mixed venous } O_2 \text{ content} = \frac{(.70 + .70 + .70 + .68)}{4} = 0.69$$
$$\times 1.36 \times 13.0 \times 10 = 122$$

$$\text{Pulmonary artery } O_2 \text{ content} = (0.83 \times 1.36 \times 13.0 \times 10) = 147$$

$$\text{Pulmonary vein } O_2 \text{ content} = (0.95 \times 1.36 \times 13.0 \times 10) = 168$$

Step 2: Compute systemic flow [Equation (1)].

$$\frac{210 \, \text{ml/min}}{163 - 122} = \frac{210}{41}$$
$$Qs = 5.12$$

Step 3: Compute pulmonary flow [Equation (2)].

$$\frac{210}{168 - 147} = \frac{210}{21}$$
$$Qp = 10$$

Step 4: Compute Qp/Qs.

$$\frac{10}{5.1} = 1.96$$

———— Example for Simplified Qp/Qs Formula Using Saturations Only: ————

$$\frac{QP}{Qs} = \frac{SAo_2 - MVo_2}{PVo_2 - PAo_2} \quad \frac{\text{Art} - \text{MV}}{\text{PV} - \text{PA}}$$

(Art, arterial; SAo_2, systemic artery o_2 saturation; PVo_2, pulmonary vein o_2 saturation; MVo_2, mixed venous o_2 saturation; PAo_2, pulmonary artery o_2 saturation)

Using saturation data from example of left-to-right ASD:

$$\frac{Qp}{Qs} = \frac{92 - 69}{95 - 83} = \frac{23}{12}$$
$$= 1.92$$

* See Fick method, p. 131.

_____ Example for Right-to-Left Shunt: _____

Data obtained at catheterization:

$$Hgb = 15\,g$$
$$O_2\ consumption = 195\ ml/min$$

Location	Saturation (%)
Arterial	89
SVC	81
RA, mid	83
RA, low	82
LA	88
PA	82
Pulmonary vein	96
IVC	70

Step 1: Compute O_2 content.

$$Arterial = (0.89 \times 15 \times 1.36 \times 10) = 181\ ml/L$$
$$= 167\ ml/L$$

$$Pulmonary\ arterial = (0.82 \times 15 \times 1.36 \times 10) = 167\ ml/L$$

$$Pulmonary\ vein = (0.96 \times 15 \times 1.36 \times 10) = 195\ ml/L$$

Step 2: Compute systemic flow [Equation (1)].

$$\frac{O_2\ consumption}{SAo_2 - PAo_2} = \frac{195}{181 - 167} = \frac{195}{14}$$
$$Qs = 13.9$$

Step 3: Compute pulmonary blood flow [Equation (2)].

$$\frac{O_2\ consumption}{PVo_2 - PAo_2} = \frac{195}{195 - 167} = \frac{195}{28}$$
$$Qp = 7.0$$

Step 4: Compute Qp/Qs.

$$\frac{7.0}{13.9} = 0.5\ (right\text{-}to\text{-}left\ shunt)$$

Limitations of the oximetric technique

1. Because of its low sensitivity, oximetry may fail to detect a small ($<20\%$) shunt.
2. The application of the Fick principle to calculate blood flow presumes a steady state during the diagnostic run

and measurement of oxygen consumption (i.e., timely collection of saturation sample within a period when the oxygen consumption and cardiac output are stable).

3. The oximetry method also assumes that complete mixing is achieved instantly and that the blood samples obtained are representative of blood in the respective compartment.

4. The rate of systemic blood flow is important in detecting a shunt by oximetry. A high systemic flow tends to equalize the arteriovenous oxygen difference across a given vascular bed. Therefore, in the presence of elevated systemic blood flow, the mixed venous oxygen saturation is higher than normal, and intrachamber variability caused by streaming is blunted. By contrast, when the systemic blood flow is reduced and the mixed venous oxygen saturation is lower, a larger step-up must be detected before a significant left-to-right shunt is diagnosed.

Dye Dilution Method

The second method for the detection of an intracardiac shunt employs dye dilution curves. This is an extremely sensitive method that can detect even very small shunts. Quantification of shunts from dye dilution curves uses several methods of measurement.

Comparison of oximetry and indicator dilution technique for the assessment of left-to-right intracardiac shunting in adults showed close approximation by both techniques. The shunt volume by oximetry exceeded the shunt volume by indocyanine green method by more than 20% to 60% of patients. In infants, indicator dye dilution yielded larger shunt values than did the oximetric method, but in adults the indicator dye dilution technique yielded consistently smaller shunt values than oximetry. Arteriovenous indocyanine green dilution curves may be relied upon in detecting shunting when the oximetry values demonstrate a left-to-right shunt in excess of 26% of the pulmonary flow. A venovenous (right side injection–right side sampling) dye dilution curve is more sensitive in this situation (see Fig. 3-14).

Angiography

Angiography is a nonquantitative method that can be used to localize either left-to-right or right-to-left shunts. The angiographic method is useful when the site of origin of the shunt cannot be entered. Contrast media can be injected into the closest proximal accessible chamber to detect the shunt. The LAO view with cranial angulation puts the interatrial and interventricular septae *en face* providing an ideal view for detection of contrast passage across the atrial and ventricular septal defects (see Table 5-4 for practical tips for angiography of shunts).

Radioactive Tracers

Radioactive tracers for shunts are administered by vein in the nuclear medicine department and provide a useful estimate of shunt flow. Radioactivity seen in the brain or kidneys after right-sided injection means the tracer has passed through an intracardiac shunt (right-to-left), escaping entrapment by the lungs.

EQUIPMENT USED FOR HEMODYNAMIC STUDY
Pressure Manifold and Hemodynamic Setup (Fig. 3-15)

The optimal set of transducers, tubing, and manifolds for any laboratory is that which is cost-efficient, familiar, accurate, and simple to use. Several varieties of manifolds exist, both disposable and reusable. A variety of transducers, positioned either on the manifold or at the side of the catheterization table, are suitable. For research studies, special transducer-tipped micromanometer pressure catheters are used for the high-fidelity pressure recordings. High-fidelity recordings are not necessary for daily clinical hemodynamic studies; accurate measurements can be obtained with fluid-filled systems if appropriate precautions in the set-up are made. Clear plastic manifolds are now equipped with four valves in which the pressure line and a zero line are connected at the first stopcock, saline flush solution at the second, contrast media at the third, and a waste flush port (to minimize contamination of personnel and laboratory) at the fourth stopcock. All injections into the arterial system are performed by hand syringes or with an appropriately cleared power syringe setup. Pressure tubing should be short and stiff. Ideally, the transducer should be as close to the catheter as possible.

For optimal pressure measurements, minimize the tubing

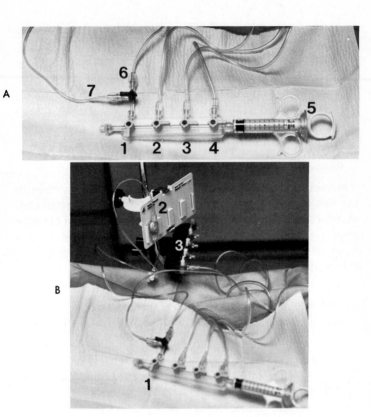

Fig. 3-15. **A,** Close-up of pressure manifold used for coronary angiography. *1,* The connection to the patient at the end of a plastic, movable, swivel connector. This also connects to *6* and *7,* which are the pressure and zero lines, respectively. *2,* Saline flush line; *3,* contrast line; *4,* waste line; *5,* control syringe. **B,** Close-up of the pressure manifold. *1* is connected to the transducer and zero lines. *2,* Tranduces on its holder; *3,* off table zero.

length from the catheter to the transducer. Longer tubing contributes to poorer quality tracings (more "fling" artifact). The zero level is set at midchest (measured anterioposterior [AP] diameter of patient divided by two). When the transducer is raised above zero level, pressure is artifically lower. When the transducer is lower than zero, pressure is artifically higher. When abnormally low pressures are seen initially, recheck the zero for proper positioning (at midchest) and detection of air bubbles or loose connections.

Physiologic Recorder (Fig. 3-16)

The physiologic monitor/recorder is the primary instrument used for the processing and recording of hemodynamic signals. The typical monitor in the cardiac catheterization laboratory is a multichannel unit that can process, display, and record ECG signals, pressure tracings, and direct current (DC) inputs from external sources (e.g., thermodilution or green dye cardiac output curves). Recorders vary from two-channel input to multichannel input (18 to 20 inputs). The number of channels determines how many indivicual signals

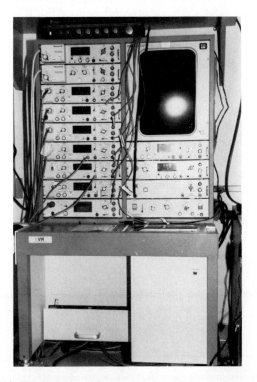

Fig. 3-16.   Typical physiologic recorder (Electronics for Medicine VR-12) showing multiple amplifiers, both electrocardiographic and hemodynamic. In addition, a green dye amplifier can be inserted into this module.

are displayed and recorded simultaneously. For routine cardiac catheterization, one ECG signal and two to three pressure signals normally are recorded. In certain complex cases such as EPS and cases with complex congenital or valvular heart disease, it is common to use 4 to 18 channels.

The physiologic recorder must be set up and calibrated to reference standards before the case for each amplifier being used, the most common being ECG and pressure amplifiers.

ECG amplifier (Fig. 3-17).   The ECG signal should be checked before the start of each case to ensure that the signal is calibrated for a 1 mV/10 mm ratio. The standard is 1 mV/10 mm of deflection on the paper or monitor. This standardization is important if the ECG is going to be used for diagnostic purposes such as measurement of the P wave, QRS, ST segment, etc. If the signal is to be used for monitoring purposes only, this standardization is less important. For monitoring purposes, increasing the gain higher than 1 mV/10 mm will display a larger QRS amplitude. Note that increasing the calculation higher than 1 mV/10 mm also will amplify and exaggerate artifact.

Some ECG amplifiers have filter switches that may aid in reducing noise. These filters may enable the technician to enhance the incoming ECG signal. Some common features of ECG amplifiers are:

1. *Lead selector switch.* This switch allows the operator to select which pair of electrodes will be displayed on the recorder/monitor. The standard configuration for lead selection is made up of the bipolar limb leads (I, II, III), the

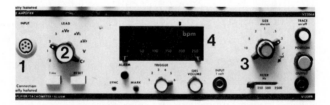

Fig. 3-17.   Close-up view of ECG amplifier. *1,* Input connection; *2,* lead selector; *3,* millivolt per centimeter scale factors; *4,* digital readout. See text for details.

augmented unipolar limb leads (aV_R, aV_L, aV_F), and the unipolar precordial leads (V_1-V_6).

2. *Calibration input.* This allows the operator to input a 1-mV signal as a reference so that the operator can set the trace size on the recorder/monitor.
3. *QRS trigger/beep.* This provides an audible "beep" to correspond to the r wave. Hearing the heart is a must. All personnel can appreciate arrhythmias or early onset of vagal reaction by the change of the beep.
4. *Rate meter.* This meter provides a digital display of the heart rate in beats per minute.
5. *Mark button/switch.* This switch allows the operator to place a mark on the recorder/monitor to indicate an event.

Pressure amplifiers (Fig. 3-18).   The pressure amplifier of the physiologic monitor connects with the pressure transducer, providing the pressure wave from the intravascular catheter. The transducer and amplifier convert the mechanical energy of a pulsatile column of fluid in the catheter to an electrical signal that is displayed on the monitor/recorder. The system should be checked at the start of each day to insure that signal deflection is accurate and calibrated to a known pressure from a blood pressure cuff.

Calibration. The transducer/amplifier of the physiologic monitor system should be calibrated daily. A common technique uses a mercury manometer and applies a known pres-

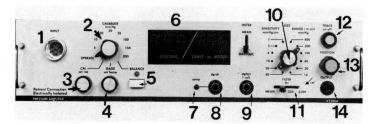

Fig. 3-18.   Close-up view of pressure amplifier. *1,* Input; *2,* calibration factors; *3,* CAL (calibration) setting; *4,* gauge factor; *5,* balance control; *6,* systolic/diastolic digital readout; *7,* ramp button for dP/dt; *8,* dP/dt output; *9,* auxiliary input channel; *10,* sensitivity and range setting; *11,* filter to obtain electronic mean of pressure; *12,* on/off switch; *13,* position of trace switch; *14,* auxillary output channel.

sure to the transducer (Fig. 3-19). The gain setting on the amplifier is adjusted so that the amplitude of the signal matches the pressure being applied.

Gauge factor. Most transducers come with a specific gauge factor. This is a number assigned from the factory to a specific

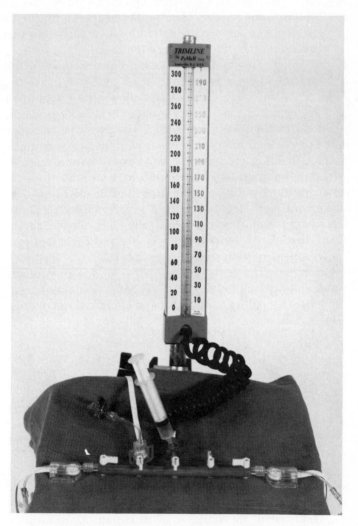

Fig. 3-19.   Close-up of mercury sphygmomanometer attached to the transducers for precise calibration before cardiac catheterization.

transducer that allows the operator to preset the amplifier as a rapid means of calibration. While this may put the amplifier gain "in the ballpark," it should not be a substitute for direct manometric calibration.

Suggested guidelines for transducer calibration using a manometer

1. Set the display of the monitoring system to a routine reference standard. A common display standard is a 10-cm deflection with 1-cm division over the range selected. For example, if the range were 100 mm Hg full scale, the full deflection (top line) of 10 cm would = 100 mm Hg. Therefore 10 divisions of each centimeter would each be equal to 10 mm Hg. For right heart pressures, 0 to 40 mm Hg scale is generally used; for left heart pressures, 0 to 200 mm Hg is used. To compare LV and PCW, 0 to 40 mm Hg scale is used. (See pressure hemodynamic protocols on pp. 112, 113, and 115.)
2. After the display is set zero to full scale, open all transducers to room air.
3. Balance the transducer by using the balance or zero button on the amplifier.
4. If the transducer signal does not appear on the zero reference line after using the balance button, place the signal on the zero line using the position knob/switch of the amplifier (i.e., move the position of the signal trace to zero line).
5. Select the range of calibration. A common range is a 100 scale with full deflection equal to 100 mm Hg.
6. Apply 100 mm Hg to the transducer. If you are using a metered amplifier, adjust the gain so that the meter reads 100. Now check the signal deflection on the display. If it does not reach the 10-cm line, adjust the gain or size control of the amplifier so that the signal is exactly on the top full scale line.
7. Open the transducer again to air and recheck the zero position. If stable, repeat steps 3 to 6 and record the calibration on the paper.
8. If more than one transducer is going to be used, all of them should be calibrated simultaneously. If a manometer is used for calibration, all transducers should be con-

nected to the same pressure source. This can be accomplished by connecting the transducers to the manometer through a manifold system, ensuring that all transducers "see" the exact same pressure input. This is especially important when using two pressures simultaneously to determine a pressure gradient between heart chambers.

Electronic calibration. Most recorders have an electronic calibration that allows the operator to input an electronic "pressure" standard. This feature provides a convenient means for simulating pressure signals to calibrate the display. The hemodynamic recording protocols in some laboratories require that the operator input a "cal" (calibration) signal at the end of each physiologic recording to document the range on which the recording was made.

Features of pressure amplifiers

1. *Mean switch.* This switch converts the phasic tracing into an averaged signal (see Fig. 3-18)
2. *dP/dt differentiator* (see Chapter 6, Fig. 6-1). This converts the pressure signal into a pressure/time signal, calculating the change in the slope of the pressure curve in relation to time. A practical use in the catheterization laboratory would be to measure the dP/dt (rate of rise) of the LV pressure. The more rapid the rise of the LV upstroke, the higher the dP/dt signal, indicating a stronger LV contraction; conversely a slower upstroke would indicate a weaker contraction with a reduced dP/dt. A high-fidelity, transducer-tipped catheter is necessary for this research-type data.
3. *Filter switch.* This switch selects the frequency response for the amplifier, ranging from 10 to 2500 Hz, depending on the recorder. For practical purposes, 10 Hz is the normal filter selection. The 250-Hz position would be used for high-fidelity recordings.
4. *Ramp slope.* This injects a rising voltage of constant slope for calibration of dP/dt.

Display settings for recording paper/video monitor. The operator has a number of choices when setting the display for physiologic monitoring. These include the following:

1. *Time lines.* The time interval at which a vertical line appears on the recording paper. The usual choices are: 0.01 second, 0.04 second, 0.1 second, 0.2 second, 0.5 second,

1 second, 5 seconds (Figs. 3-20 and 3-21). The typical setting for a routine case is 1-second time lines (i.e., a line each second). For special studies or when faster paper speed is used, a faster time line sequence should be used. It is important to know the time line interval used as certain calculations are made from the time line interval (heart rate, diastolic filling times, etc). If the paper speed is known, the time line interval can be measured and calculated. Also use a full-page inscription of time lines to assist the timing of pressure wave changes (Fig. 3-21).

2. *Paper speed.* The rate of paper speed can be changed by the operator. The paper speed choices for most recorders range from 5 to 500 mm/sec. The typical choice for most procedures is 25 mm/sec. In certain hemodynamic studies, 50 and 100 mm/sec are used. Slower paper speeds (10 and 5 mm/sec) are used when recording the mean pressure or when conserving paper in long hemodynamic studies. It should be noted that in some recorders, different paper types (photographically faster) may be necessary if paper speed >150 mm/sec is used.

3. *Sweep speed (video monitor).* This control gives the operator the choice of changing the sweep of the oscilloscope monitor. On some monitors this feature is linked to the paper speed.

4. *Calibration lines.* This switch allows the operator to set number and spacing of the horizontal calibration lines on the monitor and paper. A usual configuration is 10 cm per full scale spacing.

5. *Position button.* This control allows adjustment of the calibration lines on the paper. NOTE: Inadvertent movement of this position can shift the calibration lines and cause erroneous pressure readings (see Fig. 3-22).

HEMODYNAMIC RECORDING TECHNIQUES

Certain basic techniques are required to obtain high-quality hemodynamic recordings. The following are some suggestions that will aid in providing consistent, reliable data:

1. At the start of each procedure, place the patient's name, the date, and calibration inputs on the recording paper.

2. Zero the transducers/recorder properly. Transducers should be placed at the midchest level and opened to air

Timelines

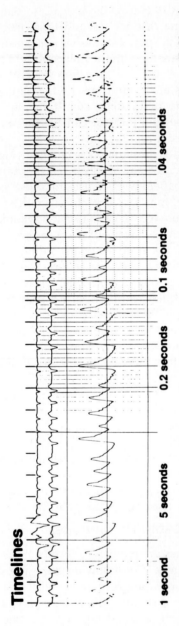

Fig. 3-20. Demonstration of time line recordings. Most tracings use 1 line/sec as a routine. (From Kern MJ: *Hemodynamic rounds: interpretation of cardiac pathophysiology from pressure waveform analysis.* St. Louis, 1993, Wiley-Liss.)

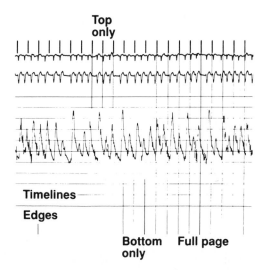

Fig. 3-21. Time lines can be inscribed differently across the recording paper. For accurate and easy timing of hemodynamic events (i.e., correlation with pressure waves), use full-page time lines (*far right side*). (From Kern MJ: *Hemodynamic rounds: interpretation of cardiac pathophysiology from pressure waveform analysis*. St. Louis, 1993, Wiley-Liss.)

before setting reference zeros. Midchest can be measured with a ruler and marked for later reference.

3. Indicate what scale is being used during the recording. If simultaneous tracings are being recorded, good technique dictates that all channels be placed on the same scale factor. This may not always be possible but should be encouraged. (Some units print the scale on the paper automatically.)

4. The recording technician should anticipate changes for recording technique as the catheter is moved to new positions. Change pressure scales and recording paper speed as needed.

EXAMPLE: When monitoring right atrial pressure in a patient with pulmonary hypertension, a full scale 0 to 50 mm Hg may be appropriate. As the catheter passes through the tricuspid valve, the RV pressure may be higher than 50 mm Hg. The technician should observe

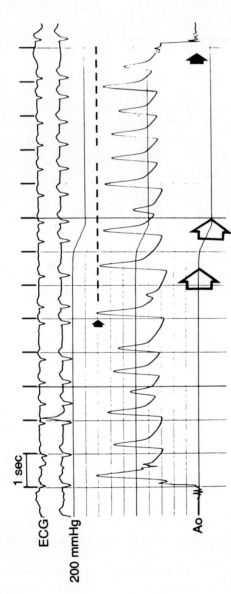

Fig. 3-22. Effect of changing position of the calibration lines. Shifting the grid downward (*two open arrows*) causes an erroneous increase in systolic aortic pressure from 160 to nearly 180 mm Hg. At low pressures this could be a critical problem. Note the confirmation of the error by the zero recheck at the far right arrow. *Ao*, aortic pressure. (From Kern MJ: *Hemodynamic rounds: interpretation of cardiac pathophysiology from pressure waveform analysis*. St. Louis, 1993, Wiley-Liss.)

this, anticipate the change, and quickly change the scale (e.g., 0 to 100 mm Hg full scale) accordingly. This is an instance when the recording paper should be marked accurately so there is no question when reviewing the tracings as to what scale was used.

5. Some recorders require adjustments to the temperature and intensity settings that control the print quality on the recording paper. If the tracings are too light, the temperature or intensity needs to be increased. If the tracings are too dark, the temperature or intensity needs to be decreased.

HEMODYNAMIC EXAMPLES AND ARTIFACTS
Normal RV and RA Pressure Waves

Simultaneous RV and RA pressures (0 to 40 mm Hg scale) are shown in Fig. 3-23. Notice the correspondence of the atrial filling wave a and ventricular filling wave v to the right ventricular pressure tracing. Following the a wave is the X descent and following the v wave is the normal Y descent. These features may be altered in the presence of disease or obscured in patients who have atrial arrhythmias. The notch (closed arrow, Fig. 3-23) on the top of the RV tracing is the "ringing" of a fluid-filled catheter. This rebound or ringing is also evident on the early diastolic part of the pressure wave (open arrow, bottom of same beat).

Fig. 3-24 shows the continuous pressure on pullback (*) across the interatrial septum from the left atrium to the right atrium of a patient with aortic stenosis showing the differences between LA and RA a and v waves. The v waves on the left atrium are very prominent with their corresponding X and Y descents. In the right atrium, the a and v waves are present but less striking. In general, RA a waves are bigger than v waves. In the left atrium, v waves are more prominent than a waves.

Respiratory influence on RA pressure (Fig. 3-25)

RA Pressure with Tricuspid Regurgitation

Unlike the normal pattern (see Fig. 3-23) the right atrial pressure rises throughout right ventricular systole as a result of tricuspid valvular regurgitation pushing blood back into the right atrium (Figs. 3-26 and 3-27). In this patient the RA

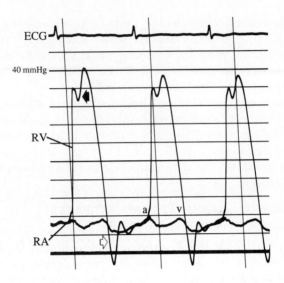

Fig. 3-23.   Right atrial (*RA*) and right ventricular (*RV*) tracings in a normal patient. *Closed arrow,* Notch of ringing or overshoot on right ventricular pressure rise; *open arrow,* ringing and overshoot of decline in right ventricular pressure at early diastole; *a,* atrial wave; *v,* ventricular filling wave.

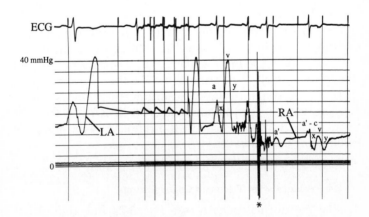

Fig. 3-24.   Hemodynamic tracing of left atrium (*LA*) with catheter pullback to right atrium (*RA*) across the intraatrial septum. See text for details of waveform analysis.

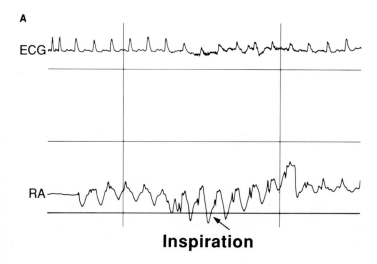

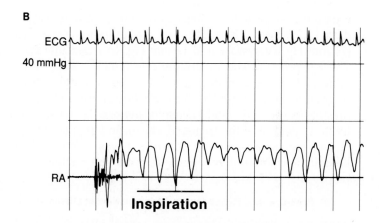

Fig. 3-25. **A,** Normal decrease in right atrial (*RA*) pressure during inspiration (scale 0 to 40 mm Hg). Note increase in Y descent (*arrow*). **B,** Abnormal response of right atrial pressure to inspiration in a patient with constrictive physiology or heart failure. Although Y descent is exaggerated, there is no corresponding fall in A or V wave height.

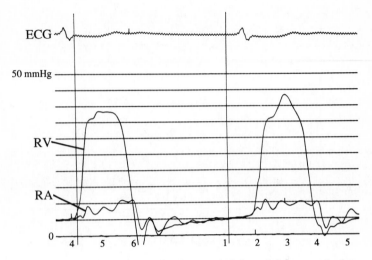

Fig. 3-26. Simultaneous right atrial (*RA*) and right ventricular (*RV*) tracings in a patient with tricuspid regurgitation.

pressure during diastole matches the RV pressure indicating no tricuspid stenosis. Tricuspid regurgitation is also evident in Fig. 3-27. Both RV and RA pressure is elevated (70 mm Hg RV systolic and 17 mm Hg RA mean pressure). The RA pressure shows striking regurgitant waves during systole. There is a small gradient between the right atrium (higher tracing) and right ventricle (lower tracing) during diastole because of mild tricuspid stenosis (a narrow and limited opening of the tricuspid valve). In patients with tricuspid regurgitation, large pulsatile waves in the jugular, hepatic, and femoral venous system may be easily seen or palpated (Fig. 3-28).

RA Pressure in a Patient with Atrioventricular Dissociation

Normal a waves (see Fig. 3-23) represent atrial contraction into the ventricle with no obstruction to in-flow. In an atrioventricular block, the atria are not contracting at the proper time in relation to the ventricles (Fig. 3-29). Immediately after the QRS the ventricles contract and the tricuspid and mital valves close. If the p wave (and atrial contraction) comes after the tricuspid valve is closed a giant C or cannon wave can be seen. When atrioventricular synchrony (normal sequence) occurs on beats 6 and 7 the a waves return, propor-

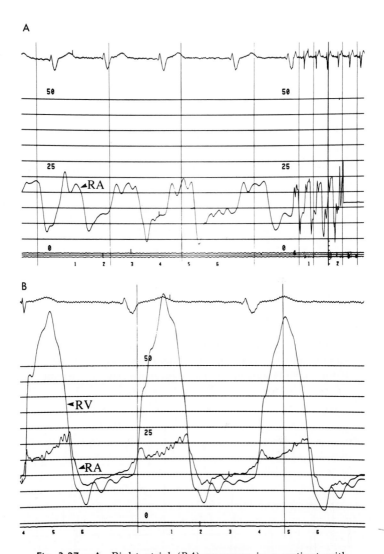

Fig. 3-27. **A,** Right atrial (*RA*) pressure in a patient with severe tricuspid regurgitation. **B,** When paired with simultaneous right ventricular (*RV*) pressure, tricuspid regurgitation can now be seen associated with tricuspid stenosis as the separation (gradient) between the right atrial-right ventricular pressures during diastole. See text for details.

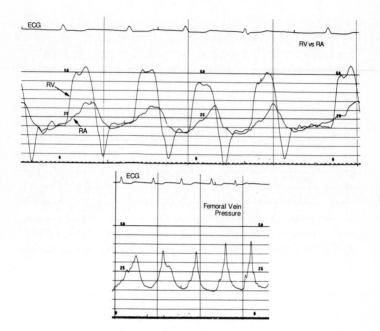

Fig. 3-28. **A,** Right ventricular (*RV*) and right atrial (*RA*) pressures (scale 0 to 50 mm Hg) showing severe tricuspid regurgitation. **B,** Note transmission of regurgitant wave to the femoral vein (sheath).

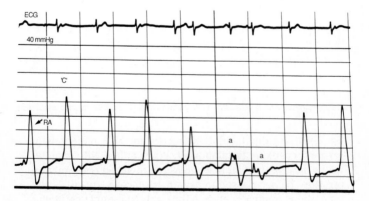

Fig. 3-29. Right atrial (*RA*) pressure during atrial-ventricular dissociation. 'C', Cannon wave; *a*, small a wave during synchrony of the atrial and ventricular activity. See text for details.

tional in size to the timing of the atrial contraction, emptying blood before ventricular systole (QRS). Similar findings may be seen when the dissociation is caused by a pacemaker. Giant C waves occur during pacing (Fig. 3-30).

PCW Pressure and LA Pressure with Simultaneous Transseptal and Right Heart Catheterization

The PCW pressure is measured through a 7 French fluid-filled balloon-tipped catheter; the LA pressure is measured through a Brockenbrough catheter (Fig. 3-31). The LA pressure rise precedes that of the PCW pressure for every waveform by approximately 100 to 150 ms. The good correspondence (generally) of these two pressures permits clinical use of PCW pressure for the majority of standard hemodynamic cases (a, a' and v, v' are the LA and PCW pressures, respectively).

Listings of pathologic changes of the atrial, systemic, and pulmonary pressure waveforms and some possible causes for the abnormalities are provided in the boxes on pp. 171–173.

Normal Femoral Arterial and Central Aortic Pressures

The femoral arterial pressure measured through the side arm of the femoral arterial sheath (8 French) is matched against pressure in the pigtail catheter (7 French) positioned above the aortic valve (Fig. 3-32). These pressures normally correspond closely. There is a slight overshoot of the more peripheral FA pressure (open arrow). Also, by observing the time of upstroke of the pressures, the central aortic pressure (first rising) can be distinguished. The mean of the two pressures is identical (closed arrow).

Fig. 3-33 demonstrates simultaneous arterial pressure with LV pressure (closed arrow). Matching of the pressures before crossing the aortic valve (see Fig. 3-32) permits satisfactory assessment of most aortic valvular lesions. Note the phase lag and normal overshoot of the arterial pressure compared to the LV pressure. The aortic and LV pressure tracings here and in Fig. 3-34 are characteristic for most patients using an 8 French femoral arterial sheath and a 7 French pigtail catheter.

The contribution of atrial filling to systemic pressure can

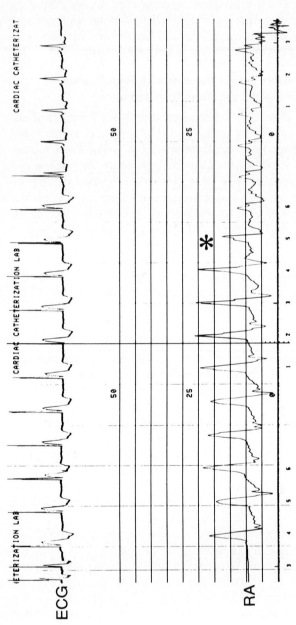

Fig. 3-30. Right atrial (*RA*) pressure during and after temporary right ventricular pacing. ECG shows large pacer spikes associated with giant C waves on right atrial pressure. Fusion beats begin at the asterisk, and the timing of an atrial contraction begins to precede ventricular activation, resulting in normal A waves.

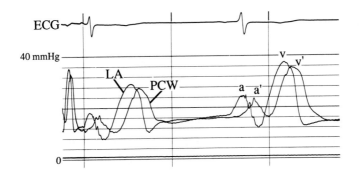

Fig. 3-31. Simultaneous left atrial (*LA*) and pulmonary capillary wedge (*PCW*) tracings. (The patient has aortic stenosis with high ventricular filling pressure.) See text for details.

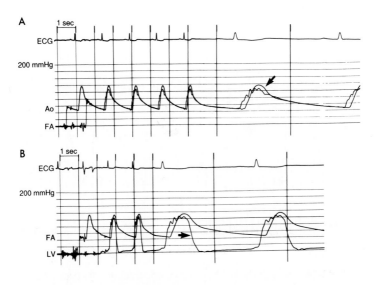

Fig. 3-32. **A,** Simultaneous hemodynamic tracings of femoral artery (*FA*) pressure, taken through the side arm of the 8 French sheath and central aortic pressures. Central aortic (*Ao*) pressure is obtained through the 7 French pigtail catheter. The overshoot of the femoral artery pressure (*arrow*) and lag in the pressure upstroke is the normal characteristic for the femoral tracings. **B,** Femoral artery and left ventricular (*LV*) pressure (*arrow*).

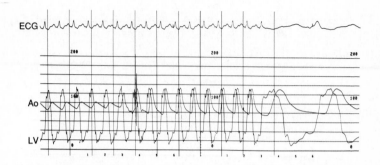

Fig. 3-33. Simultaneous aortic (*Ao*) pressure (from the femoral artery sheath) and left ventricular (*LV*) pressure from the pigtail catheter. Note the damped femoral artery tracing at the left side with the delayed upstroke. After flushing the femoral artery sheath (*right side*) systolic pressure matches the left ventricular pressure. For the clinical determination of aortic valve gradients, this technique is satisfactory in most patients.

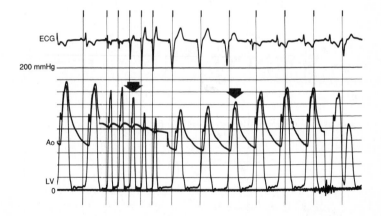

Fig. 3-34. Simultaneous hemodynamic tracings of aortic (*Ao*) and left ventricular (*LV*) pressures in a patient with a pacemaker. Loss of atrial contraction (paced beats) decreases ventricular filling with loss of systemic pressure. Left arrow shows the initiation of ventricular pacing with loss of the atrial contribution to left ventricular filling. Right arrow shows return of atrial synchrony and normal sinus rhythm. The systemic pressures are markedly increased during normal sinus rhythm.

be seen in Fig. 3-34. The normal sinus beats (1 and 2) with simultaneous aortic (femoral arterial) and left ventricular tracings show a systolic pressure of 175 mm Hg (scale 0 to 200 mm Hg); and aortic diastolic pressure of 70 mm Hg. Atrial contribution is lost because of a-v dissociation (arrow) and a pacemaker rhythm takes over. The systolic pressure falls dramatically to 118 mm Hg and gradually returns as atrial activity becomes more connected to the QRS.

Pathological Changes of the Atrial Pressure Waveforms

ELEVATED MEAN ATRIAL PRESSURE (RA > 4 TO 8 mm Hg, LA > 8 TO 12 mm Hg)

Insufficiency of the following chamber (i.e., ventricle)
Stenosis or insufficiency of the AV valve
Hypervolemia
Pericardial disease or effusion
Congestive heart failure or infarction

LOW MEAN ATRIAL PRESSURE

Hypovolemia
Zero line artifact

A (ATRIAL CONTRACTION) WAVE

Elevated a wave

Hypertrophy or decreased ventricular compliance (i.e., "Stiff Heart")
Mitral or tricuspid insufficiency
Mitral or tricuspid stenosis
Decreased atrial pressure-volume compliance curve (i.e., stiffer chamber) (CASE EXAMPLE: Fig. 3-31)

Missing a wave

Atrial arrest
Atrial fibrillation
Atrial flutter
False lowered a wave in patients with a large c-v wave

V (DIASTOLIC FILLING) WAVE

Elevated v waves in

Increased flow (e.g., atrial or ventricular septal defect)
AV valve insufficiency (in the case of severe insufficiency, the high v wave is called ventricularization of the atrial pulse curve) (mitral regurgitation; Fig. 3-46)
Atrial fibrillation

Atrial fibrillation and AV-valvular insufficiency (in cases of atrial
fibrillation, valvular insufficiency can be diagnosed on the basis
of the atrial pulse curve only if the v wave is markedly elevated)
(CASE EXAMPLE: large v wave, Fig. 3-47)

X AND Y DESCENTS (ATRIAL PRESSURE WAVES)

Missing in atrial fibrillation (NORMAL CASE EXAMPLE: LA, RA, Fig.
3-24)

SPECIAL ABNORMALITIES OF THE ATRIAL PULSE CURVE

Equalization of the right and left atrial pressures in severe atrial
septal defect or cardiac constriction
Inspiratory increase of the mean right atrial pressure in
constrictive pericarditis
Multiple pressure wave deformities of the atrial pulse curve in
patients with rhythm disturbances (e.g., pacemakers, multifocal
atrial tachycardia)
Saw tooth deformity of the atrial pressure in atrial flutter
Dissociation of atrial and ventricular chamber pressure waves and
corresponding intracardiac ECG in Ebstein's abnormality
(atrialization of right ventricle)

Pathological Changes of the Ventricular Pressure Waveforms

SYSTOLIC PRESSURE

Elevated

Pulmonary or arterial hypertension
Pulmonary stenosis, aortic stenosis, aortic insufficiency

Decreased

Hypovolemic state
Cardiac congestion, cardiac failure, tamponade, infarction

END-DIASTOLIC PRESSURE

Elevated

Hypervolemia
Hypertrophy
Decreased compliance
Cardiac failure, tamponade
Aortic insufficiency

Decreased

Hypovolemia
Tricuspid stenosis, mitral stenosis

A WAVE ON VENTRICULAR PRESSURE TRACE

Decreased or missing in

Mitral stenosis, tricuspid stenosis
Mitral insufficiency, tricuspid insufficiency (if left or right
  ventricular compliance is increased)
Atrial fibrillation
Atrial flutter
Atrial arrest
Severe aortic insufficiency

EARLY RAPID DIASTOLIC PRESSURE "DIP" WITH
MID-DIASTOLIC "PLATEAU" (FLAT WAVE)

Artifact (bradycardia)
Constrictive pericarditis with elevated diastolic plateau
Restrictive cardiomyopathy

Special Abnormalities of the Pressure Waves

PULMONARY ARTERY PRESSURE

Elevated

Primary or secondary pulmonary hypertension
Large left-to-right shunt
Peripheral pulmonary stenosis
Mitral stenosis, regurgitation, congestive heart failure

Decreased

Hypovolemia
Pulmonary stenosis (valvular, subvalvular, and peripheral)
Ebstein's anomaly
Hypoplastic right heart syndrome
Tricuspid stenosis and tricuspid atresia

AORTIC PRESSURE

Elevated

Arterial hypertension

Decreased

Aortic stenosis
Low cardiac output
Shock

WIDE AORTIC PULSE PRESSURE

Arterial hypertension
Aortic insufficiency

Large left-to-right shunt (e.g., open ductus, aortopulmonary
    window, truncus arteriosus communis, perforated sinus
valsalva-aneurysm)

NARROW AORTIC PULSE PRESSURE

Aortic stenosis
Heart failure
Cardiac tamponade
Shock

ARTERIAL PULSUS BISFERIENS (SPIKED PULSE)

Aortic insufficiency
Obstructive hypertrophic cardiomyopathy

PULSUS PARADOXUS (ABNORMALLY LARGE DECREASE IN
ARTERIAL PRESSURE SYSTOLIC PEAKS DURING
INSPIRATION [>10 mm Hg])

Cardiac tamponade

PULSUS PARVUS (WEAK) AND TARDUS (SLOW) (DELAYED
AND REDUCED ARTERIAL PRESSURE)

Aortic stenosis

PULSUS ALTERNANS (ALTERNATING STRONG/WEAK
ARTERIAL PRESSURE)

Congestive heart failure
Cardiomyopathy

Normal Right Heart Pressures on Catheter Pullback

Normal right heart pressures are demonstrated during continuous pressure recording (using balloon-tipped pulmonary
artery catheter) on catheter pullback from pulmonary artery
to right ventricle and right atrium (0 to 40 mm Hg scale)
(Fig. 3-35). Simultaneous LV and RV are compared on same
scale and fast (50 mm/sec) paper speed. Premature ventricular contractions are common when catheters contact the RV
outflow tract.

Large v Waves on the PCW Tracing

LV and PCW generally match well in diastole (0 to
40 mm Hg scale) (Fig. 3-36). The PCW a wave (a′) follows
the LV a wave by 150 ms (beat 1). The v wave is large.
There is no important diastolic PCW-LV gradient. On beat
2, because of late atrial activity loss of the LV a wave is seen

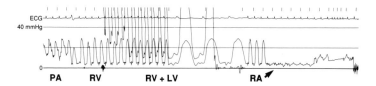

Fig. 3-35. Continuous hemodynamic tracing during catheter pullback from the pulmonary artery (*PA*) to right atrium (*RA*). Differences in left ventricular (*LV*) and right ventricular (*RV*) pressures are shown (0 to 40 mm Hg full scale).

by the different initial upstroke of the LV pressures. The PCW has large, late a and v waves. The v wave on a PCW pressure tracing usually is associated with significant mitral regurgitation. However, large v waves are not highly sensitive nor specific for mitral regurgitation. Large v waves also may be present with ventricular septal defect or any condition in which the left atrial volume (e.g., ventricular septal defect (VSD)) or left atrial pressure relationship (the stiffness or compliance) is increased (such as rheumatic heart disease, postcardiac surgery, and infiltrative heart diseases). Mitral valve obstruction from any cause and congestive heart failure

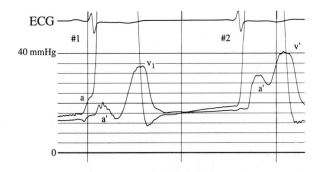

Fig. 3-36. Simultaneous pulmonary capillary wedge and left ventricular pressures in a patient who has loss of atrial activity (beat 2). On beat 1 the a wave is evident on both left ventricle (*a*) and pulmonary capillary wedge pressure (*a'*). The a wave is lost in beat 2 with no atrial activity. The a' wave is considerably higher because of its contraction against the closed mitral valve. See text for details.

in the absence of mitral regurgitation also are associated with large v waves. Giant v waves, also seen in Fig. 3-24, may be large enough to be transmitted to the PA pressure, causing a notch on the diastolic downslope (Fig. 3-37).

Aortic Stenosis

Simultaneous left ventricular and aortic pressure tracings in a patient with minimal aortic stenosis (0 to 200 mm Hg scale) are shown in Fig. 3-38. The pressures were measured with a Millar high-fidelity catheter with two transducers on the tip of the catheter (see Chapter 6). Peak-to-peak aortic-left ventricular pressure difference is only 10 mm Hg. The mean gradient (area between Ao-LV during systole) is 15 mm Hg. The rapid aortic upstroke shows the effect of the turbulent jet of the narrowed valve vibrating the catheter. There is no lag in the timing of the aortic pressure rise with respect to the LV. A higher LV pressure also may be seen after an extrasystolic beat, called postextrasystolic accentuation shown in Fig. 3-39.

The atrial contraction is important in patients with aortic

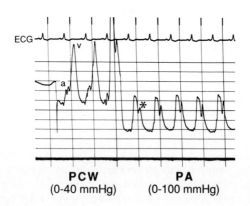

Fig. 3-37.   Giant v waves on the pulmonary capillary wedge (*PCW*) tracing can be transmitted to the pulmonary artery (*PA*) pressure, producing a notch (∗) on the pulmonary artery downslope.

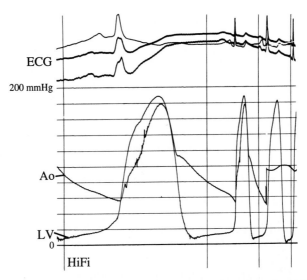

Fig. 3-38. Simultaneous aortic (*Ao*) and left ventricular (*LV*) pressures from dual micromanometer-tipped (high-fidelity, *HiFi*) catheter in a patient with mild aortic stenosis. See text for details.

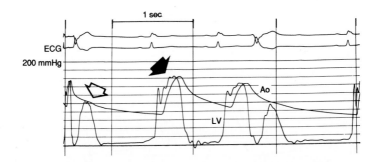

Fig. 3-39. Postextra systolic accentuation of left ventricular (*LV*) and aortic (*Ao*) pressures (*closed arrow*) after a premature ventricular contraction (*open arrow*). This patient does not have aortic stenosis. The premature ventricular contraction also does not generate pressure sufficient to open the aortic valve and, thus, results in a dropped beat when counting the peripheral pulse rate. (From Kern MJ: *Hemodynamic rounds: interpretation of cardiac pathophysiology from pressure waveform analysis.* St. Louis, 1993, Wiley-Liss.)

stenosis (Fig. 3-40). Simultaneous aortic and LV pressure (transseptal approach, 0 to 200 mm Hg scale). Atrial activity is absent in the first beat, a junctional beat (*). Without the atrial contribution, aortic systolic pressure is 132 mm Hg; an LV systolic pressure, 190 mm Hg. In the following beat, number 3 atrial activity (P wave) precedes the QRS and the aortic pressure increases to 160 mm Hg; LV pressure increases to 225 mm Hg, representing an approximately 25% increase in pressure augmentation. This effect is critically important in patients with poor LV function. Two additional features of this tracing are worthy of note; the a wave on the LV pressure tracing (arrow) can be seen on the LV beat 2, and aortic regurgitation may also be present when a very wide pulse pressure (aortic systolic-diastolic pressure) greater than 50 to 60 mm Hg is observed. The aortic pressure has fallen to less than or equal to 50 mm Hg at the end of diastole. Bradycardia also may produce a wide pulse pressure.

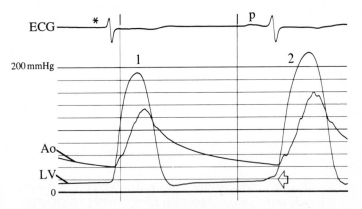

Fig. 3-40. Simultaneous left ventricular (*LV*; obtained with transseptal technique) and aortic (*Ao*) pressures from fluid-filled catheter systems. Note the contribution of atrial contraction (*arrow*) to the change in left ventricular and systemic pressures on beat 2. *p*, p wave; *, absence of p wave on this tracing. The wide pulse pressure also is indicative of aortic insufficiency. See text for details.

LV Gradient Below the Aortic Valve

Hypertrophic cardiomyopathy is a condition in which very thick heart muscle, especially inside the LV chamber, contracts so hard that it obstructs flow out of the ventricle, and thus by its own contraction produces a pressure gradient with a normal aortic valve. Fig. 3-41 depicts simultaneous LV and aortic pressure showing large aortic-LV gradient (LV = 220 mm Hg; Ao = 120 mm Hg). On pullback of the LV catheter (multipurpose) from the distal LV to a position just beneath the aortic valve the Ao-LV gradient disappears (see the LV pressure matching with aortic pressure, arrow). Table 3-5 lists provocative maneuvers to increase an outflow

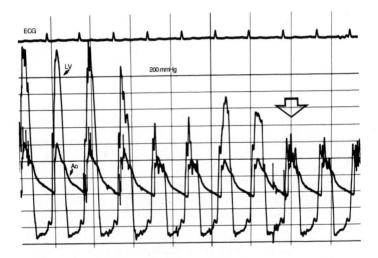

Fig. 3-41. Simultaneous left ventricular (*LV*) and aortic (*Ao*) pressures in a patient with obstructive hypertrophic cardiomyopathy during pullback of the catheter from the distal portion of the left ventricle. The pressure gradient between the aorta and left ventricle is lost. Left ventricular systolic pressure matches aortic pressure during catheter pullback before the catheter is pulled out of the left ventricle (*arrow*). There is no true aortic valve gradient. This left ventricular-aortic gradient is located in the mid-left ventricular wall beneath the aortic valve. The arrow indicates the matching of aortic and left ventricular systolic pressures in the proximal chamber. See text for details.

TABLE 3-5. Provocative tests for hypertrophic cardiomyopathy

Drug or maneuver	Mechanism increasing Ao-LV gradient
Drugs	
Isoproterenol	Increased myocardial contractility
Amyl nitrite	Decreased systemic arterial pressure (peripheral vasodilatation), reflex increasing sympathetic tone, decreased venous return and increased myocardial contractility
Nitroglycerin	Decreased venous return; decreased cardiac output and increased narrowing of LV outflow tract
Maneuver	
Extrasystole	Postextrasystolic increase in myocardial contractility
Valsalva's maneuver	Decreased venous return; decreased LV volume, increased narrowing of outflow tract

Ao, Aortic; LV, left ventricular.
Stroke volume and systemic arterial pulse pressure decrease in the postextrasystolic beat (Brockenbrough-Braunwald sign). This is in contrast with valvular aortic stenosis, in which the postextrasystolic beat is characterized by increased stroke volume and systolic gradient, as well as by increased systemic arterial pressure.

tract gradient in patients with hypertrophic cardiomyopathies.

Aortic Regurgitation

Figs. 3-42, 3-43, and 3-44 illustrate simultaneous Ao and LV pressures (0 to 200 mm Hg scale) in several patients with different degrees of aortic regurgitation. The characteristic hemodynamic feature of this condition is a wide pulse pressure. The aortic (femoral) brisk pressure upstroke can be easily seen. Often there will be marked overshoot of the femoral artery pressure. In Fig. 3-43, the large and prominent a wave shows the effect of first-degree AV block (long PR interval, arrow), on the LV pressure. Fig. 3-42 diagrams the physiology of the Ao-LV gradient in diastole. No atrial contribution of LV pressure is present.

Fig. 3-44 illustrates hemodynamically severe aortic regurgitation by rapidly increasing LV diastolic pressure and wide aortic pressure with near equilibration of aortic and LV pressure at end diastole. Note the aortic pressure overshoot.

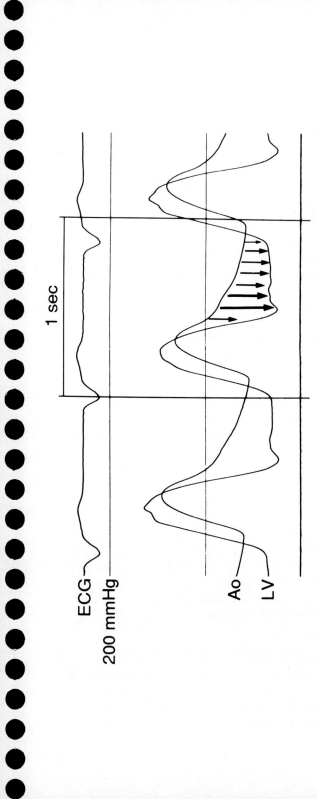

Fig. 3-42. Hemodynamic tracing in a patient with aortic insufficiency (and minimal aortic stenosis (AS)) showing the aortic-left ventricular (*LV*) diastolic gradient (*arrows*) important for coronary perfusion. (Note loss of a wave due to paced rhythm.)

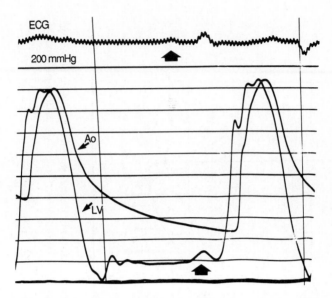

Fig. 3-43. Simultaneous aortic (*Ao*) and left ventricular (*LV*) pressures in a patient with aortic insufficiency. Note the absence of a systolic pressure gradient. The time delay in the aortic pressure upstroke indicates femoral sheath pressure is used. The presence of a large and early a wave (*bottom arrow*) occurs with PR interval prolongation (*top arrow*). See text for details.

Mitral Regurgitation

In Figs. 3-45 and 3-46 large v waves in the PCW tracing represent LV pressure transmitted backward through an incompetent mitral valve. The v wave occurs on the downstroke of the LV pressure. Fig. 3-46 shows large v waves (up to 60 mm Hg) in a patient with mitral regurgitation. However, as noted in Fig. 3-36, v waves also reflect a change in the pressure-volume filling curve of the atrium.

Mitral Stenosis

In Fig. 3-47 simultaneous LV and PCW pressures demonstrate a mitral valve gradient throughout diastole (dot). The a wave in the first beat is associated with a normal v wave. In the following beat, atrial activity is delayed and follows the QRS, contributing to large giant v wave (36 mm Hg).

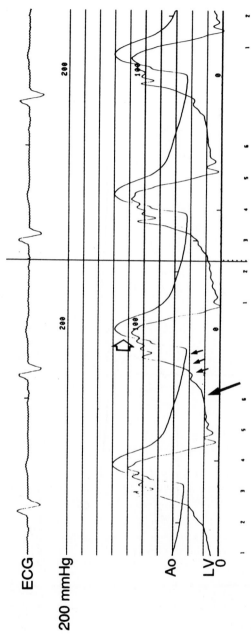

Fig. 3-44. Severe aortic regurgitation demonstrated by rapidly increasing left ventricular (*LV*) diastolic pressure (*large black arrow*) and end-diastolic equilibration of aortic (*Ao*) and left ventricular pressure (*three small arrows*). Peripheral arterial pressure overshoot or amplification is due to forceful left ventricular ejection and compliant arterial system. (In this case aortic pressure was matched with femoral artery sheath pressure.) (From Kern MJ: *Hemodynamic rounds: interpretation of cardiac pathophysiology from pressure waveform analysis.* St. Louis, 1993, Wiley-Liss.)

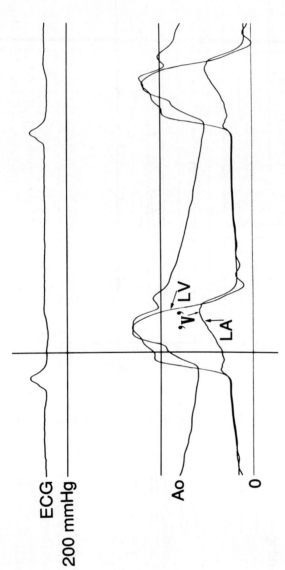

Fig. 3-45. Hemodynamic tracings in a patient with mitral regurgitation characterized by giant v wave in the left atrial (*LA*) pressure. This v wave corresponds to marked increase in flow and volume into the left atrium. See text for details.

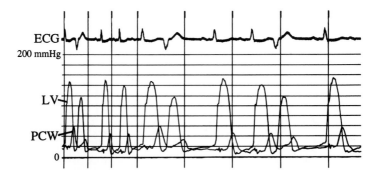

Fig. 3-46. Simultaneous left ventricular (*LV*) and pulmonary capillary wedge (*PCW*) pressures in a patient with mitral regurgitation. During ventricular ectopic activity (premature beats), large v waves (up to 60 mm Hg) on the pulmonary capillary wedge pressure are seen. Giant v waves are hallmarks of severe mitral regurgitation. See text for details.

The augmented filling increases the mitral valve gradient. In some patients with mitral stenosis balloon catheter valvuloplasty may be used to split open narrowed mitral orifice. Figs. 3-48 and 3-49 show the mitral valve gradient before and after balloon catheter valvuloplasty in two patients. Left

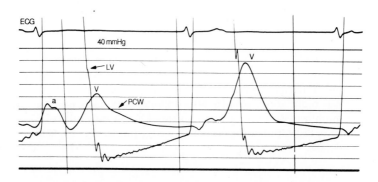

Fig. 3-47. Simultaneous pulmonary capillary wedge (*PCW*) and left ventricular (*LV*) pressures in a patient with mitral stenosis. The contribution of atrial contraction is evident on beat 1. Loss of atrial activity on beat 2 results in loss of the a wave and a giant v wave with an increased mitral valve gradient. See text for details.

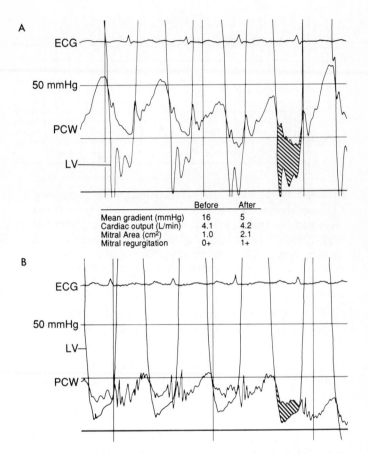

	Before	After
Mean gradient (mmHg)	16	5
Cardiac output (L/min)	4.1	4.2
Mitral Area (cm^2)	1.0	2.1
Mitral regurgitation	0+	1+

Fig. 3-48. Hemodynamic tracings in a patient with mitral stenosis before **(A)** and after **(B)** mitral valvuloplasty. The mean diastolic gradient of 16 mm Hg before valvuloplasty was reduced to 5 mm Hg after valvuloplasty, increasing the mitral valve area from 1.0 to 2.1 cm^2. LV, left venticular pressure; PCW, pulmonary capillary wedge pressure. See text for details.

atrial pressure is measured by the transseptal technique. Before valvuloplasty the large gradient of 16 mm Hg (refer to Fig. 3-48) resulted in a mitral valve area of 1.0 cm^2. After valvuloplasty the gradient is considerably less (5 mm Hg). The valve area increased to 2.1 cm^2. An even better result can be seen in Fig. 3-49.

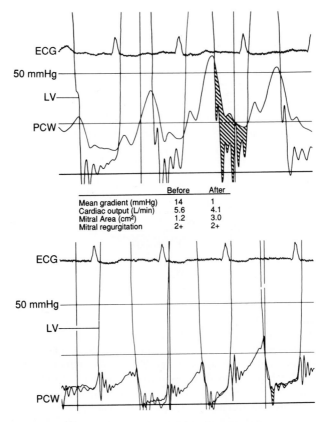

	Before	After
Mean gradient (mmHg)	14	1
Cardiac output (L/min)	5.6	4.1
Mitral Area (cm^2)	1.2	3.0
Mitral regurgitation	2+	2+

Fig. 3-49. Hemodynamic tracings in another patient undergoing balloon valvuloplasty for mitral stenosis. The mean diastolic gradient of 14 mm Hg before valvuloplasty was reduced to 1 mm Hg after valvuloplasty, increasing the mitral valve area from 1.2 to 3.0 cm^2 after valvuloplasty. LV, left ventricular pressure; PCW, pulmonary capillary wedge pressure. See text for details.

Mitral valve gradients are influenced by heart rate. When the rhythm is irregular (atrial fibrillation), calculations of gradients should be made from the average of 10 beats. Fig. 3-50 illustrates the effect of RR cycle length on the mitral stenosis gradient.

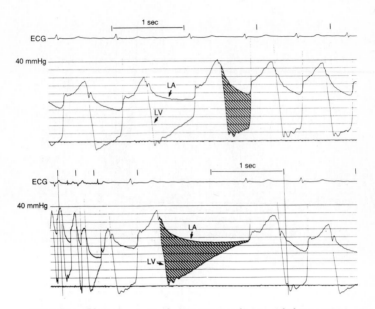

Fig. 3-50.   Changing mitral stenosis gradient with heart rate (RR interval). **A,** Short RR interval is associated with gradient (shaded area) of 22 mm Hg. **B,** The long RR interval has a mean gradient of 29 mm Hg. When computing mean valve area in atrial fibrillation, average 10 beats. *LA,* left atrial pressure; *LV,* left ventricular pressure. (From Kern MJ: *Hemodynamic rounds: interpretation of cardiac pathophysiology from pressure waveform analysis.* St. Louis, 1993, Wiley-Liss.)

Mixed Mitral Stenosis and Regurgitation

Fig. 3-51 illustrates simultaneous LV and PCW pressures (0 to 40 mm Hg scale) showing giant v waves with persistent PCW-LV gradient during diastole. Left ventriculography confirmed significant mitral regurgitation. The slope of the v waves in mitral regurgitation/stenosis is flatter than that in which large v waves are associated with isolated regurgitant flow (see Fig. 3-36).

Differences in RV and LV Pressures in Patients with Mitral Stenosis

Normal RV and LV pressures are separated by >5 mm Hg in early and late diastole, and the RV pressure tracing is usually contained completely within the LV pressure tracing

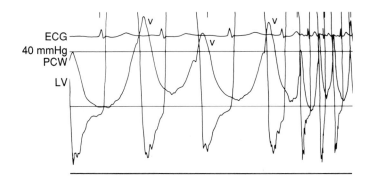

Fig. 3-51. Simultaneous left ventricular (*LV*) and pulmonary capillary wedge (*PCW*) pressures in a patient with severe mixed mitral regurgitation and mitral stenosis. The large v wave and the persistent diastolic gradient is characteristic of mixed mitral valvular disease. See text for details.

(Figure 3-52). The diastolic ventricular pressures normally differ in slope and end-diastolic pressure. The A waves also differ in size due to the lower compliance (stiffer) left ventricle. Changes in the RV-LV pressure relationship are related to ventricular septal interaction and will occur in pulmonary hypertension, bundle branch block, myocardial infarction, RV volume overload, and, most commonly, pericardial constrictive physiology.

RV and LV pressure in a patient with left bundle branch block is shown in Fig. 3-53. The timing of ventricular activation is delayed in the bundle branch block. RV pressure decline occurs outside the LV pressure. The clinical importance of this observation is unknown.

In Fig. 3-54 simultaneous LV and RV pressure (0 to 40 mm Hg scale) in a patient with mitral stenosis shows differences in filling patterns due to high PA pressure. For most beats the diastolic filling patterns correspond (i.e., increase gradually during diastole by normal filling). However, after a premature contraction (beat 2) the long (compensatory) pause shows continued filling of the LV pressure with a plateau in the RV pressure waveform, indicating different diastolic compliance (stiffness of heart muscle) between these two chambers.

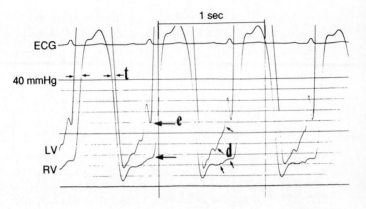

Fig. 3-52. Simultaneous right (*RV*) and left ventricular (*LV*) pressures in a patient with mild pulmonary hypertension. Note the different diastolic upslopes (*e*) and end-diastolic pressure (*d*). The right ventricular tracing is entirely within the left ventricular tracing (*t*), a normal pattern. (From Kern MJ: *Hemodynamic rounds: interpretation of cardiac pathophysiology from pressure waveform analysis.* St. Louis, 1993, Wiley-Liss.)

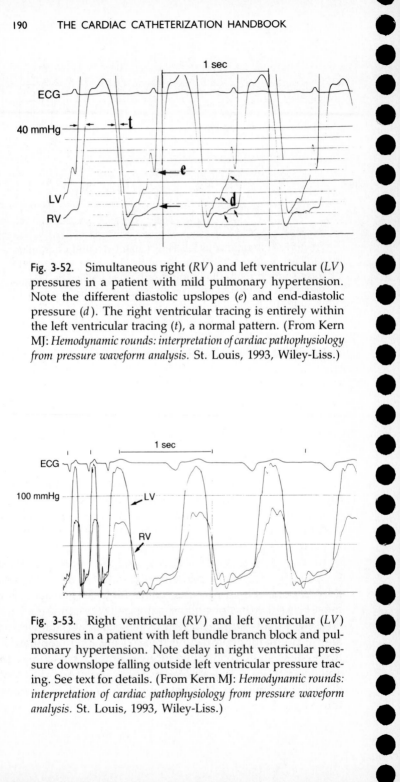

Fig. 3-53. Right ventricular (*RV*) and left ventricular (*LV*) pressures in a patient with left bundle branch block and pulmonary hypertension. Note delay in right ventricular pressure downslope falling outside left ventricular pressure tracing. See text for details. (From Kern MJ: *Hemodynamic rounds: interpretation of cardiac pathophysiology from pressure waveform analysis.* St. Louis, 1993, Wiley-Liss.)

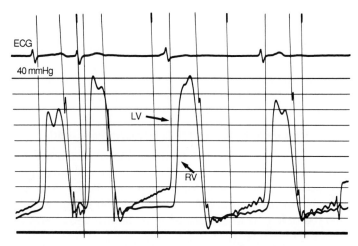

Fig. 3-54. Simultaneous right ventricular (*RV*) and left ventricular (*LV*) pressures in a patient with mitral stenosis showing different diastolic filling patterns during long diastole. The right ventricular pressure is flat and fails to rise while the left ventricular pressure continues filling during a long diastolic period. This illustration suggests different compliance between the two ventricular chambers in a patient with mitral stenosis.

Constrictive Pericarditis

Constrictive pericarditis produces abnormal hemodynamics characterized by low arterial pressure, tachycardia, Kussmaul's sign (inspiratory increase in RA pressure) "M" or "W" configuration on RA pressure, and dip and plateau of early rapid diastolic filling with abrupt cessation due to the pericardial constraint. When comparing constriction with tamponade physiology, the two are differentiated by the RA waveform (elevated and blunted in tamponade) and pulsus paradoxus (inspiratory decrease in arterial pressure in tamponade). Because these two entities are similar in their early stages, the RA pressures may also be similar. Two-dimensional echocardiography demonstrates the amount of pericardial fluid and RA and RV chamber collapse of tamponade physiology. See Chapter 8 on pericardiocentesis for details of tamponade.

In Fig. 3-55, matching of elevated diastolic pressures with an early dip followed by a plateau during diastole (first beat) is the characteristic pattern. Often, only during slow heart rates does the classic dip and plateau configuration appear. Tachycardia and respiratory effort obscure the pattern, but matching of both RV-LV pressures during diastole is consistent (see Figs. 3-56, 3-57, and 3-58).

RA Pressure in Patients with Constrictive Pericarditis

In Fig. 3-59 the characteristic pattern shows very prominent Y descent with a classic M or W configuration of constrictive physiology. These waveforms are the altered X and Y troughs resulting from impaired ventricular filling. Myocardial restrictive heart disease or heart failure also shows this pattern occasionally.

Artifacts of Hemodynamic Tracings

Normal pressure curves from fluid-filled systems are sharp without rounded contours. When examining the pressure tracings, narrow spikes or overshoot in the ventricular (both

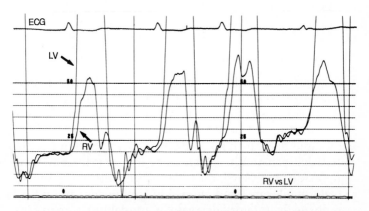

Fig. 3-55. Simultaneous left ventricular (*LV*) and right ventricular (*RV*) pressure tracing in a patient with constrictive pericarditis. Matching of diastolic pressures is one of the hallmarks of this condition. See text for details. Normal example of right ventricular and left ventricular pressures is also shown on Fig. 3-35. Note separation and increasing pressure in diastole.

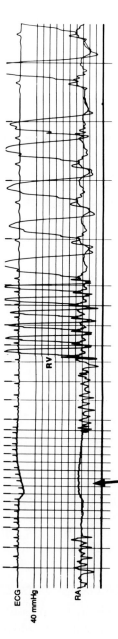

Fig. 3-56. Right atrial (*RA*) and right ventricular (*RV*) pressure tracings in a patient with constrictive pericarditis. The right atrial pressure has prominent Y descent and small X descent. There is matching of right atrial and right ventricular diastolic pressures (*right side*) and of right ventricular and left ventricular diastolic pressures (not shown). Note right atrial Kussmaul's sign during inspiration (*arrow*). (From Kern MJ: *Hemodynamic rounds: interpretation of cardiac pathophysiology from pressure waveform analysis.* St. Louis, 1993, Wiley-Liss.)

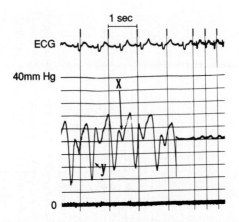

Fig. 3-57.   Right atrial pressure showing pattern of constrictive physiology with large Y descent and smaller X descent. Mean right atrial pressure is 20 mm Hg.

right and left) pressure suggests underdamping (i.e., too sensitive a pressure system). Wide, rounded waves indicate overdamping (i.e., not sensitive enough), usually produced by a problem in the fluid path to the transducer or a transducer that is not calibrated correctly.

_____ Artifact Example 1 _____

An air bubble in an LV pressure line (Fig. 3-60) produces a tracing with exaggerated systolic and diastolic overshoot (arrow), suggesting underdamping. After flushing the air bubble out the sharp, crisp upstroke of the ventricular pressure demonstrates a normal pressure rise. The short "ring" artifact of the pressure wave at peak LV pressure and during diastole should remain visible but occurs at a much higher frequency (i.e., shorter deflections). This pattern is an accurate waveform for a properly flushed fluid-filled catheter system.

_____ Artifact Example 2 _____

Contrast media or a bubble in the pressure line also can *correct* an underdamped tracing. Fig. 3-61 demonstrates a suitable LV pressure with normal (or only slightly rounded) waveform. This tracing is acutally a damped version of an

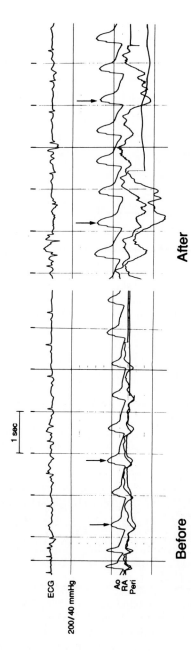

Before

After

Fig. 3-58. Right atrial (*RA*), pericardial (*peri*), and aortic (*Ao*) pressures in a patient with pericardial tamponade. Before pericardiocentesis, right atrial pressure has blunted X and Y descents. Arterial pressure shows pulsus paradoxus (inspiratory decrease > 10 mm Hg of systolic pressure, *arrow*). After pericardiocentesis, pulsus paradoxus is absent and right atrial waveform is more phasic. (From Kern MJ: *Hemodynamic rounds: interpretation of cardiac pathophysiology from pressure waveform analysis.* St. Louis, 1993, Wiley-Liss.)

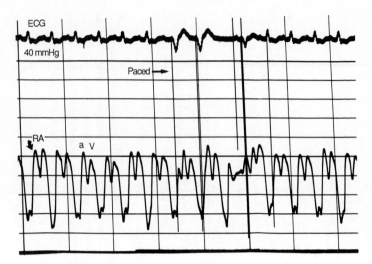

Fig. 3-59. Right atrial (*RA*) pressure in a patient with constrictive pericarditis demonstrating abnormally elevated pressure with a classic M configuration. The elevated pressure with exaggerated Y descent is also seen in cardiomyopathy. See text for details.

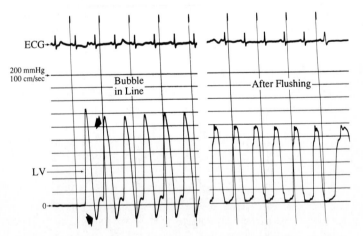

Fig. 3-60. Hemodynamic tracing demonstrating the effect of an air bubble in pressure line. Note the change in hemodynamic waveform after flushing the bubble. The "ringing" artifact (*sharp points at arrows*) is eliminated and fine detail of precise pressure is restored after flushing.

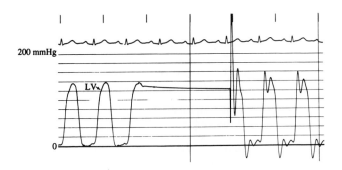

Fig. 3-61. *Left*, Left ventricular (*LV*) pressure tracing normally "damped" with viscous contrast media in the fluid path. *Right*, After flushing with saline, the tracing is now seen as underdamped with exaggerated ringing artifact.

underdamped signal that is apparent after flushing the line (right side of tracing). Both early diastolic and systolic portions of the pressure wave on the right show striking overshoot underdamping. Table 3-6 lists common problems and solutions for hemodynamic waveforms.

Underdamping produces a "noisy" PCW pressure (see Fig. 3-62). With instillation of contrast media into the catheter, underdamping is corrected yielding a tracing with clearly interpretable waveforms (Fig. 3-63).

_____ Artifact Example 3 _____

False aortic stenosis gradient (Fig. 3-64).   When measuring LV-Ao pressures, all the side holes of the pigtail catheter must be under the aortic valve. In Fig. 3-64, **B,** the pigtail catheter is partly out of the left ventricle. The LV pressure is contaminated partly by aortic pressure, reducing the LV-Ao gradient. This artifact is also evident by the abnormal diastolic waveform—a continued decline in diastolic pressure throughout the cycle. (LV diastolic pressure should be lowest in the first part of diastole with a rising pressure across the diastolic period). Fig. 3-64, **A** shows the true gradient when the pigtail catheter is advanced slightly. This artifact is important and may lead to a conclusion of only minimal aortic valve disease if not appreciated (see Figs. 3-65, 3-66, and 3-67).

TABLE 3-6. Common hemodynamic recording problems

Problem	Possible cause	Solution
Overdamping*	Bubble or clot in line or transducer	Reflush system
	Small lumen of tubing system	Increase internal diameter of tubing
	Soft/compliant tubing	Use stiffer tubing
	Loose catheter connection	Tighten catheter
	Kink in catheter	Unkink catheter
Underdamping*	System tubing too stiff	Softer tubing
	System tubing too long	Shorten tubing
	Hyperdynamic state	Increase filter on amplifier
		Introduce small bubble or contrast media
	Catheter tip in turbulent jet	Reposition catheter
Loss of signal	Bad transducer	Change transducer
	Bad cable	Change cable
	Bad amplifier	Switch amplifier
	Catheter disconnected	Check connections
	Catheter obstructed/ "kinked"	Flush/change catheter
Pressures do not return to zero	Same as above	Readjust zero line
		Recalibrate
		Check zero at midchest

*Overdamping system is not sensitive enough and yields flat or rounded tracings. Underdamping system is too sensitive and produces too much "ringing" or overshoot of tracings.

Modified from Tilkian AG, Daily EK: *Cardiovascular procedures: diagnostic techniques and therapeutic procedures*, St. Louis, 1986, Mosby.

——————————— Artifact Example 4 ———————————

Inspiratory increases in RA mean pressure is Kussmaul's sign (Fig. 3-68) for constrictive pericarditis. However, on phasic examination of this waveform the RA pressure was elevated artifactually during inspiration by RV pressure as shown on the lower panel. The catheter inadvertently

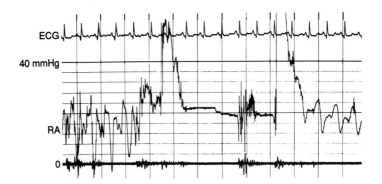

Fig. 3-62. Right atrial (*RA*) pressure showing marked under-damped ringing artifact. Instillation of viscous contrast media damps the system, producing excellent waveforms.

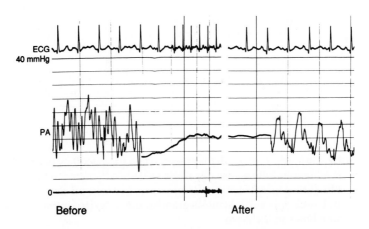

Before   After

Fig. 3-63. Pulmonary (*PA*) pressure after contrast has been instilled to produce some damping of the previously under-damped tracing, now demonstrating excellent waveforms. See text for details.

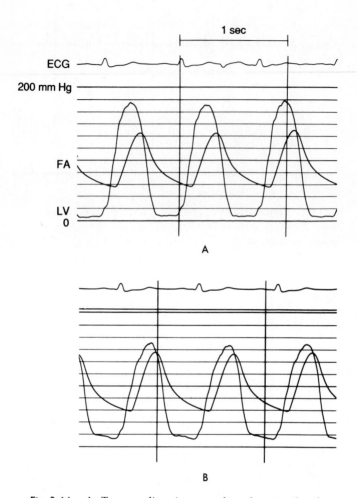

Fig. 3-64. **A,** True gradient is seen when the pigtail catheter is advanced fully across the aortic valve. *FA,* Femoral artery pressure; *LV,* left ventricular pressure. See text for details. **B,** Falsely low aortic stenosis gradient due to pigtail catheter side holes in the aorta.

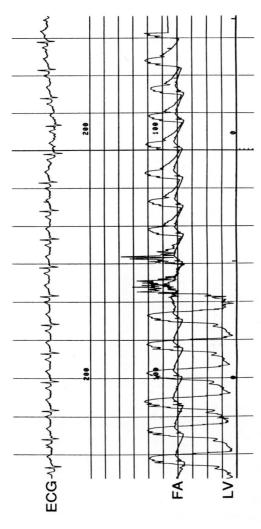

Fig. 3-65. Femoral artery (*FA*) and left ventricular (*LV*) pressures show systolic gradient with damped arterial tracing despite flushing arterial sheath. On pullback, the arterial pressure is unchanged and central aortic pressures show no differences in systole. Damped femoral artery pressure is due to sheath kink or, in this case, severe peripheral vascular disease in the iliac artery. A long sheath, second arterial catheter or transseptal route, would prove the presence of a gradient if clinically necessary.

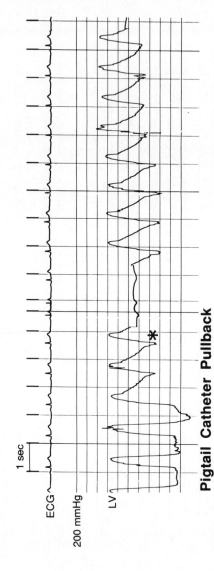

Pigtail Catheter Pullback

Fig. 3-66. A falsely wide aortic pulse pressure (*) using a pigtail catheter is caused by incomplete withdrawal of all side holes outside the left ventricle (*LV*). On final catheter positioning (*far right*), aortic pressure is normal.

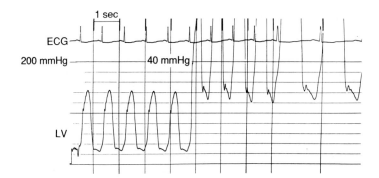

Fig. 3-67. Left ventricular (*LV*) diastolic pressure appears to fall during mid- and late diastole. This pattern is seen in patients with hypertrophic cardiomyopathy. However, when one or more of the side holes of the pigtail catheter are in the aorta, the early diastolic pressure may be high and the pattern confused for pathology.

flipped into the RV during inspiration. In a patient without clinical signs of constrictive or restrictive physiology, this artifact should be suspected and fluoroscopy or phasic pressure recording during inspiratory effort will identify this error.

_____ Artifact Example 5 _____

The PCW pressure is satisfactory in most hemodynamic studies. However, in mitral valve disease, especially in patients who have had prosthetic mitral valves in place, the PCW may not reflect LA pressure accurately. This difference is not a true artifact, but the difference in the two pressures may be clinically important. Fig. 3-69 shows simultaneous LA, PCW, and LV pressure tracings. The PCW is delayed as compared with directly measured LA pressure. Larger LA v waves without delay in downslope, unlike the PCW tracing, demonstrate a major difference in the mitral valve gradient. The PCW-LV gradient may be much greater than the LA-LV in some patients with mitral valve disease.

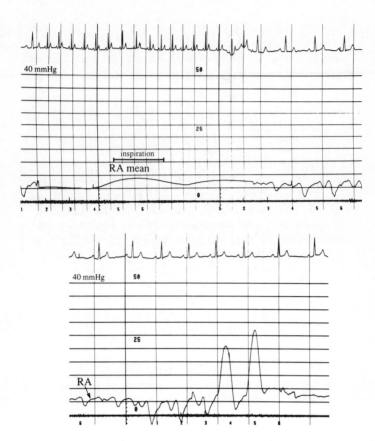

Fig. 3-68. **A,** Right atrial (*RA*) mean pressure increasing during inspiration. The artifact occurs when the catheter has moved accidentally into the right ventricular pressure. **B,** If not observed on phasic waveform, this artifact may be missed. See text for details.

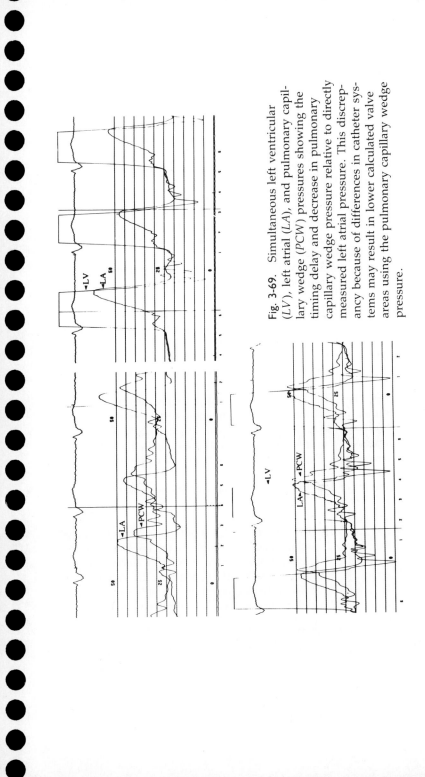

Fig. 3-69. Simultaneous left ventricular (*LV*), left atrial (*LA*), and pulmonary capillary wedge (*PCW*) pressures showing the timing delay and decrease in pulmonary capillary wedge pressure relative to directly measured left atrial pressure. This discrepancy because of differences in catheter systems may result in lower calculated valve areas using the pulmonary capillary wedge pressure.

SUGGESTED READINGS

Angel J, Soler JS, Anivarro I, Domingo E: Hemodynamic evaluation of stenotic cardiac valves: II. modification of the simplified valve formula for mitral and aortic valve area calculation, *Cathet Cardiovasc Diagn* 11:127–138, 1985.

Cannon SR, Richards KL, Crawford M: Hydraulic estimation of stenotic orifice area: a correction of the Gorlin formula, *Circulation* 71:1170–1178, 1985.

Carabello BA: Advances in the hemodynamic assessment of stenotic cardiac valves, *J Am Coll Cardiol* 10:912–919, 1987.

Damen J, Bolton D: A prospective analysis of 1400 pulmonary artery catheterizations in patients undergoing cardiac surgery, *Acta Anaesthesiol Scand* 30:386–392, 1986.

Elliot CG, Zimmerman GA, Glemmer TP: Complications of pulmonary artery catheterization in the care of critically ill patients, *Chest* 76:647–652, 1979.

Feldman T, Ford L, Chiu YC, Carroll J: Changes in valvular resistance, power dissipation and myocardial reserve with aortic valvuloplasty, *J Heart Valve Dis* 1:55–64, 1992.

Flamm JD, Cohn KE, Hancock EW: Measurement of systemic cardiac output at rest and exercise in patients with atrial septal defect, *Am J Cardiol* 23:258–265, 1969.

Ford L, Feldman T, Chiu YC, Carroll J: Hemodynamic resistance as a measure of functional impairment in aortic valvular stenosis, *Circ Res* 66:1–7, 1990.

Fuchs RM, Heuser RR, Yin FCP, Brinker JA: Limitations of pulmonary wedge V waves in diagnosing mitral regurgitation, *Am J Cardiol* 49:849–854, 1982.

Grose R, Strain J, Cohen MV: Pulmonary arterial V waves in mitral regurgitation: clinical and experimental observations, *Circulation* 69:214–222, 1984.

Hakki AH, Iskandrian AS, Bemis CE, Kimbiris D, Mintz GS, Segal BL, Brice C: A simplified valve formula for the calculation of stenotic cardiac valve areas, *Circulation* 63:1050–1055, 1981.

Halperin JL, Brooks KM, Rothlauf EB, Mindich BP, Ambrose JA, Teichholz LE: Effect of nitroglycerin on the pulmonary venous gradient in patients after mitral valve replacement, *J Am Coll Cardiol* 5:34–39, 1985.

Haskell RJ, French WJ: Accuracy of left atrial and pulmonary artery wedge pressure in pure mitral regurgitation in predicting left ventricular end-diastolic pressure, *Am J Cardiol* 61:136–141, 1988.

Henriques AH, Schrijen FV, Redondo J, Delorme N: Local variations of pulmonary arterial wedge pressure and wedge angiograms in patients with chronic lung disease, *Chest* 94:491–495, 1988.

Hillis LD, Firth BG, Winniford MD: Analysis of factors affecting the variability of Fick versus indicator dilution measurements of cardiac output, *Am J Cardiol* 56:764–768, 1985.

Hillis LD, Firth BG, Winniford MD: Comparison of thermodilution and indocyanine green dye in low cardiac output or left-sided regurgitation, *Am J Cardiol* 57:1201–1202, 1986.

Hillis LD, Winniford MD, Jackson JA, Firth BG: Measurement of left-to-right intracardiac shunting in adults: oximetric versus indicator dilution techniques, *Cathet Cardiovasc Diagn* 11:467–472, 1985.

Lange RA, Moore EM Jr, Cigarroa RG, Hillis LD: Use of pulmonary capillary wedge pressure to assess severity of mitral stenosis: is true left atrial pressure needed in this condition? *J Am Coll Cardiol* 13:825–829, 1989.

Matthay MA, Chatterjee K: Bedside catheterization of the pulmonary artery: risks compared with benefits, *Ann Intern Med* 109:826–834, 1988.

Niggemann EH, Ma PTS, Sunnergren KP, Winniford MD, Hillis LD: Detection of intracardiac left-to-right shunting in adults: a prospective analysis of the variability of the standard indocyanine green technique in patients without shunting, *Am J Cardiol* 60:355–357, 1987.

Nigri A, Martuscelli E, Mangieri E, Voci P, Danesi A, Sardella R, Feroci L, Reale A: Nomogram for calculation of stenotic cardiac valve areas from cardiac output and mean transvalvular gradient, *Cathet Cardiovasc Diagn* 10:613–618, 1984.

Pichard AD, Kay R, Smith H, Rentrop P, Holt J, Gorlin R: Large V waves in the pulmonary wedge pressure tracing in the absence of mitral regurgitation, *Am J Cardiol* 50:1044–1050, 1982.

Sandler H, Dodge HT: The use of single plane angiocardiograms for the calculation of left ventricular volume in man, *Am Heart J* 80:343–352, 1970.

Schoenfeld MH, Palacios IF, Hutter AM Jr, Jacoby SS, Block PC: Underestimation of prosthetic mitral valve areas: role of transseptal catheterization in avoiding unnecessary repeat mitral valve surgery, *J Am Coll Cardiol* 5:1387–1392, 1985.

Segal J, Lerner DJ, Miller DC, Mitchell RS, Alderman EA, Popp RL: When should Doppler-determined valve area be better than the Gorlin formula? Variation in hydraulic constants in low flow states, *J Am Coll Cardiol* 9:1294–1305, 1987.

Smucker ML, Lipscomb K: A fluoroscopic method to confirm proper catheter position to measure pulmonary artery wedge pressure, *Cathet Cardiovasc Diagn* 8:83–87, 1982.

Strunk BL, Cheitlin MD, Stulbarg MS, Schiller NB: Right-to-left interatrial shunting through a patent foramen ovale despite normal intracardiac pressures, *Am J Cardiol* 60:413–415, 1987.

4

ELECTROPHYSIOLOGIC STUDIES AND ABLATION TECHNIQUES

Denise L. Janosik and M. Carolyn Gamache

The electrophysiology study (EPS) is an invasive procedure that involves the placement of multipolar catheter electrodes at various intracardiac sites. Electrode catheters are routinely placed in the right atrium, across the tricuspid valve annulus in the area of the AV node and His bundle (a special part of the conduction system), the right ventricle, the coronary sinus, and sometimes the left ventricle (Fig. 4-1). The general purposes of EPS are to characterize the electrophysiologic properties of the conduction system, induce and analyze the mechanism of arrhythmias, and evaluate the effects of therapeutic interventions. When EPS was introduced in the early 1970s, it was utilized primarily for diagnostic purposes. Over the past two decades, the indications and applications of EPSs have greatly expanded. Currently, EPS is a technique routinely utilized in the clinical management of patients with both supraventricular and ventricular arrhythmias (Table 4-1). With the development of safe and effective catheter ablation techniques, an exciting new area of interventional electrophysiology has evolved. The field of electrophysiology is a complex subspecialty of cardiology, which is introduced

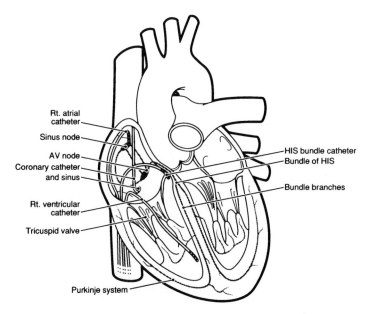

Rt. atrial
catheter

Sinus node

AV node

Coronary catheter
and sinus

Rt. ventricular
catheter

Tricuspid valve

HIS bundle catheter

Bundle of HIS

Bundle branches

Purkinje system

Fig. 4-1. The catheter positions for routine electrophysiologic study are demonstrated. Multipolar catheters are positioned in the high right atrium near the sinus node, in the area of the atrioventricular *(AV)* node and His bundle, in the right ventricular apex, and in the coronary sinus.

in this section. Individuals seeking a more in-depth discussion of the procedures and concepts described should refer to the suggested reading section.

TECHNICAL ASPECTS
Personnel

It is imperative that EPS be performed by appropriately trained personnel. The physician responsible for the performance and analysis of the EPS should be fully trained in clinical cardiology and should have spent a minimum of one or preferably 2 additional years training in the subspeciality of electrophysiology. A thorough knowledge of normal and abnormal conduction, refractory periods, activation sequences, and the significance of various responses to programmed electrical stimulation are necessary before clinical judgments can be based on information obtained from the

TABLE 4-1.   Clinical applications of electrophysiologic studies

Diagnostic

Diagnose sinus node dysfunction
Determine site of AV nodal block
Define cause of syncope of unclear etiology
Differentiate VT from SVT in cases of wide complex tachycardia
Define mechanism of SVT or VT and map site of origin of tachycardia

Therapeutic

Guide drug therapy for sustained VT, aborted sudden death or SVT
Select appropriate candidates for antitachycardic pacemakers and
   cardioverter-defibrillator therapy
Test efficacy of device therapy for ventricular tachyarrhythmias
Select appropriate candidates for catheter ablative and surgical therapy
Test efficacy of ablative and surgical therapies

Interventional

AV nodal ablation for atrial fibrillation
Ablation for atrial tachycardia and atrial flutter
AV nodal modification (slow-pathway ablation)
Accessory pathway ablation in WPW
Ablation of ventricular tachycardia

Prognostic*

Risk stratification in asymptomatic WPW
Risk stratification in patients post myocardial infarction
Risk stratification in patients with nonsustained VT

VT, ventricular tachycardia; SVT, supraventricular tachycardia; WPW, Wolff-Parkinson-White syndrome.
* Clinical utility not established or indication controversial.

EPS. A well-trained nurse or technician is essential to the performance of safe and comprehensive EPSs. Because the physician's attention is often focused on the stimulator and electrograms, he or she relies heavily upon the nurse to monitor the patient's condition and communicate significant changes in the patient's condition to the physician. The nurse usually sits between the patient and the cardioverter-defibrillator and crash cart. The nurse monitors the patient's blood pressure, heart rate, rhythm, and, often, oxygen saturation via a pulse oximeter. It is the nurse's responsibility to obtain a 12-lead ECG and perform cardioversion/defibrillation in response to an induced hemodynamically unstable arrhythmia. Optimally, a second nurse is available during procedures to administer medications and/or to assist in technical aspects of the procedure. Specific guidelines have been published for the training necessary for the physicians and nurses involved in electrophysiologic procedures. In laboratories performing mapping and catheter ablation procedures, an anesthesiologist and cardiothoracic surgeon should be available in case of need for general anesthesia or a rare complication requiring emergency surgery. A biomedical engineer should be readily available to repair equipment that may malfunction and compromise the ability to perform an optimal EPS.

Equipment

The quality of the data collected during an EPS is partially dependent on the equipment utilized. An electrophysiology laboratory must be equipped with radiographic equipment, a recording and monitoring system, a stimulator, and all drugs and equipment required for complete cardiopulmonary resuscitation (Fig. 4-2). The reproduction of intracardiac electrical events requires a signal processing system that contains filters and amplifiers that optimize the electrical signals. At least eight amplifiers should be available to display several surface electrocardiographic leads simultaneously with multiple intracardiac electrograms. The number of surface electrocardiographic leads and intracardiac electrograms displayed will vary depending on the type of study being performed. The recent development of computerized digital

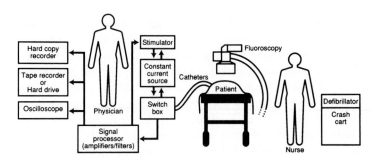

Fig. 4-2.   General setup of the equipment utilized for electrophysiologic studies.

recording systems with optical disk storage facilitates collection of large quantities of data that may later be analyzed on system-specific software. Older analog recording systems may be interfaced to a tape recorder or VHS system for storage of data. The recorder must be able to print hard copy at a variety of paper speeds (10 to 300 mm/sec). Selected segments of the study are printed on hard copy for on-line analysis and interpretation or for inclusion in the patient's medical record. Some method of obtaining a 12-lead ECG should be available either by standard electrocardiography or through the recording system. Radiographic equipment with a permanent image intensifier capable of a high-quality image is required. It is optimal to have the capacity for multiple views either with a biplane system or a fluoroscopy unit equipped with a rotating C arm. Electrical interference may distort intracardiac electrograms and make interpretation of data more difficult. A biomedical/electrical engineer should be involved in the initial design of the electrophysiology laboratory to assure appropriate shielding and suspension of wires and cables and proper grounding of equipment.

A programmable stimulator is necessary to perform an EPS. The stimulator is equipped with dials or switches by which the pacing intervals and coupling intervals of the extrastimuli may be adjusted (Fig. 4-3). The stimulator is able to pace over a wide range of rates from two sites simultaneously. It has the ability to introduce a minimum of three extrastimuli (premature beats) coupled to a train of pacing or synchronized to sinus rhythm. A junction box which interfaces with the recording system and stimulator facilitates changes in pacing site without disconnecting catheters.

A cardioverter-defibrillator should be close to the patient at all times. A back-up defibrillator is optimal in case of a rare, but potentially disastrous failure of one defibrillator. The defibrillators should be tested prior to each study and equipped with an emergency power source. Many laboratories utilize commercially available R-2 pads. One pad is placed under the right scapula and the other on the anterior chest over the left ventricular apex and connected via an adaptor to the defibrillator. In rare instances in which transthoracic defibrillation fails to convert induced ventricular fibrillation, emergency defibrillation through an intracardiac

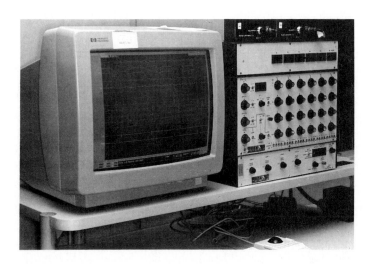

Fig. 4-3.   A recording system and monitor *(left)* and commercially available stimulator *(right).*

electrode catheter may be effective in terminating the arrhythmia (Fig. 4-4).

Catheters

There are a variety of catheter electrodes available for the performance of EPSs and catheter-guided ablation (Fig. 4-5). There are many different types of catheters designed for specific purposes, such as steerable and deflectable tip catheters, which facilitate mapping of the atria, AV ring, and ventricles. Special large-tip catheters have been designed for delivery of radiofrequency energy. The catheters are constructed of woven Dacron or synthetic material such as polyurethane and contain 2 to 20 electrodes with 1- to 10-mm spacing between electrodes. The majority of catheters utilized in adult patients are 5 to 7 French in size. The type of catheter selected may vary depending upon the intracardiac position desired and the type of data being collected. The preference of catheters may vary between operators and is dependent upon properties of the catheter such as torque, durability, flexibility, and experience of the operator.

Bipolar pacing is performed from the distal pair of elec-

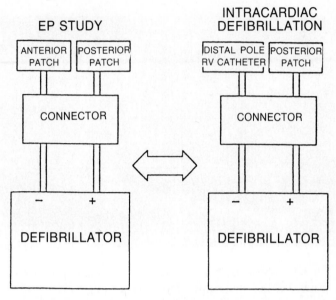

Fig. 4-4.   Diagram of intracardiac defibrillation, which may be utilized when ventricular fibrillation is refractory to multiple transthoracic defibrillations. During the routine electrophysiologic *(EP)* study, anterior and posterior skin patches are attached by a connector to a standard defibrillator. When multiple transthoracic high-energy shocks fail to terminate ventricular fibrillation, the anterior patch may be disconnected and the distal pole of the right ventricular *(RV)* catheter attached to the defibrillator. High-energy shocks are then delivered from the right ventricular catheter to the posterior patch. (From Cohen TJ, Scheinman MM, Pullen BT, Chiesa NA, Gonzalez R, Herre JM, Griffin JC: Emergency intracardiac defibrillation for refractory ventricular fibrillation during routine electrophysiologic study. *J Am Cell Cardiol* 18:1280–1284, 1991.)

trodes, and simultaneous recording of intracardiac electrograms can be performed from more proximal electrode pairs. For most routine studies a catheter with two pairs of electrodes (quadripolar catheter) with 5-mm spacing between electrodes is sufficient; pacing is performed from the distal pair of electrodes while the intracardiac electrogram is recorded from the proximal pair of electrodes. In mapping

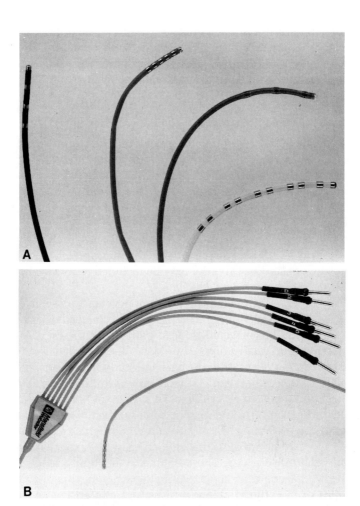

Fig. 4-5. **A,** Several types of multipolar catheters utilized in routine electrophysiologic studies are displayed. Note the difference in the number of electrodes and the differences in spacing between the electrodes between the various catheters. **B,** The proximal end of a hexipolar electrode catheter. The number on each pin corresponds to the electrode position at the tip of the catheter with D representing the most distal electrode.

studies where it is important to precisely localize the area of earliest electrical activation, catheters with a greater number of electrodes (up to 12) and smaller inner electrode distances (as little as 1 mm) are optimal.

PROCEDURES

Evaluation and Preparation of the Patient Prior to EPS

The results of the EPS must be considered in the context of the patient's clinical presentation and underlying cardiac substrate. Thus, the physician performing the EPS must perform a comprehensive evaluation of the patient prior to the EPS and plan the procedure based on the information being sought in the individual patient. Whenever possible, electrocardiographic documentation of the clinical event, preferably by 12-lead ECG, should be obtained. Some or all of the procedures listed in Table 4-2 may be included in this evaluation.

Any potentially reversible arrhythmogenic factors such as electrolyte abnormalities or decompensated congestive heart failure should be corrected prior to performing the EPS. All antiarrhythmic medications should be discontinued for at least five half-lives prior to the baseline study. For supraventricular tachycardia studies, medications influencing AV nodal conduction (e.g., beta-blockers, digoxin, and calcium channel blockers) should also be discontinued. The patient should have nothing by mouth after midnight except for essential cardiac medications, which may be taken with a small amount of water. The patient may be lightly sedated with IV diazepam or midazolam. In very long diagnostic studies or in catheter ablation cases, more intensive levels of sedation are usually required. We routinely utilize IV fentanyl and midazolam to achieve somulence during lengthy ablation procedures. However, it should be kept in mind that excessive sedation may influence the ability to induce arrhythmias in some individuals.

Venous Access

Routine diagnostic EPSs involve stimulation and recording of electrical activity from the right heart. Venous access may be obtained from the femoral, subclavian, internal jugular, or antecubital veins. A routine initial diagnostic EPS usually

TABLE 4-2. Evaluation prior to electrophysiologic testing*

Procedure	Purpose
History and physical	Identify signs/symptoms of cardiac or neurologic disease
	Identify factors known to exacerbate arrhythmias
	Details of syncopal events
Neurological evaluation (if history and physical suggest)	
EEG	Rule out seizure disorder
CT/MRI	Identify focal lesion
Carotid ultrasound	Identify significant cerebrovascular disease
12-lead ECG	Previous myocardial infarction
	Intraventricular conduction delays
	Prolonged QT interval
	Preexcitation syndromes
24- to 48-hr ambulatory electrocardiography	Correlation of symptoms with electrocardiographic events
	Quantitation of ambient ectopy
	Diurinal variation in arrhythmia
Event recorder	Correlation of symptoms with electrocardiographic events
Head-up tilt table testing	Diagnose vasovagal/vasodepressor syncope
Echocardiogram/radionuclide ventriculography	Assessment of left ventricular and right ventricular size and function
	Detect valvular pathology
Stress test (with or without perfusion scanning)	Detect reversible ischemia
	Assess effects of catecholamines on arrhythmia induction
Cardiac catheterization	Define coronary anatomy

ECG, Electrocardiogram; EEG, electroencephalogram; CT, computerized tomography; MRI, magnetic resonance imaging.
* Selected procedures may vary depending on the clinical presentation.

involves insertion of at least three catheters, most commonly inserted via the femoral veins. These large veins easily permit the introduction of two 5 to 7 French catheters per vein. The number of catheters required and venous access selected depends on the type of study being performed and the data being collected. For example, a follow-up study to assess drug efficacy for ventricular tachycardia may be accomplished by the placement of a single quadripolar catheter in the right ventricular apex via the internal jugular access. However, mapping of a left-sided bypass tract may require the insertion of five multipolar catheters and even necessitate catheterization of the left heart for precise mapping.

For patients requiring beat-to-beat assessment of the hemodynamic effects of an induced arrhythmia, an arterial line may be placed. To evaluate completely a patient with Wolff-Parkinson-White syndrome, it may be necessary to access the left ventricle for stimulation and/or recording of intracardiac electrical activity. If arterial catheterization is necessary, administration of IV heparin is mandatory. Patients undergoing prolonged studies involving venous access or with a history of venous thromboembolism should also receive heparin.

Positioning of Catheters

The right atrium is easily accessible by any venous access. The most common site for stimulation and recording is the high posterior lateral wall in the region of the sinus node. Recording of the His potential is most easily achieved from a catheter introduced by the femoral approach and passed into the right atrium across the tricuspid valve and into the right ventricle. The catheter is then withdrawn across the tricuspid valve with the application of a slight degree of clockwise torque that tends to keep the catheter in contact with the septum (Fig. 4-6). A hexapolar or octapolar catheter in the His position may be used so that electrical activity from multiple electrode pairs can be recorded and the one demonstrating the most stable and consistent His potential may be displayed. If multiple attempts to record a His potential with one catheter are unsuccessful, a differently shaped or steerable catheter with a deflectable tip may be utilized. In the overwhelming majority of patients, a His potential can be successfully recorded.

The left atrium is usually indirectly approached by recording from the coronary sinus. Cannulation of the coronary sinus os is most often successful from the left subclavian or antecubital approach. Catheters introduced through these approaches are more easily deflected off the lateral RA wall toward the coronary sinus os, which lies posteromedially

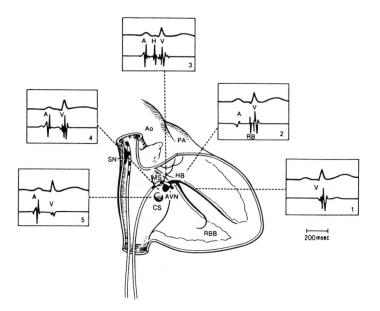

Fig. 4-6. Intracardiac electrograms recorded from various positions on a multipolar catheter positioned across the tricuspid valve. The numbers 1 to 5 refer to the intracardiac location of the catheters along with the corresponding electrograms. 1 represents the most distal location recording a large ventricular electrogram and no atrial electrogram while 5 represents the most proximal location displaying a large atrial electrogram with a very small ventricular electrogram. The His potential is observed when the catheter is in the area of the tricuspid annulus and the atrial and ventricular electrograms recorded are approximately of equal size (position 3). (From Grossman W: Cardiac catheterization and angiography, 2nd edition. p. 285, Philadelphia, 1974, Lea and Febiger.)

above the tricuspid annulus. Fluoroscopically, successful cannulation of the coronary sinus is suspected when advancement of the catheter curves upward toward the left shoulder in the LAO projection and is posteriorly oriented in the lateral projection. Electrocardiographically, atrial and ventricular electrograms are recorded with the timing of the atrial electrogram appearing later than the high RA electrogram. Direct recording of electrical activity from the left atrium is possible in individuals with a patent foramen ovale or atrial septal defect.

The placement of the catheter in the right ventricle is readily achieved by any venous approach. In most studies, the catheter is placed in the RV apex. For ventricular stimulation protocols, a second ventricular catheter is often placed in the RV outflow tract although some operators prefer to reposition the catheter from the apex to the outflow tract. The order in which the right-side catheters are placed varies between operators and no particular order is mandatory. In patients with a preexisting left bundle branch block, it is recommended that the RV apical catheter be positioned first to assure adequate ventricular pacing in the event of catheter-induced trauma to the right bundle, which may result in complete heart block while positioning the His catheter.

Catheterization of the left ventricle may be necessary in patients with ventricular tachycardia or preexcitation syndromes. The left ventricle is most commonly accessed by the retrograde arterial approach for mapping procedures. Fluoroscopy permitting views in multiple planes is essential to ensure accurate positioning of the catheter. Stimulation may also be performed from the left ventricle in cases in which patients are with clinically documented sustained ventricular tachycardia are noninducible using the standard protocol from the right ventricle. The left ventricle may be entered and mapped by the retrograde arterial approach or through the left atrium and mitral valve in patients with atrial septal defects or patent foramen ovale or in those undergoing transseptal punctures.

Complications

The complications associated with EPSs are very low, and mortality is extremely rare. The complications of the procedure are usually secondary to catheterization and catheter manipulation rather than stimulation and the induction of arrhythmias. The reported complications include hemorrhage, venous thromboembolism (less than 1%), phlebitis (less than 1%), cardiac perforation and tamponade, and refractory ventricular fibrillation. Hemothorax and pneumothorax are recognized complications when utilizing the subclavian or internal jugular venous approaches. Arterial catheterization increases the associated morbidity of the procedure including vascular complications, stroke, systemic embolism, and protamine reactions. The mortality associated with EPSs is extremely rare, occurring in less than 1 per 25,000 procedures. Most reported deaths have been secondary to incessant ventricular fibrillation and have occurred in patients with severe LV dysfunction, active myocardial ischemia, or hypertrophic obstructive cardiomyopathy or due to proarrhythmic effect of drugs administered during the evaluation. Defibrillation through an intracardiac electrode has been reported to be effective in situations when transthoracic defibrillation fails and mortality may have otherwise resulted (see Fig. 4-4).

Study Protocol

Although details of the protocol may vary depending on the indication for the EPS and the information being obtained, most studies involve the recording and measuring of spontaneous intracardiac events and observing the effects of programmed electrical stimulation. An initial study usually takes several hours and depends on the complexity of the case. The possible components of the initial comprehensive EPS are listed in Table 4-3.

TABLE 4-3. Possible components of comprehensive initial EPS*

Measurement of basic intervals
Determination of sinus node function
Determination of atrial, AV nodal, His-Purkinje, and ventricular
  conduction and refractoriness
Identification of presence of dual AV nodal pathways
Identification of presence, location, and electrical properties of accessory
  atrioventricular pathways
Attempts to induce supraventricular tachycardia
Attempts to induce ventricular tachycardia
Determine mechanism of induced arrhythmias
Map site of origin of induced arrhythmias
Determine effect of intravenous antiarrhythmic drugs on induced
  tachycardia
Determine efficacy of antitachycardic pacing for induced tachycardia

* The actual procedure will vary depending on the individual case; not all parameters
will be assessed in all cases.

Measurement of Conduction Intervals

After positioning of the catheters, basic conduction intervals are measured, including the basic sinus cycle length (the A to A interval), the AH interval, His spike duration, and HV interval (Fig. 4-7). In addition, measurements from the surface ECG including the PR interval, the QRS interval, and QT interval are measured. Conduction interval measurements and refractory period measurements should be made at a paper speed of at least 100 mm/sec in routine cases and in detailed mapping procedures at speeds of 200 to 300 mm/sec. All measurements of rate and conduction times are made in terms of milliseconds. The pacing interval can be converted to heart rate by the following formula:

$$\text{Interval (ms)} = \frac{60,000}{\text{heart rate}} \text{ (Table 4-4)}$$

The AH interval represents conduction time from the low right atrium at the interatrial septum through the atrioventricular node to the His bundle and approximates atrioventricular nodal conduction time. The measurement is made from the earliest reproducible rapid deflection of the atrial electrogram on the His bundle recording to the onset of the

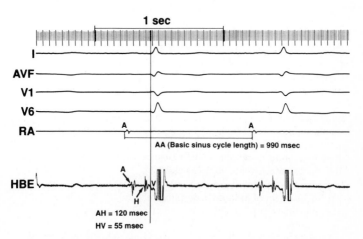

Fig. 4-7. The measurement of the basic sinus cycle length and the AH interval and HV interval is demonstrated. *RA*, right atrium; *HBE*, His bundle electrogram.

TABLE 4-4. Pacing interval conversion chart*

Pacing interval (ms)	Heart rate (bpm)
200	300
222	270
231	260
240	250
250	240
261	230
273	220
286	210
300	200
311	193
316	190
333	180
353	170
375	160
400	150
429	140
462	130
500	120
545	110
550	109
600	100
667	90
750	80
857	70
1000	60
1200	50
1500	40
2000	30

* Pulse-to-pulse interval (ms) to beats per minute (bpm).

His deflection on that electrogram (Fig. 4-7). Normal values for adults are reported to range from 50 to 140 ms. It is important to realize that the AH interval is strongly influenced by the patient's autonomic tone and may vary by up to 50 ms during a study in a given patient. The AH interval normally increases in response to increases in atrial pacing rates. It also may be altered by drugs that affect AV conduction, and the measurement may be artificially influenced by factors such as gain setting and position of the atrial catheter.

The HV interval represents conduction time from the proximal His bundle to the ventricular myocardium. The measurement is made from the earliest deflection of the His spike on the His bundle recording to the earliest onset of ventricular activation recorded from any intracardiac electrogram or surface ECG. Normal values range from 30 to 55 ms. In contrast to the AH interval, the HV interval normally remains relatively constant and is not significantly affected by variations in autonomic tone or atrial pacing rates.

Sequence of Activation

Determination of the sequence of antegrade and retrograde atrial activation during spontaneous rhythms, atrial pacing, ventricular pacing, and induced rhythms is essential in differentiation of ventricular tachycardia from supraventricular tachycardia and in defining the reentrant circuit in supraventricular tachycardias. Normally, the atrial activation begins in the high right atrium, spreads to the low right atrium and His bundle with left atrial activation, recorded from the coronary sinus catheter, occurring significantly later. When ventriculoatrial conduction is present during ventricular pacing, the earliest retrograde atrial activity is recorded in the His bundle electrogram followed by the RA and coronary sinus recordings. Abnormal or eccentric sequences of retrograde atrial activation occur in the presence of atrioventricular accessory pathways (Fig. 4-8). This is discussed in more detail in subsequent sections dealing with supraventricular tachycardia and catheter ablation.

Programmed Electrical Stimulation

Programmed electrical stimulation involves observing the electrophysiologic effects of incremental pacing and the introduction of programmed extrastimuli coupled to normal sinus rhythm or paced rhythms. The major purposes of programmed electrical stimulation are to characterize the electrophysiologic properties of cardiac tissue and to induce and analyze the mechanism of arrhythmias. The two most commonly employed types of pacing during the EPS are burst or incremental pacing and programmed stimulation. Fixed burst pacing involves the delivery of a series of impulses at a constant rate. A decremental burst consists of a series of impulses at progressively increasing rates. Programmed stimulation involves the coupling of premature extrastimuli

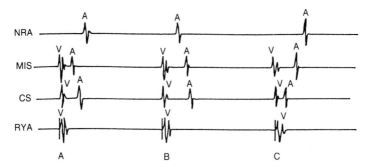

Fig. 4-8. Patterns of retrograde atrial activation. The figure shows electrograms from the high right atrium *(HRA),* the His bundle, the coronary sinus *(CS),* and the right ventricular apex *(RVA)* during ventricular pacing. **A,** Normal pattern of retrograde atrial activation through the atrioventricular conducting system is demonstrated. The atrial septum is activated first (His) followed by the left atrium (CS) and right atrium (HRA). **B,** Sequence of retrograde activation with a right-sided accessory pathway. The earliest retrograde activation occurs in the high right atrium since retrograde conduction occurs over a right-sided accessory pathway. **C,** Sequence of retrograde atrial activation with a left-sided accessory pathway. The left atrium is activated first (CS) since retrograde conduction over a left-sided accessory pathway occurs. A = atrial electrogram; V = ventricular electrogram. (From Forgoros RN: Electrophysiologic testing. Oxford, 1991, Blackwell.)

to a short train (six to eight beats) of burst pacing or to sinus rhythm. The number of extrastimuli may vary from one to four. The pacing train is referred to as S1, first extrastimulus as S2, second extrastimulus as S3, etc. The coupling intervals are progressively and systematically decreased until an arrhythmia is induced or the first extrastimulus loses capture (the cardiac tissue is refractory).

Assessment of Sinus Node Function

Many studies begin with an evaluation of sinus node and AV node function and assessment of atrial and AV nodal refractoriness. Measurement of sinus node recovery time is performed by pacing the right atrium (most commonly the high right atrium in the region of the sinus node) at a rate slightly faster than the intrinsic sinus rate for approximately 30 seconds and abruptly terminating pacing. The sinus node recovery time is defined as the time from the last paced atrial complex on the RA recording to the return of the first sinus complex (Fig. 4-9). Generally, the slower the intrinsic sinus rate, the longer the sinus node recovery time. The absolute sinus node recovery time may be corrected for heart rate by subtracting the basic sinus cycle length. Normal values for absolute sinus node recovery time are approximately 1.5 seconds and for corrected sinus node recovery time, 550 ms. For most routine studies, several measurements of sinus node recovery time are sufficient for assessment of sinus node function. The interested reader may consult the suggested reading for further description of techniques utilized in the assessment of sinus node function.

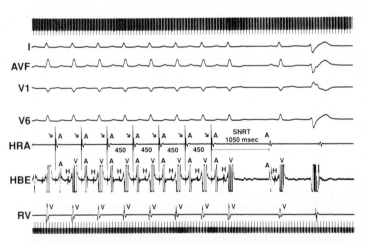

Fig. 4-9. Demonstration of a normal sinus node recovery time in a patient undergoing electrophysiologic study for the evaluation of syncope of unknown etiology. Following a train of atrial pacing at a cycle length of 450 (approximately 133 bpm), 1050 ms elapse before return of sinus node activity. Thus, the absolute sinus node recovery time is 1050 ms *HRA*, high right atrium; *HBE*, His bundle electrogram; *RV*, Right ventricle; *SNRT*, Sinus node recovery time.

Assessment of AV Nodal and His Purkinje System Function

Atrioventricular nodal function is assessed by determining the point at which 1 : 1 atrioventricular conduction ceases and AV nodal Wenckebach begins. The normal response to incremental atrial pacing at progressively faster rates is to develop a longer AH interval and, ultimately, block in the AV node (Fig. 4-10). Most normal individuals develop AV nodal Wenckebach at paced atrial cycle lengths of 500 to 350 ms (heart rates of 120 to 170 bpm). AV nodal Wenckebach does not normally occur during exercise when similar heart rates are achieved because catecholamines enhance conduction through the AV node. The point at which Wenckebach occurs in response to atrial pacing may be influenced by

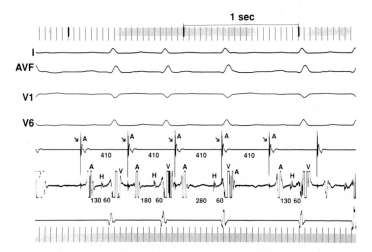

Fig. 4-10. Type I second degree atrioventricular block (Wenckebach) in the atrioventricular node induced by atrial pacing at a cycle length of 410 ms. Each paced atrial depolarization is followed by a progressively longer AH interval until the fourth atrial depolarization is blocked in the atrioventricular node (no His depolarization is seen following the atrial electrogram). The AH interval following the blocked atrial depolarization is shorter (130 ms) compared to the AH interval preceding the block beat (280 ms). Note that the HV interval remains constant despite the progressive increase in AH interval during the Wenckebach sequence.

drugs that affect AV nodal conduction and by autonomic tone. Wenckebach occurs at longer cycle lengths (slower pacing rates) in patients with enhanced vagal tone and at shorter cycle lengths (faster pacing rates) in patients with enhanced sympathetic tone. In contrast to the AH interval, the HV interval remains relatively constant during decremental atrial pacing and block below His (infra-Hisian block) is considered pathologic at pacing cycle lengths of greater than 350 ms (rates <170 bpm).

Determination of Refractory Periods

The refractoriness of cardiac tissue is defined by the response of the tissue to the introduction of premature stimuli. For most routine EPSs, the effective refractory period is defined as the longest coupling interval between the basic drive and the premature stimulus that fails to propagate through the tissue. Normal values for AV nodal, atrial, and ventricular refractory periods have been established (Table 4-5). The effective refractory period of cardiac tissue may be effected by the current strength used, the pacing rate, medications, and the AV nodal refractory period by autonomic tone.

AV Nodal Function Curves

AV nodal function curves can be constructed by plotting the coupling interval of the premature stimulus (A_1A_2 interval) on the horizontal axis versus the AH interval (AV nodal conduction time) of the premature stimulus (A_2H_2 interval) on the vertical axis. In individuals without dual AV nodal pathways, there is a progressive and gradual increase in the

TABLE 4-5. Normal intervals and refractory periods

Parameter	Normal Duration (ms)
AH	50-150
HV	30-55
His	10-25
Atrial ERP	150-360
AV nodal ERP	230-430
HPS ERP	330-450
Ventricular ERP	170-290

ERP, Effective refractory period; AV, atrioventricular; HPS, His-Purkinje system.

AH interval prior to the premature stimulus blocking in the AV node and the function curve is continuous (Fig. 4-11**A**). A sudden large increase in the AH interval (often referred to as a jump) in response to a small decrement in the coupling interval of the premature is evidence of functional dual AV nodal pathways (Fig. 4-12). This represents a shift from conduction over the fast AV nodal pathway to conduction over the slow AV nodal pathway (with a longer AH interval) and the AV nodal function curve is discontinuous (see Fig. 4-11**B**). In patients with AV nodal reentrant tachycardia, supraventricular tachycardia is often initiated when the jump to the slow pathway occurs. In patients with suspected or

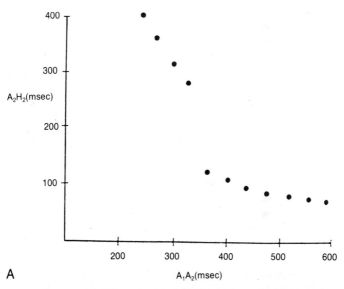

A

Fig. 4-11. **A,** Normal atrioventricular nodal function curve in a patient without functional dual atrioventricular nodal pathways. In this graph, the conduction intervals (A_1A_2) are displayed on the X axis and the resulting AH interval (A_2H_2) on the Y axis. With progressively shorter coupling intervals, premature atrial beats are followed by progressively longer AH intervals (A_2H_2), which represents progressive conduction delay in the atrioventricular node. The normal atrioventricular nodal conduction curve is smooth and continuous. *Continued on page 230.*

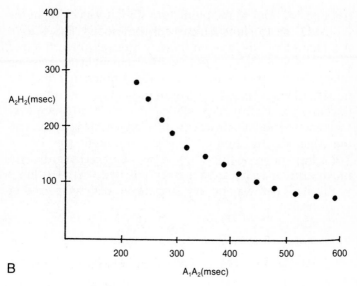

Fig. 4-11. *Continued from page 229.* **B,** A typical atrioventricular nodal function curve in a patient with functional dual atrioventricular nodal pathways. Premature atrial impulses with longer coupling intervals conduct down the fast pathway and therefore have short AH intervals. With progressively earlier premature atrial impulses, the refractory period of the fast pathway is reached and conduction shifts to the slow pathway. The jump from the fast pathway to the slow pathway is manifested by a sudden lengthening of the A_2H_2 interval and discontinuity in the atrioventricular nodal function curve. (From Forgoros RN: Electrophysiologic testing, Oxford, 1991, Blackwell.)

known supraventricular tachycardia, multiple extrastimuli may be utilized in an attempt to induce a clinically significant tachycardia. In some circumstances, isoproterenol or atropine may be given in attempts to induce a clinically significant supraventricular tachycardia.

Ventricular Stimulation

The safety and efficacy of programmed electrical stimulation in the diagnosis and treatment of patients with ventricular arrhythmias has been well established. The reported sensitivity and specificity of ventricular stimulation may vary de-

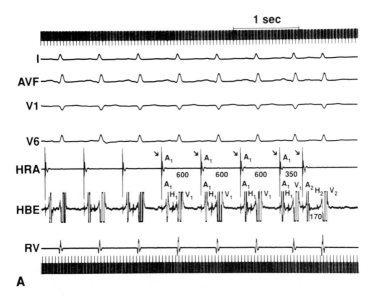

Fig. 4-12. **A,** 130-ms jump in atrioventricular nodal conduction is demonstrated in a patient with functional dual atrioventricular nodal pathways. Premature atrial stimuli are coupled to a train of atrial pacing at a cycle length of 600 ms. **A,** At a coupling interval of 350 ms, the premature atrial stimulous has an AH interval of 170 ms. *Continued on page 232.*

pending on the stimulation protocol utilized and differences in patient population in terms of presenting arrhythmia and underlying cardiac disease. The sensitivity and specificity of programmed electrical stimulation has been best defined in patients with coronary artery disease who present with spontaneous sustained monomorphic ventricular tachycardia. In these individuals, the yield (and sensitivity) of the EPS increases with the addition of up to three extrastimulis with little or no added benefit from more extrastimuli. In the vast majority of patients, the clinical ventricular tachycardia will be reproducibly initiated by programmed electrical stimulation. The clinical significance of arrhythmias induced by programmed electrical stimulation must be interpreted with regard to the specific arrhythmia for which a patient is being evaluated. With more aggressive stimulation protocols, poly-

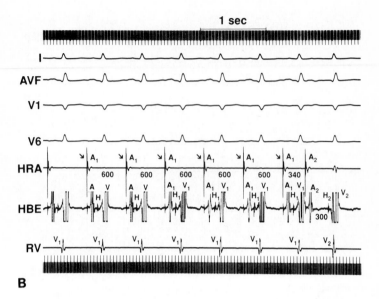

Fig. 4-12. *Continued from page 231.* **B,** At a coupling interval of 340 ms, the AH interval of the premature impulse suddenly increases to 300 ms representing a shift to the slow pathway. *HRA,* high right atrium; *HBE,* His bundle electrogram *RV,* right ventricle.

morphic ventricular tachycardia or ventricular fibrillation that may represent a nonclinical (or false positive) response may be initiated. Even in normal individuals, at very close coupling intervals of the extrastimuli (usually less than 180 ms), ventricular fibrillation or polymorphic ventricular tachycardia may be induced. In contrast, sustained mono-morphic ventricular tachycardia is considered a very specific response to programmed electrical stimulation and generally occurs only in patients with previous spontaneous ventricu-lar tachycardia or a pathologic substrate known to predispose to ventricular tachycardia.

Although ventricular stimulation protocols may vary slightly between different laboratories, the minimal complete protocol usually involves the introduction of up to three extrastimuli coupled to ventricular pacing at two cycle lengths from two RV sites (Table 4-6). LV stimulation may be

TABLE 4-6. Ventricular stimulation protocol

Standard protocol

Single extrastimuli coupled to ventricular pacing at cycle lengths of 600 and 400 ms from RV apex and RV outflow tract

Double extrastimuli coupled to ventricular pacing at cycle lengths of 600 and 400 ms from RV apex and RV outflow tract

Rapid ventricular pacing (400 ms to loss of 1 : 1 ventricular capture)

Triple extrastimuli coupled to ventricular pacing at cycle lengths of 600 and 400 ms from RV apex and RV outflow tract

Additional maneuvers may be performed

Extrastimuli may be coupled to sinus rhythm or other paced cycle lengths

A fourth extrastimuli may be coupled to ventricular pacing at cycle lengths of 600 and 400 ms from both RV sites

Stimulation may be performed at additional RV sites or from the left ventricle

Isoproterenol may be infused and the stimulation protocol repeated

Intravenous procainamide may be infused and the stimulation protocol repeated

RV, right ventricular.

performed in some individuals with documented sustained monomorphic ventricular tachycardia who are noninducible from the right ventricle. The yield is relatively low and may increase the morbidity of the procedure. In individuals with exercise-induced ventricular tachycardia or catecholamine-dependent ventricular tachycardia, isoproterenol may be infused.

The stimulation protocol is performed by systematically decreasing the coupling interval between the last beat of the pacing train and the extrastimuli until the tissue reaches refractoriness (the first extrastimuli fails to capture) or an arrhythmia is induced (Fig. 4-13). If the patient is hemodynamically stable, a 12-lead ECG of the induced ventricular tachycardia is recorded prior to attempts to terminate the tachycardia. The morphology of the ventricular tachycardia is noted and the cycle length is obtained. The most common method of terminating the ventricular tachycardia is ventricular burst pacing at a cycle length less than that of the tachycardia. The cycle length of the burst pacing is gradually decreased until the tachycardia either terminates (Fig. 4-

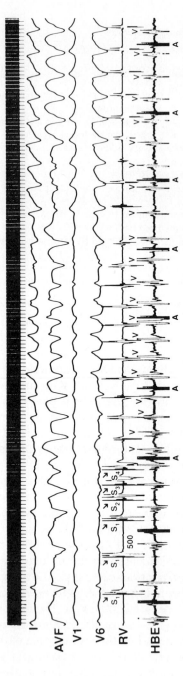

Fig. 4-13. Induction of sustained ventricular tachycardia with triple extrastimuli coupled to a train of ventricular pacing at 500 ms S_1 refers to the train; S_2, to the first extrastimulus; S_3 refers to the second extrastimulus; and S_4, to the third extrastimulus. During the induced ventricular tachycardia, the atrial activity is dissociated from the ventricular activity. This may be observed on the His channel (HBE) by the atrial electrogram (A) marching randomly through the tachycardia. RV, right ventricle; HBE, His bundle electrogram.

14) or accelerates, resulting in hemodynamic compromise at which point the patient is cardioverted or defibrillated. An initial 200-J shock is routinely utilized for sustained ventricular tachycardia and 360 J for subsequent shocks. The arrhythmia is often induced at least twice to assure reproducibility. This is particularly important if drug therapy is to be guided by serial electrophysiological testing.

The most specific end point of the ventricular stimulation protocol is the induction of a sustained monomorphic ventricular tachycardia which is identical to a patient's clinical ventricular tachycardia. Sustained ventricular tachycardia is commonly defined as ventricular tachycardia lasting at least 30 seconds or requiring termination due to hemodynamic collapse prior to 30 seconds. Noninducibility by ventricular stimulation refers to the failure to induced sustained ventricular tachycardia after utilizing at least three extrastimuli at two pacing rates from two RV pacing sites. A patient may be noninducible on the initial EPS or may be rendered noninducible by antiarrhythmic drug therapy. Partial drug efficacy refers to significant lengthening (>100 ms) of the cycle length of the induced tachycardia and/or rendering a previously intolerable tachycardia hemodynamically stable.

UTILITY OF EPS FOR SPECIFIC DIAGNOSIS
Sinus Node Disease

The clinical applications of electrophysiologic testing in sinus node disease are limited. Although abnormal sinus node recovery times and sinus atrial conduction times have been reported to have a specificity of 90% to 100% in patients documented to have spontaneous sinus node dysfunction, the sensitivity is significantly less. Unlike most induced tachyarrhythmias on electrophysiologic testing, it is difficult to correlate symptoms with an abnormal sinus node recovery time. In symptomatic patients with sinus bradycardia, an abnormal sinus node recovery time has been reported to predict which patients may benefit from cardiac pacing. An abnormal sinus node recovery time in an asymptomatic patient who is being studied for tachyarrhythmias, may influence one's decision to utilize certain medications or in device candidates, to select a cardioverter defibrillator with backup pacing for bradycardia.

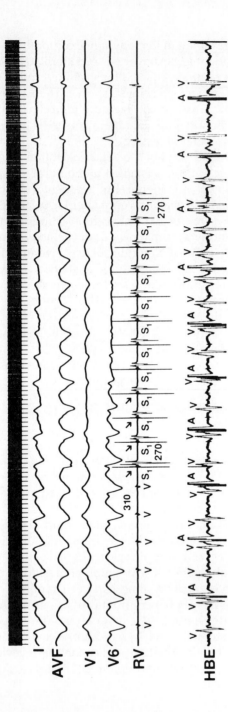

Fig. 4-14. Termination of monomorphic ventricular tachycardia with ventricular burst pacing at a rate faster than that of the tachycardia. On the right ventricular channel (*RV*) the cycle length of the monomorphic ventricular tachycardia is measured at 310 ms. Ventricular burst pacing (indicated by the arrow and label S_1) at a cycle length of 270 ms terminates the tachycardia. *HBE,* His bundle electrogram.

Disorders of Atrioventricular Conduction

Abnormalities of atrioventricular conduction are classified as first, second- or third-degree AV block (Table 4-7). Clues to the site of atrioventricular block can be derived by observing serial changes in PR interval in sequences of block that are less than $2:1$ (i.e., $3:2$ or $4:3$.), the rate and duration of the QRS of the escape rhythm, and the presence or absence of underlying intraventricular conduction delays on ECG. Compared to prolonged conduction in the AV node, conduction disease within or below the His bundle is associated with a high likelihood of developing complete AV block. Complete AV block that occurs within or below the His bundle is associated with a slower and less stable escape rhythm than complete AV block in which the site of block is within the AV node. EPSs can confirm the site of spontaneous AV block or conduction delay and assess the response of the conduction system to various pacing rates and the introduction of premature impulses. EPSs may identify indications for permanent pacemaker implantation in individuals with syncope of unknown etiology. Very long HV intervals (>100 ms) and block below His at atrial pacing rates of

TABLE 4-7. Types of atrioventricular block

Type	Characteristics	Site of block
First-degree AV block	All P waves conducted, prolonged conduction manifested by long PR interval	Delay may be above, within, or below His
Second-degree AV block	P waves are intermittently blocked	
Type I	Progressive prolongation of PR interval prior to blocked P wave	Usually within AV node
Type II	Sudden failure of conduction with no change in PR interval	Usually within or below His bundle
Third-degree AV block	None of P waves are conducted to ventricle, ventricular escape rhythm may occur	May be within AV node, within or below His

AV, atrioventricular.

less than 170 bpm are indicative of disease in the His-Purkinje system and associated with a relatively high incidence of subsequent complete heart block.

Malignant Ventricular Arrhythmias

The use of electrophysiologic testing to guide the treatment of ventricular arrhythmias is based on (1) the supposition that the induced arrhythmia represents the patient's clinical arrhythmia and (2) inability to induce tachycardia in a patient on drug therapy who was inducible on baseline EPS correlates with freedom from clinical reoccurrence. The ability of programmed electrical stimulation to induce the patient's clinical arrhythmia and, therefore, serve as a reliable end point for guiding drug therapy is greater in patients with coronary artery disease compared to other subgroups of patients such as those with idiopathic dilated cardiomyopathy or valvular heart disease. Several studies indicate that the predictive accuracy of drug therapy guided by serial electrophysiologic testing in patients with coronary artery disease and sustained monomorphic ventricular tachycardia is very good. If a patient who has inducible monomorphic ventricular tachycardia on baseline EPS becomes noninducible on an antiarrhythmic agent, there is approximately a 90% likelihood that that patient will remain free of arrhythmia recurrence over a subsequent 2-year period. Prior to the wide availability of implantable cardioverter-defibrillator (ICD) devices, studies indicated that patients who remain inducible despite multiple drug trials have a poor prognosis and a very high incidence of sudden death. Patients whose ventricular tachycardia remains refractory to antiarrhythmic drug therapy by serial electrophysiologic testing and those who are noninducible on initial study (have no end point by which to guide medical therapy) are candidates for an implantable internal cardioverter-defibrillator.

Differential Diagnosis of Wide Complex Tachycardia

Although criteria exists for differentiation of SVT with aberrancy from ventricular tachycardia on 12-lead ECGs, there are no criteria that are 100% sensitive or specific. Induction of a wide complex tachycardia while recording the His bundle electrogram is the gold standard for differentiation of SVT from ventricular tachycardia. In cases of SVT, the electrical impulse travels over the His bundle to reach the ventricle; therefore, a His deflection precedes the QRS with a normal or prolonged HV interval.

Patients with ICD

Discussion regarding the function of the ICD is beyond the scope of this chapter and interested readers are referred to comprehensive textbooks on this subject. Briefly, the ICD is a device capable of sensing ventricular tachycardia or fibrillation and rapidly delivering a shock. Recently, devices that also incorporate antitachycardic and antibradycardic pacing are available. The prototype device is connected to two lead systems, a rate-sensing lead system consisting of two epicardial bipolar leads or an endocardial lead and a defibrillation lead system that consists of two epicardial patches or an epicardial patch combined with an endocardial spring electrode. Recently, nonthoracotomy lead systems, which consist entirely of endocardial or subcutaneously leads, have been released and eliminate the need for a thoracotomy in many patients. The role of electrophysiologic testing in patients with devices includes selection of appropriate patients, intraoperative testing of the lead systems assuring appropriate rate sensing and defibrillation threshold, and, frequently, postoperative testing to ensure adequate function of the device for all induced arrhythmias. Postoperative testing of devices is particularly important for the newer third-generation defibrillators that incorporate the capability of antitachycardic pacing and have complicated detection and termination alogorithms. When a patient with an ICD undergoes a change in his or her antiarrhythmic drug regimen, it is recommended that the device be retested since changes in rate of the tachycardia may necessitate reprogramming of the device's rate detection criteria, and changes in defibrillation threshold may be caused by certain medications.

Syncope of Unknown Etiology

Syncope is a common clinical disorder, the workup of which can be expensive and nonproductive. The diagnostic utility of electrophysiologic testing in patients with recurrent syncope has been reported to be as low as 12% and as high as

79%. The reported abnormalities are displayed in Table 4-8. The yield is highly dependent on the prevalence of structural heart disease in the population being studied. In patients with structurally normal hearts and no suggestion of ischemia, electrophysiologic testing has a low yield and an increased likelihood of false-positive results. In patients with a history of coronary artery disease and segmental wall abnormality or conduction disease on ECG, the EPS has a relatively high yield and may rule out potentially life-threatening causes of syncope such as sustained ventricular arrhythmia. It is important to realize that in an unwitnessed syncope, the etiology of the patient's syncope is never certain. Thus, there is always the potential for inaccurately attributing the patient's syncope to an abnormality detected on electrophysiologic testing. It is desirable that patient's symptoms be reproduced by the induced arrhythmia.

Supraventricular Tachycardia

The treatment of supraventricular tachycardia has undergone dramatic change since radiofrequency catheter ablation offers a high probability of cure with a negligible complication rate for many reentrant tachycardias. Although the relationship between the QRS complex and P waves on the 12-lead ECG may suggest the mechanism of supraventricular tachycardia, performance of a detailed EPS is the only

TABLE 4-8.   Reported abnormalities in patients with syncope on EPSs

Sinus node dysfunction
Prolonged sinus node recovery period
Prolonged sinus atrial conduction time
Secondary pauses

Abnormalities of AV conduction
Prolonged AV nodal refractory period
Early AV nodal Wenckebach
Prolonged HV interval
Block induced within or below the His bundle

Induced tachyarrhythmias
Rapid supraventricular tachycardia
Sustained ventricular tachycardia

AV, atrioventricular.

method of accurately characterizing the mechanism of tachycardia and defining the anatomic substrate.

The most frequent mechanism of narrow complex supraventricular tachycardia is AV nodal reentrant tachycardia, which usually involves slow- and fast-conducting pathways within or near the AV node. Although it was once thought that AV nodal reentry occurred entirely within the compact AV node, experience from radiofrequency catheter ablation indicates that extranodal tissue may be involved in the reentrant circuit. Dual AV nodal pathways are characterized by discontinuous AV nodal conduction curves (see Fig. 4-10**B**). In typical AV nodal tachycardia, which constitutes over 90% of AV nodal reentrant tachycardia, antegrade conduction occurs over the slow pathway and retrograde conduction occurs up the fast pathway (slow-fast tachycardia) (Fig. 4-15). Therefore, the retrograde ventriculoatrial (VA) conduc-

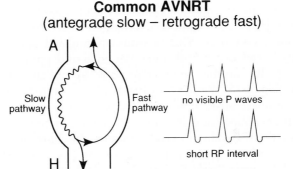

Common AVNRT
(antegrade slow – retrograde fast)

Fig. 4-15. Schematic representation of the common form of atrioventricular nodal reentrant tachycardia. In the typical form of atrioventricular nodal tachycardia, antegrade block occurs in the fast pathway, thus forcing antegrade conduction down the slow pathway. If antegrade conduction down the slow pathway is slow enough to allow retrograde conduction to occur up the previously refractory fast pathway, reentrant tachycardia ensues. Although it was once felt that the limbs of the tachycardic circuit were contained within the compact atrioventricular node, recent studies utilizing radiofrequency ablation for atrioventricular nodal tachycardia suggest that perinodal tissue is contained in the reentrant circuit.

tion time is usually very short, and the atrial depolarization often occurs simultaneously with or immediately following the ventricular depolarization. On surface electrocardiogram the P waves are either not visible or occur in the ST segment with a very short RP interval.

Another common mechanism of supraventricular tachycardia is atrioventricular reciprocating tachycardia, using an extranodal atrioventricular bypass tract (also referred to as an accessory pathway). The most common type of accessory pathway is the bundle of Kent, which occurs in Wolff-Parkinson-White syndrome. The accessory pathway may be between the right atrium and ventricle or left atrium and ventricle. In an individual patient, an accessory pathway may be capable of antegrade, retrograde conduction, or both. Individuals with antegrade conduction over an accessory pathway exhibit a short PR interval and a wide QRS complex due to ventricular preexitation (this is also referred to as a delta wave). The axis of the delta wave and morphology of the QRS is dependent upon the position of the accessory pathway and the amount of tissue depolarized through accessory pathway conduction compared to conduction over the normal AV node. During sinus rhythm, activation of the ventricle can occur both over the accessory pathway and through the normal conduction pathway utilizing the AV node (Fig. 4-16). Pathways capable of only retrograde conduction are referred to as concealed pathways and no ventricular preexitation (or delta wave) will be present on the ECG.

The Wolff-Parkinson-White syndrome is characterized by the presence of ventricular preexcitation (short PR interval and delta wave in ECG) and the clinical occurrence of arrhythmias. In patients with Wolff-Parkinson-White syndrome, the most common type of supraventricular tachycardia is orthodromic tachycardia in which antegrade block occurs in the accessory pathway and a reentrant circuit is established with antegrade conduction occurring over the AV node and retrograde conduction up the accessory pathway (Fig. 4-16B). In orthodromic tachycardia, the QRS is narrow unless aberrancy occurs, and there is a short RP interval on the surface ECG. A less common type of tachycardia in patients with Wolff-Parkinson-White syndrome is antidromic tachycardia, which is a reentrant tachycardia with antegrade conduction occurring over the accessory pathway and retrograde conduction through the AV node (Fig. 4-16C). Antidromic tachycardia is a regular wide complex tachycardia that may resemble ventricular tachycardia on surface ECG. Compared to the general population, patients with Wolff-Parkinson-White syndrome have an increased incidence of atrial fibrillation and conduction to the ventricle may occur over both the accessory pathway and the AV node (Fig. 4-16D). The QRS morphology will depend on the relative amount of conduction occurring through the accessory pathway compared to the normal conduction system. In patients with pathways capable of antegrade conduction and atrial fibrillation, very rapid ventricular responses may occur with a potential for degeneration to ventricular fibrillation.

CATHETER ABLATION

Catheter ablation is a new interventional discipline within electrophysiology whereby an arrhythmogenic focus or critical portion of an arrhythmia circuit is identified, localized, and subsequently destroyed utilizing a percutaneous transcatheter technique. Arrhythmias that are currently amenable to ablative therapy include atrial fibrillation, atrial flutter, ectopic atrial tachycardias, supraventricular tachycardias secondary to AV nodal reentry or accessory bypass tracts, and ventricular tachycardia. A number of modalities have been utilized for ablative therapy; however, currently, the most commonly used energy sources for ablation are radiofrequency energy and direct current (DC) energy. Historically, DC energy was the initial energy source utilized for ablative procedures dating back to the early 1980s and continues to be used on a smaller scale in electrophysiology laboratories. During DC ablation, a defibrillator is interfaced with a standard transvenous catheter and energy pulses ranging between 50 and 500 J are applied to the distal pole of a standard recording catheter. The system is grounded utilizing a large surface skin electrode applied to the patient's back. Barotrauma and thermal injury result in extensive tissue damage and scar formation as far as 3 cm away from the catheter tip. This large area of tissue destruction is difficult to control, but this can be advantageous when the arrhythmogenic site is diffuse or difficult to localize. Complications to DC energy include tamponade, pericarditis, coronary sinus rupture and

Possible Rhythms in WPW Syndrome

Sinus Rhythm

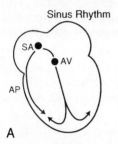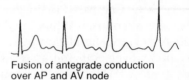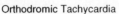

Fusion of antegrade conduction
over AP and AV node

A

Orthodromic Tachycardia

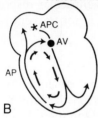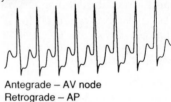

Antegrade – AV node
Retrograde – AP
Narrow QRS complex

B

Antidromic Tachycardia

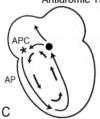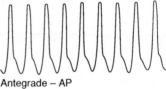

Antegrade – AP
Retrograde – AV node
Wide QRS complex

C

Atrial Fibrillation

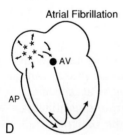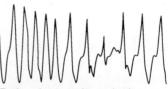

Fusion of antegrade conduction
over AP and AV node
Varying QRS morphology

D

thrombosis, circumflex artery lesions, ventricular dysfunction, cardiac perforation, and sudden cardiac death.

More recently, the use of radiofrequency energy has become the energy source of choice for ablative therapy. Radiofrequency energy utilizes a frequency range from 200 to 1200 kHz. Application of radiofrequency current results in tissue desiccation in a well-localized region at the point of catheter contact, resulting in a small discreet lesion approximately $0.5 \times 0.5 \, cm^2$. The localized nature of radiofrequency energy-induced lesions has made it the energy source of choice for most ablative procedures.

Indications for Ablative Therapy

Atrial fibrillation.   Catheter destruction of the AV junction has been utilized to treat patients who present with atrial fibrillation and rapid ventricular responses refractory

---

Fig. 4-16.   Possible rhythms in WPW syndrome. Schematic representation of possible rhythms in a patient with an accessory atrioventricular bypass tract. **A,** During sinus rhythm the ventricle may be activated by conduction over both the accessory pathway *(AP)* in a normal atrioventricular *(AV)* conduction system. The QRS complex may be narrow if the ventricle is activated primarily by conduction through the atrioventricular node. The QRS complex will be wide and preexcited if activation of the ventricle occurs primarily via the accessory pathway. **B,** During orthodromic reentrant tachycardia, antegrade conduction occurs through the atrioventricular node and normal conduction system while retrograde conduction occurs via the accessory pathway. The resulting tachycardia has a narrow QRS morphology. **C,** Antidromic tachycardia utilizes the accessory pathway as the antegrade limb of the reentrant circuit and the atrioventricular node and normal conduction system as the retrograde limb. The resulting tachycardia has a wide QRS complex. **D,** When atrial fibrillation occurs in a patient with manifest accessory pathway, antegrade conduction to the ventricle may occur through the atrioventricular node or over the accessory pathway. Morphology of the QRS complex may be narrow, which occurs primarily through the atrioventricular node or wide and preexcited if conduction occurs over the accessory pathway. The morphology of the QRS complex may vary beat by beat during atrial fibrillation.

to medical therapy. In this procedure, complete heart block is created and a permanent ventricular pacemaker is required to normalize the heart rate. For patients presenting with symptomatic atrial fibrillation and a controlled ventricular response, this procedure offers little symptomatic improvement.

Atrial flutter.   Mapping and ablative techniques have recently been used to identify and interrupt critical portions of the flutter circuit in patients presenting with symptomatic medically refractory atrial flutter. This is a new application of radiofrequency ablation and initial reports demonstrate an efficacy rate of greater than 50% in patients with lone atrial flutter. Increased clinical experience with atrial flutter ablative therapy should improve the success rate of this procedure.

Ectopic atrial tachycardias.   Ectopic atrial tachycardia, also known as automatic atrial tachycardia, is currently being mapped and ablated. Initial reports of safety and efficacy are encouraging. This procedure shows clinical promise as a front-line therapy for medically resistant ectopic atrial tachycardias as a more economical and less invasive alternative to the traditional therapy of surgical isolation procedures.

Atrioventricular reciprocating tachycardias.   The utility of catheter ablation is best described in this category of reentrant tachycardias, which include the more common mechanisms of supraventricular tachycardias: AV nodal reentrant tachycardia and those tachycardias associated with accessory bypass tracts. The indication for catheter ablation in this group of arrhythmias includes recurrent symptomatic tachycardias that are medically refractory or in situations where medical management is not well tolerated by the patient. In the recent past, ablation therapy has become a front-line therapeutic option for patients presenting with paroxysmal supraventricular tachycardia, foregoing therapy with antiarrhythmic agents. Another important indication for radiofrequency ablation is atrial fibrillation in the setting of an accessory pathway capable of conducting in an antegrade manner. These pathways have the potential of conducting extremely rapidly, resulting in dangerously rapid ventricular responses with rates exceeding 250 bpm. In this clinical setting, degeneration to ventricular fibrillation is possible. Patients presenting with a history of syncope and accessory pathway capable of antegrade conduction comprise another indication for curative ablation therapy.

Ventricular tachycardia. Ventricular tachycardia presents a challenge to the interventional electrophysiologist in terms of applications of catheter ablation techniques. The extremely variable site of tachycardia origin and the diffuse nature of the arrhythmia circuit make localizing successful sites for energy application difficult. Initial applications of ablation therapy in ventricular tachycardia were undertaken in patients presenting with recurrent ventricular tachycardia and structurally normal hearts. Catheter mapping and ablation has successfully abolished recurrent ventricular tachycardia with a remarkably low recurrence rate. However, idiopathic ventricular tachycardia represents only a small portion of patients presenting with sustained recurrent ventricular tachycardia.

Patients presenting with coronary artery disease represent the vast majority of patients with recurrent ventricular tachycardia. Patients presenting with sustained hemodynamically stable ventricular tachycardia and relatively well-maintained LV function appear to be the best candidates for mapping and ablation procedures. Nonsustained ventricular tachycardia or hemodynamically unstable ventricular tachycardia are contraindications in that the mapping procedure can only be performed while the patient is in sustained ventricular tachycardia. Another relative contraindication to ablative therapy is the induction of multiple ventricular tachycardia morphologies during initial electrophysiologic testing.

Technical Aspects of Specific Ablation Procedures

General aspects. Prior to ablation procedures, the patient is prepared in a similar manner as a general EPS. All antiarrhythmic drugs are discontinued. Catheters are placed in the same manner as described earlier in this chapter. Systemic heparinization during the ablation procedure is required. Many laboratories administer prophylactic broad-spectrum IV antibiotics prior to and during the procedure.

In addition to the standard catheters, special steerable tip catheters have been designed to facilitate mapping and ablating procedures (Fig. 4-17). They are constructed with a large platinum tip measuring 4 mm that has been proven to

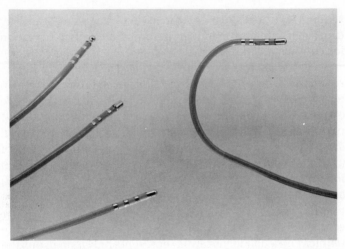

Fig. 4-17.   Specialized large-tip catheter electrodes designed for ablative procedures.

produce the largest ablation lesion in myocardium. An energy source is also necessary. In DC ablations, a standard defibrillator can be connected to the ablating catheter. In radiofrequency energy ablations, a generator that is capable of delivering a continuous unmodulated sine wave at approximately 500 kHz is standard. These generators also continuously monitor energy output and catheter impedance. The circuit is completed by a large indifferent skin electrode usually positioned in the infrascapular region on the patient's back. A sophisticated electrogram monitoring and storage system is necessary for mapping and ablation procedures. There are multiple computer-based multichannel recording systems available that allow for real-time data analysis and facilitate the mapping-ablation procedure. Radiologic equipment capable of multiplane views is necessary for optimal catheter placement.

Once the patient has been properly prepared and catheters are placed, a baseline EPS is undertaken to document the properties of the tachycardia and the inducibility of the tachycardia. After the characteristics of the tachycardia have been fully evaluated, the mapping and ablation procedures are undertaken. Techniques used in this part of the procedure are unique to the tachycardia to be studied. Specific mapping techniques are discussed as follows. When the optimal site for ablation has been localized, radiofrequency current is applied to the distal pole of the mapping catheter. Typically 15 to 35 W of current is applied over a duration of 30 to 60 seconds while the rhythm and intracardiac electrograms are monitored closely (Fig. 4-18).

Postablation there is typically a 15- to 60-minute waiting period during which repeat electrophysiologic testing is undertaken. This is used to document successful ablation or signs of early recurrence. If after approximately 60 minutes postablation, there is no evidence of recurrent tachycardia, the procedure can be terminated and the patient returned to his or her hospital room. Postprocedure, the patient should be hospitalized and observed with cardiac monitoring for approximately 24 hours. During this time, early recur-

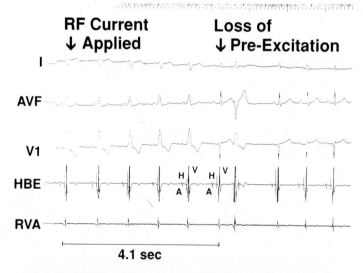

Fig. 4-18. Loss of preexcitation (delta wave) during application of radiofrequency current. Surface leads 1, aVF, and V_1 are displayed. *HBE,* His bundle electrogram; *RVA,* right ventricular apex electrogram. Note the loss of the delta wave and lengthening of the PR interval after 4.1 seconds of radiofrequency *(RF)* energy application signifying successful ablation of the accessory pathway.

rence can be detected or iatrogenic conduction abnormalities observed. Additionally, the patient can be watched for late complications from the procedure including development of postoperative fever or vascular injury associated with the ablation procedure. The patient can typically be discharged the morning after the procedure with few physical limitations.

Atrial fibrillation.   A temporary pacing wire is placed in the RV apex for pacing support during the procedure. A 4-mm deflectable tip electrode is placed across the tricuspid annulus and positioned where a prominent His potential is recorded. The catheter is then slowly withdrawn into the atrium (Fig. 4-19). When the ablation catheter is positioned so that equal atrial and ventricular electrograms are recorded with a small His potential present, radiofrequency energy can be applied. Success is indicated by an accelerated junc-

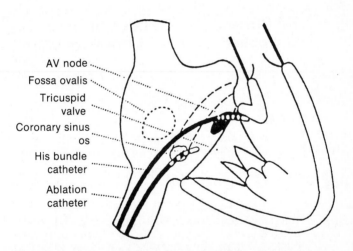

Fig. 4-19. Catheter position during atrioventricular *(AV)* junction ablation represented in the right anterior oblique view. The position of the His bundle recording catheter is used as a reference. The ablation catheter is positioned on the atrial side of the tricuspid valve just below the diagnostic catheter. (From Haines DE, Di Marco JP: Current therapy for supraventricular tachycardia. *Curr Probl Cardiol* 27:409–477, 1992.)

tional rhythm that is observed soon after the onset of radio-frequency energy delivery and followed by high-degree AV block. Immediately following AV nodal ablation, a permanent ventricular pacemaker must be implanted to ensure an adequate ventricular rate. The efficacy of radiofrequency induced AV block is approximately 90% with a 5% to 10% recurrence rate of AV conduction. DC ablation of the AV node has been associated with a 65% success rate and an approximate 10% recurrence rate of AV conduction. The complications associated with DC ablation including hypotension, pericarditis, ventricular perforation with tamponade, stroke, ventricular arrhythmia, and late sudden death make this energy source less appealing than radiofrequency energy, which carries a much lower complication rate and to date has had no documented association with late sudden cardiac death.

Atrial flutter.   Early reports have localized a critical segment of the reentrant circuit of atrial flutter to the low posterior septum of the right atrium. Radiofrequency application to the atrial septum near the os of the coronary sinus and the isthmus of atrial tissue between the inferior vena cava and the tricuspid annulus has been successful in terminating atrial flutter and preventing its clinical recurrence in a small number of patients.

Ectopic atrial tachycardia.   Extensive mapping of the atria is crucial in this procedure. A coronary sinus catheter is necessary for initial mapping of the left atrium. At least two multipolar catheters (octapolar or decapolar) are positioned in opposing regions of the right atrium. Activation mapping is performed to localize the region of earliest atrial activation. More precise mapping is undertaken with a deflectable tip mapping catheter until the earliest site of atrial activation is located. If during initial testing the tachycardia is localized to the left atrium, mapping is then undertaken with a transseptal approach via a patent foramen ovale or transseptal puncture using the Brochenbrough technique. In this situation, fewer catheters are able to be utilized for detailed mapping. When mapping the left side, meticulous anticoagulation must be maintained to reduce the risk of procedure-related embolic events.

Radiofrequency energy application to atrial endocardium

can be painful for the patient. Comfort can be maximized by using the lowest energy output capable of terminating the tachycardia.

AV nodal reentrant tachycardia. In AV nodal reentry, the circuit consists of a slowly conducting pathway and a rapidly conducting pathway. Anatomically, these pathways are located in the perinodal interatrial septum and compact AV node, respectively. The current approach to ablation for AV nodal reentry, termed *AV nodal modification,* is selective ablation of the slow pathway.

Mapping of the slow pathway is performed around the inferior and posterior perinodal area in the posterior septal region of the right atrium extending inferiorly to the os of the coronary sinus. Radiofrequency energy is delivered along the tricuspid annulus where low-amplitude fragmented atrial electrograms are recorded (Fig. 4-20). Radiofrequency energy can be delivered during AV nodal reentrant

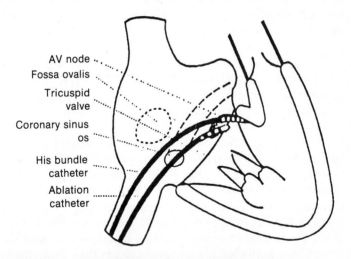

Fig. 4-20. Typical catheter position for ablation of the slow pathway for atrioventricular *(AV)* nodal reentry tachycardia. The ablation catheter is positioned on the atrial side of the tricuspid valve in the vicinity of the coronary sinus os. The ablation catheter is inferior and posterior to the His bundle catheter. (From Haines DE, Di Marco JP: Current therapy for supraventricular tachycardia. *Curr Probl Cardiol* 27:409–477, 1992.)

tachycardia or in sinus rhythm. Successful ablation is heralded by termination of the tachycardia when energy is delivered during SVT or development of accelerated junctional rhythm when ablating in sinus rhythm.

Complete elimination of this slow pathway results in the inability to induce AV nodal reentrant tachycardia or demonstrate conduction along the slow AV pathway. Postablation routine stimulation is repeated to evaluate for the presence of slow pathway conduction or inducible AV nodal reentry. If the slow pathway is not functional in the drug-free state, isoproterenol is often infused to validate noninducibility. Success rates for AV nodal modification approach greater than 95% with a risk of major complication estimated to be 1% to 5%. Potential complications include iatrogenic high-degree AV block, pericarditis, cardiac perforation with tamponade, and vascular complications related to access. The estimated recurrence rate is 5%.

Accessory pathways.   The technique used for ablating accessory pathways is different depending on the location and the conduction properties of the accessory pathways. Prior to the ablation, the patient undergoes a comprehensive EPS to determine the presence and electrical properties of the accessory pathway(s). The pathways that conduct antegrade in sinus rhythm and exhibit a delta wave (manifest preexitation) can be mapped during sinus rhythm. The general location of the accessory pathway can be identified by the axis of the delta wave on the 12-lead ECG (Fig. 4-21). However, EPS and mapping are required to precisely localize the site of the accessory pathway. With a manifest accessory pathway, the mapping catheter is slowly maneuvered along the valve annulus to locate the optimal electrode placement that will result in the earliest ventricular activation during sinus rhythm or atrial pacing (Fig. 4-22). Discreet electrical potentials from the accessory pathway have frequently been recorded at the successful ablation site and referred to as *pathway potentials*. In pathways capable of only retrograde conduction, mapping is performed by determining the site of earliest retrograde atrial activity during ventricular pacing or induced orthodromic supraventricular tachycardia.

Left-side accessory pathways can be ablated by a transseptal approach utilizing a patent foramen ovale, the Bro-

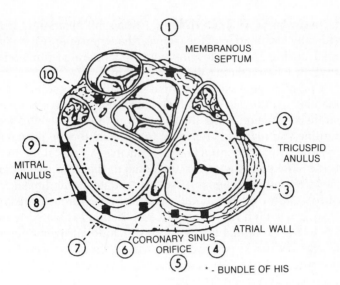

Fig. 4-21. Schematic representation of potential positions of accessory pathways. *1,* right anterior paraseptal; *2,* right anterior; *3,* right lateral; *4,* right posterior; *5,* right paraseptal; *6,* left posterior paraseptal; *7,* left posterior; *8,* left lateral; *9,* left anterior; *10,* left anterior paraseptal. (From Gallagher JJ, Pritchett EL, Sealy WC, Kasell J Wallace AG: The preexcitation syndrome. *Prog Cardiovascular Dis* 20:285–327, 1978.)

chenbrough technique (Fig. 4-23), or the more conventional retrograde approach in which the ablating catheter is prolapsed across the aortic valve (Fig. 4-24).

The overall success of radiofrequency ablation for accessory pathways is dependent upon operator experience and the location of the accessory pathway. Success rates of greater than 95% are reported for left-sided pathways. Right-sided pathways are usually reported to be less successful with efficacy rates of greater than 80%. The complication rate for accessory pathway ablation is estimated to be 1% to 2%, and most complications result from catheter manipulation and not from the delivery of the radiofrequency energy. Complications include iatrogenic high-degree AV block (most commonly seen with anteroseptal accessory pathway ablations), pericarditis, cardiac perforation with tamponade, and vascular complications related to access. The estimated

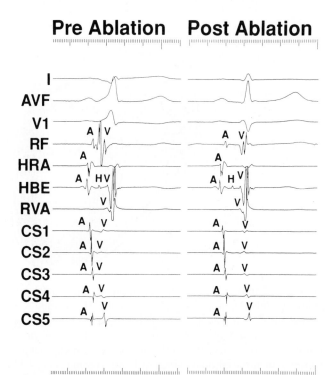

Fig. 4-22. Sequence of antegrade ventricular activation pre-radiofrequency and post-radiofrequency ablation of a left-sided accessory pathway. Surface leads 1, aVF, and V₁ are displayed. *HRA,* High right atrial electrogram; *HBE,* His bundle electrogram; *RVA,* right ventricular apex electrogram; *CS₁* to *CS₅,* recordings from the coronary sinus with CS₁ representing the most proximal coronary sinus recording and CS₅, the most distal. Note that the earliest ventricular activation during sinus rhythm occurs in the mid-coronary sinus (CS₂ to CS₃) region. Electrograms recorded from the ablating catheter at the successful ablation site *(RF)* demonstrate very early ventricular activation and a short AV interval. Post-ablation, a normal sequence of antegrade activation is demonstrated. Note lengthening of the A to V interval in the coronary sinus electrograms as well as the electrogram recorded from the ablation catheter.

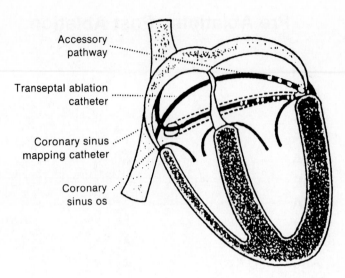

Fig. 4-23. Catheter postion for ablation of a left free wall pathway utilizing a transeptal approach. The catheter is passed through a sheath that has been placed through the atrial septum and then positioned above the mitral valve annulus in close proximity to the accessory pathway, which is located near the coronary sinus catheter. (From Haines DE, Di Marco JP: Current therapy for supraventricular tachycardia. *Curr Probl Cardiol* 27:409–477, 1992.)

recurrence rate postablation for an accessory pathway is between 5% and 10%; the higher recurrence rates are seen with right-sided accessory pathways. Patients who remain asymptomatic for three months postprocedure have an extremely low incidence of recurrence thereafter.

Ventricular tachycardia. Several mapping techniques are used to target radiofrequency application during treatment for ventricular tachycardia. These techniques are usually used in combination to locate the optimal site of energy delivery. As noted under Indications for Ablative Therapy, the tachycardia needs to be sustained and hemodynamically tolerated in order to allow adequate mapping. These techniques can be used for idiopathic ventricular tachycardias or those ventricular tachycardia associated with coronary artery disease. Initially, a gross estimation of tachycardia origin can

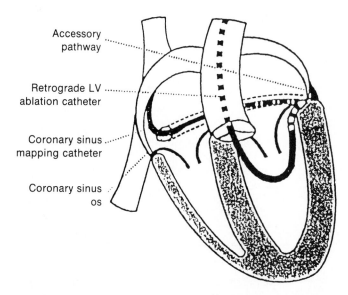

Fig. 4-24. Catheter position for ablation of left free wall accessory pathway via the retrograde approach. The ablation catheter is prolapsed across the aortic valve and positioned under the mitral valve leaflet in close proximity to the accessory pathway located near the coronary sinus catheter. *LV*, Left ventricular. (From Haines DE, Di Marco JP: Current therapy for supraventricular tachycardia. *Curr Probl Cardiol* 27:409–477, 1992.)

be made from the 12-lead ECG of ventricular tachycardia. This will help to direct mapping efforts to the right or left ventricle and specific regions within the appropriate ventricle.

During activation time mapping, the mapping catheter is maneuvered to an endocardial location that demonstrates the earliest activation time in tachycardia (Fig. 4-25). The presence of middiastolic potentials identifies optimal ablation sites. Pace mapping, in which pacing from the ablation catheter duplicates the QRS morphology of the clinical ventricular tachycardia, is also used to identify the appropriate site for ablation energy application. Following the ablation procedure, ventricular stimulation is once again undertaken to ensure that the tachycardia is no longer inducible. Abla-

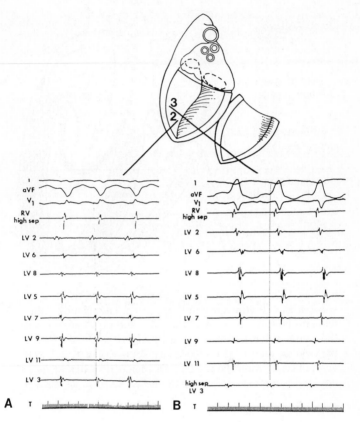

Fig. 4-25.   Endocardial catheter mapping of two different ventricular tachycardia morphologies. **A,** A ventricular tachycardia with a right bundle branch morphology and right superior access is shown. A reference right ventricular catheter *(RV)* is shown along with multiple ventricular recordings. The earliest ventricular activation is recorded at LV_2, which corresponds with the right ventricular apex. **B,** A ventricular tachycardia with a left bundle branch block pattern in right inferior access is shown. The earliest ventricular activation occurs near LV_3, which corresponds to the high septal area. *T,* time line. (From Josephson ME: Clinical cardiac electrophysiology: techniques and interpretations. Philadelphia, 1993, Lea and Febiger.)

tion therapy for ventricular tachycardia is a relatively new technique. The reported numbers of cases are few; therefore, an accurate success rate is difficult to report. Initially, idiopathic ventricular tachycardia appears to have a higher success rate than ventricular-associated coronary artery disease. Ventricular tachycardia associated with ischemic heart disease is an extremely variable entity and therefore needs to be assessed on an individual basis.

ELECTROCARDIOGRAPHY IN THE CARDIAC CATHETERIZATION LABORATORY

Basic electrocardiography may be unfamiliar to the new catheterization laboratory technician/nurse. This section is designed to review the fundamentals of electrocardiography as used in the cardiac catheterization laboratory for monitoring of patients.

The Cardiac Electrical System

Myocardial contraction is triggered by electrical activity. Therefore, for every beat on the ECG, there is usually a corresponding pressure pulse resulting from myocardial contraction. The heart's electrical system has specialized tissue for the origination and transmission of electrical impulses. The normal sequence of electrical activation is displayed in Fig. AIX-1 and consists of the following: SA node → atrial tissue → AV node → bundle of His → bundle branches → Purkinje fibers → ventricular myocardium.

The ECG

The ECG is a graphic recording of electrical impulses that are generated by depolarization (contraction) and repolarization (relaxation) of the myocardium. The standard ECG includes six limb leads and six chest leads. The proper placement of electrodes for recording the 12-lead ECG is displayed in Figs. AIX-2 and AIX-3.

The ECG displays 12 leads that reflect different electrical views of the heart depolarization and repolarization. Typically certain leads are associated with electrical activity from specific parts of the myocardium. The leads II, III, and aVF reflect electrical activity in the inferior wall of the heart; leads

I and aVL and chest leads V_5 and V_6, the lateral wall of the heart; chest leads V_1 and V_2, the septal region of the heart; and V_3 and V_4, the anterior wall of the heart. Electrical activity from the posterior wall of the heart is not directly recorded and therefore ischemia, injury, and necrosis are reflected by depolarization and repolarization abnormalities on the anterior surface of the heart (leads V_1 through V_3). Thus, in inferior-posterior myocardial infarction, ST segment, T wave changes, and Q waves are opposite in direction from an anterior myocardial infarction. For example, during ischemia instead of seeing ST depression, ST elevation occurs in V_1 to V_3. During acute injury, ST depression occurs and during infarction, a pathologic R wave rather than Q wave occurs in these leads.

COMPONENTS OF THE ECG (see Figs. AIX-4 and AIX-5)

P Wave

The sinus node is normally the pacemaker of the heart because the cells of the sinus node possess the greatest spontaneous automoticity (ability to initiate an impulse). As the electrical waves travel through the atrium, a P wave is produced with surface ECG, which represents an electrical contraction (depolarization) of the atria. Mechanical contraction of the atria follow, which contributes to ventricular filling. From the atria, the impulse travels through the AV node, through the His-Purkinje system, and results in electrical activation of the ventricle. The PR interval is the interval from the beginning of the P wave to the onset of the QRS and reflects conduction time from the sinus node through the atria, the AV node, and His-Purkinje system.

QRS Complex

Following the P wave, the next electrogram on the ECG is usually the QRS complex, which represents ventricular depolarization. The electrical activation of the ventricle results in myocardial contraction (systole).

ST Segment and T Wave

The QRS is followed by the ST segment and T wave, which represent repolarization of the ventricles and correspond to myocardial relaxation (diastole). The period from the end of the QRS complex to the beginning of the T wave is called the ST segment. Depression or elevation of this segment from baseline may be produced by ischemia (depression) or acute injury (elevation).

Abnormal Rhythms

During sinus rhythm, there is usually a regular rhythm with a normal sequence of activation. Premature beats are those that occur before the next expected beat. Premature ventricular contractions (PVCs) arise from abnormal electrical activity in the ventricles. The configuration of a PVC is usually a wide, bizarre QRS complex (see Fig. AIX-6A). PVCs that occur from a single focus are referred to as *univocal PVCs.* PVCs that arise from different areas of the ventricles have different morphologies and are referred to as *multivocal PVCs.* Ventricular tachycardia is defined as the occurrence of three or more PVCs in a row (see Fig. AIX-6B). A PVC may result in a reduced pressure pulse due to the abnormal activation sequence of the ventricle and the lack of coordination between atrial and ventricular contraction. During sustained ventricular tachycardia, the blood pressure may drop dramatically. Ventricular fibrillation is the most disorganized and hemodynamically compromising arrhythmia that can occur (see Fig. AIX4-6C). During ventricular fibrillation there is chaotic and uncoordinated electrical activities so that there is no effective ventricular contraction. As a result, there is no pulse or cardiac output and clinical death results.

Typical Electrocardiographic Changes Seen in the Cardiac Catheterization Laboratory

Changes in the ST segment and T wave of the ECG may indicate a lack of blood flow to the myocardium through the coronary arteries. This lack of blood flow, referred to as **ischemia,** results in oxygen deprivation to the myocardium. If ischemia persists, tissue damage or death (necrosis) may occur. Dead tissue is referred to as *infarcted.* The electrocardiographic changes of ischemia and infarction are illustrated in Figs. AIX-7 and AIX-8.

Ischemia can result in a number of different electrocardiographic changes. Ischemia effecting the entire depth of the myocardium (transmural) is detected as deep symmectric T wave inversion. However, T wave inversion can be seen in a number of conditions unrelated to ischemia (intracranial trauma, pulmonary embolism, myocardial contusion). Acute T wave changes occurring during anginal symptoms are specific for ischemia. Horizontal ST depression or downsloping ST segments are the hallmarks of subendocardial ischemia or infarction in many cases. Reversible depression, however, does favor ischemia. Nonspecific ST and T wave changes as well as normalization of T wave abnormalities over baseline pain-free electrocardiographic findings are also electrocardiographic findings consistent with ischemia.

The electrocardiographic findings of acute infarction occur in a stepwise temporal fashion. The earliest phase of infarction is associated with tall upright T waves that are referred to as *hyperacute T waves*. These T wave changes are usually followed shortly thereafter by the development of ST segment elevation in the region where myocardial damage is occurring. Conversely, reciprocal ST segment depression can be noted in the electrocardiographic leads recording from the opposing surface of the heart. That is to say, in an acute inferior MI, ST segment elevation will be present in the inferior leads (II, III, and aVF) while ST segment depression will be simultaneously recorded in the anterior leads (I, aVL, V, and V_2). Within hours of the onset of MI, Q waves appear as a result of damage that occurs throughout all layers of the myocardium, thus resulting in a transmural or Q wave MI. Myocardial necrosis results in an electrically silent segment that fails to contribute to the normal electrical forces of the heart during cardiac depolarization. An electrocardiographic lead recording over a segment of infarcted myocardium will detect electrical forces moving away from the dead region, resulting in a negative Q wave. Infarctions that are confined to the subendocardial region do not result in Q wave formation and are termed *non-Q wave MIs*.

Prior to performing a cardiac catheterization, a baseline 12-lead ECG is obtained. The ECG can then be used for comparison if the patient develops symptoms during the procedure. During the catheterization, one to three electrocardiographic leads are monitored continuously to evaluate for rhythm disturbances or ST segment and T wave changes that may indicate alterations in myocardial blood supply.

During coronary angioplasty, balloon inflation temporarily interrupts the blood supply to the downstream myocardium. This may result in reversible ischemia and transient ST and T wave changes. Persistent ST segment elevation or depression may indicate ongoing ischemia or acute myocardial injury. Other situations encountered in the cardiac catheterization laboratory that may result in ST segment or T wave changes include (1) injection of contrast media into a coronary artery, (2) occlusion of an artery with a diagnostic catheter (engaging the ostium of the left main or the right coronary artery), (3) improper or incomplete deflation of an angioplasty balloon catheter, (4) dissection of a coronary artery, (5) coronary artery spasm, and (6) blockage of a side branch by the balloon catheter or thrombus.

Rhythm disturbances are commonly encountered during cardiac catheterization. During right heart catheterization, atrial arrhythmias and PVCs can occur secondary to catheter irritation. Catheter trauma to the right bundle branch can occur while attempting to float a catheter into the RV outflow tract. While this often results in transient right bundle branch block, complete heart block can be induced if preexisting left bundle branch block is present. In this situation, one must be prepared to emergently pace the right ventricle until such time that the right bundle recovers its function. PVCs and ventricular tachycardia can be induced by LV irritation with the ventriculography catheter or during contrast injection. Bradycardia, sinus arrest, ventricular tachycardia and ventricular fibrillation can result from contrast injection of the coronary arteries (especially the right coronary artery). Catheter-induced coronary spasm can result in ventricular fibrillation secondary to impaired coronary blood flow. The treatment of catheter-induced arrhythmias is straightforward; removing the catheter from the LV cavity or the coronary artery ostium is often enough to terminate the arrhythmia. Ventricular tachycardia or fibrillation that persists, however, requires immediate resuscitation. If arrhythmias persist, one must investigate other underlying etiologies including ischemia or electrolyte abnormalities. Prophylactic use of antiarrhythmic drugs to suppress arrhythmias during cardiac catheterization is not recommended. Coronary spasm during cardiac catheterization may be reversed by intracoronary infusion of nitroglycerin. Bradycardia and sinus node dysfunction can be typically reversed with vigorous coughing or the administration of atropine (see Chapter 5). Knowledge and experience with the defibrillator in the cardiac catheterization laboratory is critically important (see Chapter 11).

SUGGESTED READINGS

Cohen TJ, Scheinman MM, Pullen BT, Chiesa NA, Gonzalez R, Herre JM, Griffin JC: Emergency intracardiac defibrillation for refractory ventricular fibrillation during routine electrophysiologic study, *J Am Coll Cardiol* 18:1280–1284, 1991.

Feld GK, Fleck RP, Chen PS, Boyce K, Bahnson TD, Stein JB, Calisi CM, Ibarra M: Radiofrequency catheter ablation for the treatment of human type 1 atrial flutter: identification of a critical zone in the reentrant circuit by endocardial mapping techniques, *Circulation* 86:1233–1240, 1992.

Fogoros RN: *Electrophysiologic testing,* Oxford, 1991, Blackwell.

Forcinito M: Guidelines for clinical intracardiac electrophysiologic studies: a report of the American College of Cardiology/American Heart Association Task Force on Assessment of Diagnostic and Therapeutic Cardiovascular Procedures (Subcommittee to Assess Clinical Intracardiac Electrophysiologic Studies), *J Am Coll Cardiol* 14:1827–1842, 1989.

Haines DE, DiMarco JP: Current therapy for supraventricular tachycardia, *Curr Probl Cardiol* 27:409–477, 1992.

Horowitz LN, Kay HR, Kutalek SP, Discigil KF, Webb CR, Greenspan AM, Spielman SR: Risks and complications of clinical cardiac electrophysiologic studies: a prospective analysis of 1,000 consecutive patients, *J Am Coll Cardiol* 9:1261–1268, 1987.

Jackman WM, Beckman KJ, McClelland JH, Wang X, Friday KJ, Roman CA, Moulton KP, Twidale N, Hazlitt HA, Prior MI, Oren J, Overholt ED, Lazzara R: Treatment of supraventricular tachycardia due to atrioventricular nodal reentry by radiofrequency catheter ablation of slow-pathway conduction, *N Engl J Med* 327:313–318, 1992.

Jackman WM, Wang X, Friday KJ, Roman CA, Moulton KP, Beckman KJ, McClelland JH, Twidale N, Hazlitt HA, Prior MI, Margolis PD, Calame JD, Overholt ED, Lazzara R: Catheter ablation of accessory atrioventricular pathways (Wolff-Parkinson-White syndrome) by radiofrequency current, *N Engl J Med* 324:1605–1611, 1991.

Josephson ME: *Clinical cardiac electrophysiology: techniques and interpretations,* Philadelphia, 1993, Lea & Febiger.

Morady F, Harvey M, Kalbfleisch SJ, El-Atassi R, Calkins H, Langberg JJ: Radiofrequency catheter ablation of ventricular tachycardia in patients with coronary artery disease, *Circulation* 87:363–372, 1993.

Scheidt S: *Basic electrocardiography*, West Caldwell, NJ, 1986, CIBA-GEIGY Pharmaceuticals.

Waller TJ, Kay HR, Spielman SR, Kutalek SP, Greenspan AM, Horowitz LN: Reduction in sudden death and total mortality by antiarrhythmic therapy evaluated by electrophysiologic drug testing: criteria of efficacy in patients with sustained ventricular tachyarrhythmia, *J Am Coll Cardiol* 10:83–89, 1987.

---------------- 5 ----------------

ANGIOGRAPHIC DATA

Ubeydullah Deligonul, Morton J. Kern, and Robert Roth

Angiograms are the most important product of cardiac catheterization. This procedure may be the most important test to which a patient with cardiac disease can be subjected. Currently the risks of angiography are minimal, but operators must take special care in the performance of coronary and ventricular angiography. The attitude of the expert angiographer can be observed in the face of Dr. Goffredo Gensini at the Monsignor Toomey Cardiovascular Laboratory in Syracuse, New York (Fig. 5-1). Dr. Gensini epitomizes the concerned, competent, and experienced angiographer.

Optimal angiographic data collection is a process made up of linked steps. Failure of any link breaks the chain and may cause loss of all or part of the data. The chain begins with the positioning of the patient on the table and involves performing the study, developing the cineangiographic film, and finally displaying it for review on the cineangiographic projector. The box on p. 268 summarizes the causes of poor angiograms.

The radiographic images provide the visual representation of the vascular network to internal structures and, at times, the function of the circulation. Obtaining quality images should not necessitate increasing the ordinary procedural radiation exposure to either the patient or catheterization personnel.

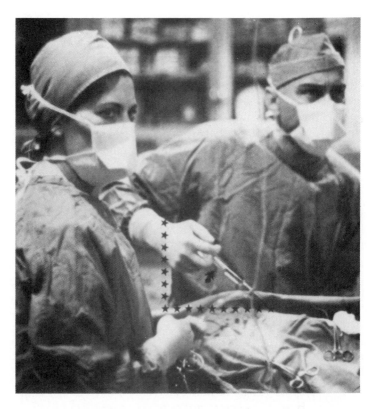

Fig. 5-1. Goffredo Gensini doing coronary arteriography. Note the raised angle (30°) of the injection syringe to keep out air bubbles. (From Gensini GG: *Coronary arteriography,* Mount Kisco, NY, 1975, Futura.)

SECTION I: CARDIAC ANGIOGRAPHY
CORONARY ARTERIOGRAPHY

The goal of coronary angiography is to visualize the coronary arteries, branches, and anomalies with enough detail to make a precise diagnosis of and plan the treatment strategy for coronary artery disease. With the introduction of percutaneous transluminal coronary balloon angioplasty (PTCA, see Chapter 9) the coronary angiographer is expected to document not only the presence of disease, but also its precise location and concomitant involvement of major and minor side branches, thrombi, and areas of calcification in more detail than was necessary for angiograms used for bypass surgery alone. For PTCA, visualization of vessel bifurcations, origin of side branches, the portion of the vessel proximal to a significant lesion, and previously "unimportant" lesion characteristics (length, eccentricity, calcium, and the like) are critical. In the case of a total vessel occlusion the distal vessel should be visualized as clearly as possible by injecting the coronary arteries that supply collaterals and taking cineangiograms with panning long enough to visualize late collateral vessel filling.

Causes for Poor Angiograms

PATIENT FACTORS
Size
Movement
Hardware (pacemaker, Harrison rods, multiple surgery with clips)
Anatomic conditions (scoliosis, scarred lungs, large heart [fluid])

ANGIOGRAPHER FACTORS

Poor catheter seating (wrong catheter shape, size, anomalous origin, subselective cannulation)
Poor contrast opacification (weak injection, volume too small, diluted contrast)

EQUIPMENT FACTORS

X-ray generator problems (high heat, quantum mottle, too high kV, too short pulse width, too long pulse width)
X-ray tube problems (anode pitting, wrong focal spot, beam geometry, proximity to image intensifier, poor collimation)

Image intensifier problems

Optical chain to TV (mirror malalignment, f-stop aperture control, overframing, focal length)
Cineangiographic camera (film gate malfunction, film travel misalignment, restricted travel)
Cineangiographic film/processing (poor sensitivity, latitude, poor exposure, poor development)
Cineangiographic projector (poor optical components)

The routine coronary angiographic views described as follows should include visualization of the origin and course of the major vessel and their branches in at least two different planes. Naturally there is a wide variation in coronary anatomy and appropriately modified views will need to be individualized.

Techniques

Hand injections for coronary arteriography.   Contrast media, an iodinated solution used to opacify the coronary arteries, is injected by hand through a multivalve manifold (see Fig. 3-1). Keep the tip of the syringe pointed down so any small bubbles float up and are not injected (see Fig. 5-1). Flow rates are usually 2 to 4 ml/sec with volumes of 4 to 8 ml in the right coronary artery and 7 to 10 ml for the left coronary artery. The use of disposable manifolds, syringes, and tubing is cost-effective, safe, and appropriate for conducting daily clinical studies.

Power injections for coronary arteriography.   Power injection of the coronary arteries has been utilized in thousands of cases in many laboratories and is equal in safety to hand injection. However, hand injection of the coronary arteries offers advantages in ease of administration of intracoronary drugs and rapid successive injections with varying degrees of opacification for either severely diseased or high-flow coronary arteries. In the latter case, a power injector at a fixed setting might require several injections to find the optimal contrast delivery flow rate.

Typical settings for power injections are as follows:
Right coronary artery: 4 ml at 3 ml/sec; maximal psi 150
Left coronary artery: 8 ml at 4 ml/sec; maximal psi 150

Filming frame rates.   Filming frame rates are usually 30 frames/sec unless heart rate is greater than 95 bpm, when the rate of 60 frames/sec is used.

Panning techniques.   Many laboratories use x-ray image screen sizes of less than 7 inches diameter, which precludes having the entire coronary artery course visualized without panning over the heart to include late filling portions of the arterial segments. In addition, in most views some degree of panning will be necessary to identify regions that are not seen from the initial setup positioning. Some branches unexpectedly may appear later from collateral filling or other unusual anatomic sources.

The key to accurate, optimal coronary cineangiography, obtaining the most information for the least amount of movement, is the initial setup of the catheter relative to the artery locations. Fig. 5-2 shows the catheter–left main artery setup keys for LAO views in the straight, cranial, and caudally angled projections. When the patient is positioned correctly and the setup key followed, only minimal panning will be necessary for these views. In the LAO view, pan down the anterior descending artery and then leftward to identify collaterals going to the right coronary artery (RCA) or, if the circumflex is occluded, rightward to include collaterals going to the distal circumflex. For the RCA in the LAO position, pan downward and to the right toward the LAD to include late filling collaterals from the right to the LAD artery. These motions have been diagrammed in Fig. 5-2.

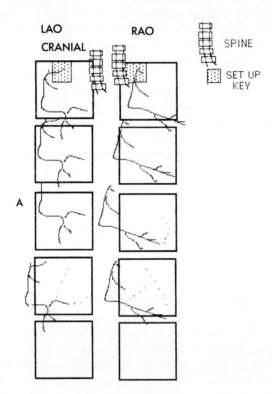

Fig. 5-2. Setup keys for panning during coronary arteriography. *LAO,* left anterior oblique view. *RAO,* right anterior oblique view. **A,** Right coronary artery (*RCA*); **B,** left coronary artery (*LCA*); **C,** lateral views.

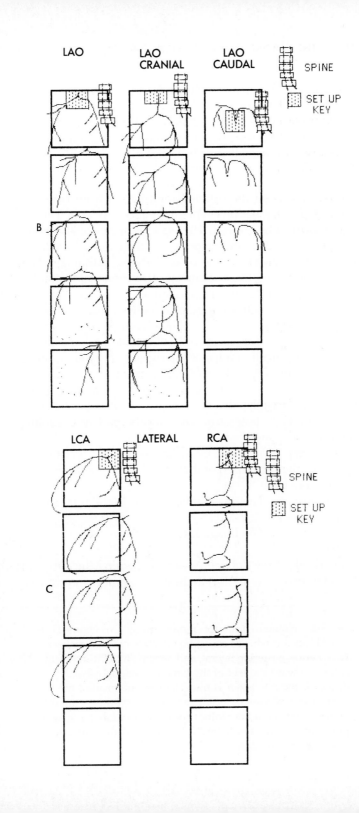

LAO   LAO CRANIAL   LAO CAUDAL   SPINE   SET UP KEY

B

LCA LATERAL RCA   SPINE   SET UP KEY

C

In the RAO projections for both the left and right coronary arteries, pan downward to the apex to identify late filling, left-to-left or right-to-left collaterals. These setup keys to panning will help the operator include all critical important information for coronary arteriography.

Views

In order to obtain the optimal information from coronary cineangiography, various views unveiling overlapped vessel segments must be utilized. These views or projections highlight specific and distinct segments of the coronary anatomy and permit a discrete view of underlying pathology. This understanding of the usefulness of various radiographic views (and nomenclature) is essential.

Nomenclature for angiographic views (Figs. 5-3 to 5-5, Table 5-1, and box on p. 287).   For all catheterization laboratories, the x-ray source is *under* the table and the image intensifier is directly on *top* of the patient. They are moving in opposite directions in an imaginary circle in which the patient is positioned in the center. The body surface of the patient that faces the observer determines the specific view. This relationship holds true whether the patient is supine, standing, or rotated.

AP position. The image intensifier is directly over the patient with the beam perpendicular to the patient lying flat on the x-ray table.

RAO position. The image intensifier is to the right side of the patient.

LAO position. The image intensifier is to the left side of the patient.

NOTE: Think of the "oblique" view as turning the left/right shoulder forward (anterior) to the camera (image intensifier).

Fig. 5-3. Nomenclature for radiographic projections. The small black arrowheads show the direction of the x-ray beam. **A,** Anterior, posterior, lateral, and oblique. **B,** If the intensifier is tilted toward the feet of the patient, a caudal view is produced. If the intensifier is tilted toward the head of the patient, a cranial view is produced. (Redrawn from Paulin S: Terminology for radiographic projections in cardiac angiography, *Cathet Cardiovasc Diagn* 7:341, 1981, with permission.) *Continued on page 274.*

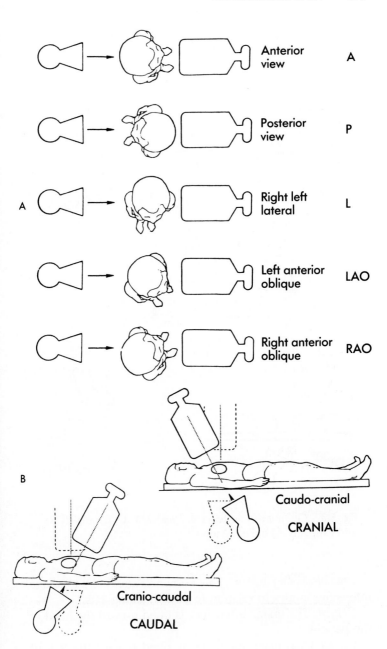

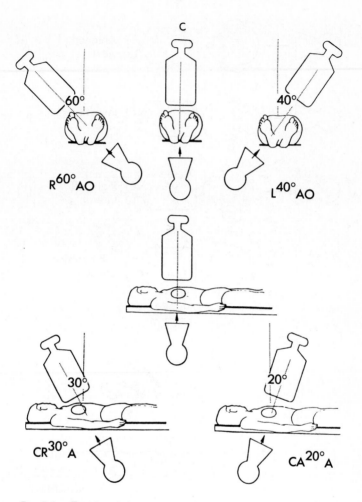

Fig. 5-3. *Continued from pages 272 and 273.* **C,** Cranial (CR) and caudal (CA) oblique views.

Cranial/caudal position. This nomenclature refers to image intensifier angles in relation to patient's long axis.

Cranial. The image intensifier is tilted toward the head of the patient.

Caudal. The image intensifier is tilted toward the feet of the patient.

Cranial and caudal views are "open" overlapped coronary segments that are foreshortened in regular views (Fig. 5-5).

A

A-P PROJECTION

The A-P projection allows a good visualization of the left main coronary artery :

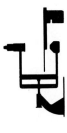

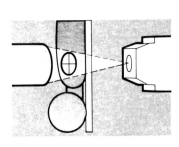

1. Left main coronary
2. Proximal part of LAD
3. Mid part of LAD
4. Distal part of LAD
5. Proximal circumflex artery
6. Distal circumflex artery
7. Left obtuse marginal artery
8. First diagonal artery
9. First septal perforating artery
10. Septal arteries
11. Auricular branch of the circumflex artery
12. Obtuse marginal artery n° 2.

Fig. 5-4. **A** to **E,** Left coronary artery. **F** to **I,** Right coronary artery. *AP,* Anteroposterior; *LAD,* left anterior descending artery; *LAO,* left anterior oblique; *RAO,* right anterior oblique. (From Bertrand ME, editor: *Coronary arteriography,* Lille, France, 1979, French Society of Cardiology.) *Continued on pages 276–283.*

B | RIGHT ANTERIOR OBLIQUE PROJECTION AT 30° (R.A.O. 30°)

The R.A.O. projection at 30° permits the entire circumflex system to be studied, as well as the first centimetres of the anterior interventricular artery.

1. Left main coronary
2. Proximal part of LAD
3. Mid. part of LAD
4. Distal part of LAD
5. Proximal circumflex artery
6. Distal circumflex artery
7. Obtuse marginal artery
8. First diagonal artery
9. Second diagonal artery
10. First septal perforating artery
11. Septal arteries
12. Auricular branch of the circumflex artery

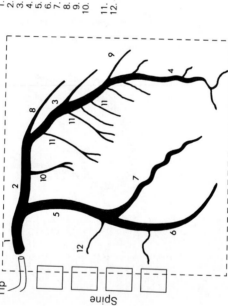

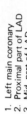

276

C LEFT ANTERIOR OBLIQUE PROJECTION AT 55/60° (L.A.O. 55/60°)

The LAO projection at 55/60° mainly studies the diagonal arteries and the mid and distal parts of the LAD. On the other hand, the circumflex system is not well defined.

1. Left main coronary
2. Proximal part of LAD
3. Middle part of LAD
4. Distal part of LAD
5. Proximal circumflex artery
6. Distal circumflex artery
7. Left obtuse marginal artery
8. First diagonal artery
9. Second diagonal artery
10. First septal perforating artery
11 and 12. Septal arteries

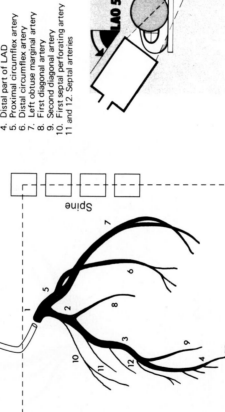

Fig. 5-4. *Continued.* **B** and **C,** Left coronary artery.

D LEFT ANTERIOR OBLIQUE PROJECTION AT 55/60° COMBINED WITH A CRANIAL ANGULATION OF 20°

The cranial angulation of 20° combined with the LAO projection at 55/60° is especially useful to study the left main coronary artery

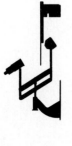

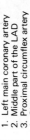

1. Left main coronary artery
2. Middle part of the LAD
3. Proximal circumflex artery
4. Obtuse marginal artery
5. First diagonal artery
6. Septal perforating artery

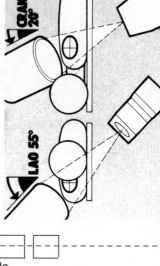

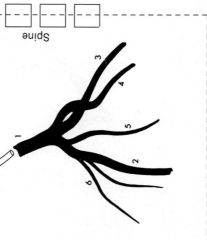

CRANIAL 20°

LAO 55°

Spine

Tip

E LEFT LATERAL PROJECTION

The left lateral projection, allows the study of the different segments of the anterior interventricular artery, the first diagonal artery and the left marginal artery.

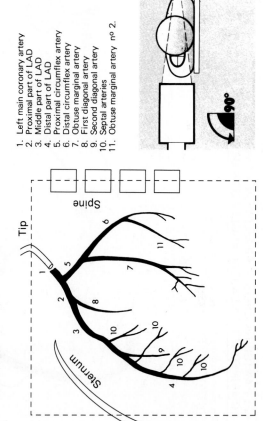

1. Left main coronary artery
2. Proximal part of LAD
3. Middle part of LAD
4. Distal part of LAD
5. Proximal circumflex artery
6. Distal circumflex artery
7. Obtuse marginal artery
8. First diagonal artery
9. Second diagonal artery
10. Septal arteries
11. Obtuse marginal artery no 2.

Fig. 5-4. *Continued.* **D** and **E**, Left coronary artery.

F LEFT ANTERIOR OBLIQUE PROJECTION AT 45° COMBINED WITH A CAUDAL ANGULATION OF 15°

This projection allows the whole study of the R.C.A. and, especially, clearly defines the region of the crux of the heart.

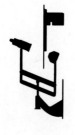

1. First (horizontal) segment of the right coronary artery
2. Second (vertical) segment of the right coronary artery
3. Third (horizontal) segment of the right coronary artery
4. Posterior interventricular

5. Retroventricular artery
6. Conus branch
7. Artery of the sinus node
8. Right ventricular artery
9. Right marginal artery
10. Artery of the A-V node
11. Diaphragmatic artery

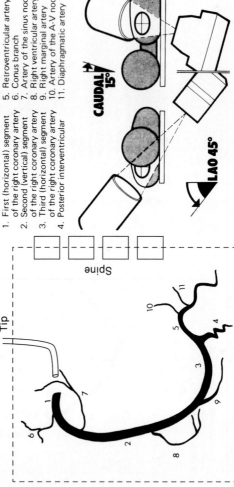

G | RIGHT ANTERIOR OBLIQUE PROJECTION AT 45°

The RAO projection at 45° permits the survey of the second (vertical) segment of the right coronary artery, the posterior interventricular artery and the collateral branches (right ventricular and right marginal arteries). On the other hand, the first segment and the third segment as well as the retroventricular artery are not clearly defined. This projection also allows the visualization of the retrograde reopacification of the distal part of LAD proximally occluded.

1. First (horizontal) segment of the right coronary artery
2. Second (vertical) segment of the right coronary artery
3. Third (horizontal) segment of the right coronary artery
4. Posterior descending artery
5. Retroventricular artery
6. Conus branch
7. Artery of the sinus node
8. Right ventricular artery
9. Right marginal artery
10. Artery of the A-V node
11. Inferior septal arteries

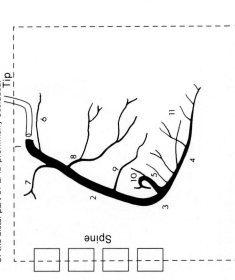

Continued.

Fig. 5-4. *Continued.* **F** and **G**, Right coronary artery.

H RIGHT ANTERIOR OBLIQUE PROJECTION AT 120° COMBINED WITH A CRANIAL ANGULATION OF 10°

This projection is very useful for studying the third horizontal segment, the crux of the heart and the retroventricular artery and its branches.

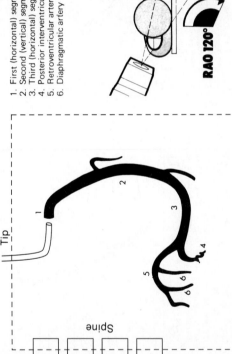

1. First (horizontal) segment of the right coronary artery
2. Second (vertical) segment of the right coronary artery
3. Third (horizontal) segment of the right coronary artery
4. Posterior interventricular artery
5. Retroventricular artery
6. Diaphragmatic artery

LEFT LATERAL PROJECTION

This projection permits the study of the second (vertical) segment of the right coronary artery and the collateral branches (conus branch, right ventricular artery, right marginal artery).

1. First (horizontal) segment of the right coronary artery
2. Second (vertical) segment of the right coronary artery
3. Third (horizontal) segment of the right coronary artery
4. Posterior interventricular artery
5. Retroventricular artery
6. Conus branch
7. Artery of the sinus node
8. Right ventricular artery
9. Right marginal artery
10. Artery of the A-V node
11. Diaphragmatic artery
12. Inferior septal arteries

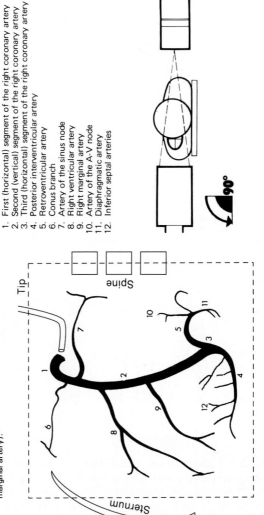

Fig. 5-4. *Continued.* **H** and **I**, Right coronary artery.

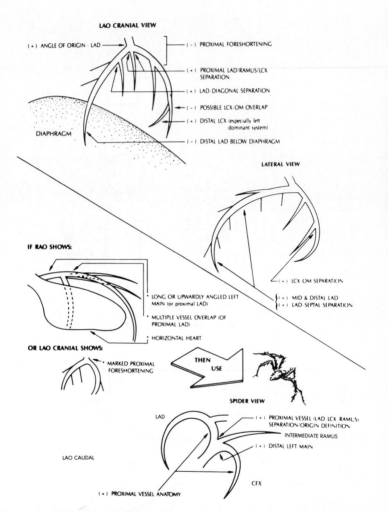

Fig. 5-5. Diagrammatic views of left coronary arteries demonstrating special positioning to best observe branch segments. LAD, left anterior descending coronary artery; LCX-OM, left circumflex-obtuse marginal branch; LAO, left anterior oblique; RAO, right anterior oblique. See text for details. (From Boucher RA, and others: Coronary angiography and angioplasty, *Cathet Cardiovasc Diagn* 14:269–285, 1988.) *Continued on page 285.*

ADDENDUM:

EFFECTS OF ANGULATION ON DEFINING CORONARY ANATOMY

[(+) denotes aspect of vessel definition advantaged by selected view;
(–) denotes disadvantage of view]

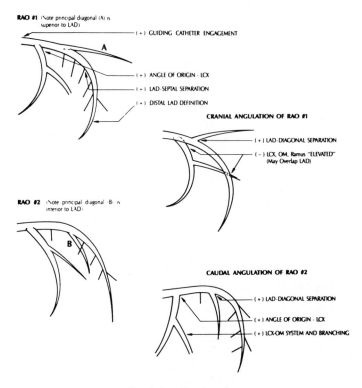

RAO #1 (Note principal diagonal (A) is superior to LAD)

(+) GUIDING CATHETER ENGAGEMENT

(+) ANGLE OF ORIGIN - LCX
(+) LAD-SEPTAL SEPARATION
(+) DISTAL LAD DEFINITION

CRANIAL ANGULATION OF RAO #1

(+) LAD-DIAGONAL SEPARATION
(–) LCX, OM, Ramus "ELEVATED"
(May Overlap LAD)

RAO #2 (Note principal diagonal (B) is inferior to LAD)

CAUDAL ANGULATION OF RAO #2

(+) LAD-DIAGONAL SEPARATION
(+) ANGLE OF ORIGIN - LCX
(+) LCX-OM SYSTEM AND BRANCHING

Fig. 5-5. *Continued.*

REMEMBER: Cranial views for the LAD; caudal views for the CFX.

The rationale for these routine angiographic views are as follows:

Left coronary artery

1. The AP view or shallow RAO displays the left main coronary artery (LMCA) in its entire perpendicular length. In this view the LAD and left circumflex (LCX) arteries branches are overlapped. Slight RAO or LAO angulation may be necessary to clear the density of the vertebrae and the catheter shaft in the thoracic descending aorta.

TABLE 5-1. Recommended "key" angiographic view for specific coronary artery segments

Coronary segment	Origin/bifurcation	Course/body
Left main	AP	AP
	LAO cranial	LAO cranial
	LAO caudal*	
Proximal LAD	LAO cranial	LAO cranial
	RAO caudal	RAO caudal
Mid-LAD	LAO cranial	
	RAO cranial	
	Lateral	
Distal LAD	AP	
	RAO cranial	
	Lateral	
Diagonal	LAO cranial	RAO cranial, caudal
	RAO cranial	or straight
Proximal circumflex	RAO caudal	LAO caudal
	LAO caudal	
Intermediate	RAO caudal	RAO caudal
	LAO caudal	Lateral
Obtuse marginal	RAO caudal	RAO caudal
	LAO caudal	
	RAO cranial (distal marginals)	
Proximal RCA	LAO	
	Lateral	
Mid-RCA	LAO	LAO
	Lateral	Lateral
	RAO	RAO
Distal RCA	LAO cranial	LAO cranial
	Lateral	Lateral
PDA	LAO cranial	RAO
Posterolateral	LAO cranial	RAO
	RAO cranial	RAO cranial

AP, anterioposterior; LAD, left anterior descending artery; LAO, left anterior oblique; PDA, posterior descending artery (from RCA); RAO, right anterior oblique; RCA, right coronary artery.
* Horizontal hearts.

2. The LAO/cranial view also shows LMCA (slightly fore-shortened but perpendicular to the RAO view), LAD, and diagonal branches. Septal and diagonal branches are separated clearly. The CFX and marginals are foreshort-ened and overlapped. Deep inspiration, moving the den-sity of the diaphragm out of the field, is essential for this view. The LAO angle should be set so that the LAD course

Routine Coronary Angiographic Views

LEFT CORONARY ARTERY

For concentration on vessel segment

Straight AP or 5° to 10° RAO — Left main
30° to 45° LAO and 20° to 30° cranial — LAD/CFX bifurcation
30° to 40° RAO and 20° to 30° caudal — CFX + marginals
5° to 30° RAO and 20° to 45° cranial — LAD + diagonals
50° to 60° LAO and 10° to 20° caudal (spider view) — LAD/CFX bifurcation, CFX, marginals
Lateral (optional) — Bypass conduits to LAD

RIGHT CORONARY ARTERY

For concentration on vessel segment

30° to 45° LAO and 15° to 20° cranial — Proximal, mid, PDA
30° to 45° RAO — Proximal, mid, PDA
Lateral (optional)

AP, anterioposterior; CFX, circumflex artery; LAD, left anterior descending artery; LAO, left anterior oblique; PDA, posterior descending artery (from right coronary artery); RAO, right anterior oblique.

NOTE: The lateral view is a very useful addition to these views for both coronary arteries. Also, the four most common views for the left coronary artery when performed LAO cranial, RAO cranial, RAO caudal, and LAO caudal form a box around the patient. Look first at the LAD (cranial views) and then at the CFX (caudal views). This box should be on every study with rare exceptions.

is parallel to the spine and stays in the "lucent wedge" bordered by the spine and the curve of the diaphragm. Cranial angulation tilts the LMCA down and permits view of the LAD/CFX bifurcation. Too steep LAO/cranial angulation or a shallow inspiration produces considerable overlapping with the diaphragm and liver, degrading the image.

3. The RAO caudal view shows the LMCA bifurcation from a view perpendicular to the LAO/cranial angle. The origin and course of the CFX/obtuse marginals, intermediate branch, and proximal LAD segment are well seen. This view is one of the best two views for visualization of the CFX artery. The LAD beyond the proximal segment is obscured by overlapped diagonals.

4. The RAO/cranial view is used to open the diagonal along the mid and distal LAD. Diagonal branch bifurcations are well visualized. The diagonal branches are projected upward. The proximal LAD and CFX usually are overlapped. Marginals may overlap and the CFX is foreshortened.

5. The LAO/caudal view ("spider" view) shows the LMCA (foreshortened) and bifurcation of the LMCA into the CFX and LAD. Proximal and mid portions of the CFX are usually seen excellently with the origins of obtuse marginal branches. Poor image quality may be due to overlapping of diaphragm and spine. The LAD is considerably foreshortened in this view.

6. A *lateral* view shows the mid and distal LAD best. The LAD and the CFX are well separated. Diagonals usually are overlapped. The (ramus) intermediate branch course is well visualized.

Right coronary artery

1. The LAO/cranial view shows the origin of the RCA, the entire length of the RCA, and the posterior descending artery (PDA) bifurcation (crux). Cranial angulation tilts the PDA down to see vessel contour and reduce foreshortening. Deep inspiration is necessary to clear the diaphragm. The PDA and posterolateral branches are foreshortened.

2. The RAO view shows the mid-RCA and the length of the PDA and posterolateral branches. Septals, supplying

occluded LAD via collaterals, may be clearly identified. The posterolateral branches are overlapped and may need the addition of the cranial view.

3. The lateral view also shows the RCA origin (especially in those with more anteriorly oriented orifices) and mid-RCA well. The PDA and posterolateral branches are foreshortened.

TECHNICAL NOTE: Because of the individual variations in anatomy, performing small (1- to 2-ml) test injections in inspiration is very helpful in obtaining the appropriate oblique and axial angulations and set-up for panning.

Coronary artery saphenous vein grafts are visualized in at least two views (LAO and RAO). It is important to show the aortic anastomosis, the body of the graft, and the distal anastomosis. The distal runoff and continued flow or collateral channels are also critical. The graft-vessel anastomosis is best seen in the view that depicts the native vessel best. Therefore the graft views can be summarized as follows:

1. *RCA graft*—LAO cranial, RAO, and lateral
2. *LAD graft* (or internal mammary artery)—lateral, RAO cranial, LAO cranial, and AP (the lateral view is especially useful to visualize the anastomosis to the left anterior descending)
3. *CFX (and obtuse marginals) grafts*—LAO and RAO caudal

GENERAL STRATEGY: Perform the standard views while assessing the vessel key views for specific coronary artery segments (see Table 5-1) to determine the need for contingency views or an alteration/addition of special views.

Assessment of coronary stenoses (Figs. 5-6 to 5-9)

Assessment of the degree of narrowing. The evaluation of the degree of a stenosis relates to the percentage reduction in the diameter of the vessel. This is calculated in the projection where the greatest narrowing can be observed. Exact evaluation is almost impossible and, in fact, the lesions are roughly classified. Six categories can be distinguished in this way:

0. Normal coronary artery
1. Irregularities of the vessel
2. Narrowing of less than 50%
3. Stenosis between 50% and 75%
4. Stenosis between 75% and 95%
5. Total occlusion

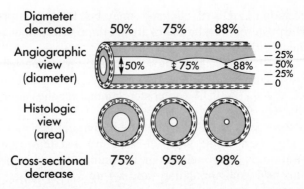

Fig. 5-6. Diagrammatic representation of angiographic versus postmortem analysis of coronary artery stenosis. (From Roberts WC: Coronary heart disease: a review of abnormalities observed in the coronary arteries. *Cardiovasc Med* 2(1):29–38, 1977.)

The length of a stenosis is simply mentioned (e.g., LAD proximal segment stenosis 25%, long or short).

Classification of distal runoff. The distal runoff is classified into four stages:

1. Normal distal runoff
2. Good distal runoff

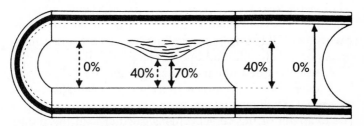

Fig. 5-7. Drawing of artery showing the effect of diffuse intimal thickening upon the evaluation of a localized stenosis. The vessel's original wall and lumen (0% narrowing; *arrow with solid line at right*). A diffuse thickening of the intima at left. If we gauge the narrowing against the diffusely stenosed lumen, a 40% narrowing (*arrow with broken line*) is measured. If it is compared against the original lumen, a 70% narrowing is seen. (From Pujadas G: *Coronary angiography: in the medical and surgical treatment of ischemic heart disease*, New York, 1980, McGraw-Hill.)

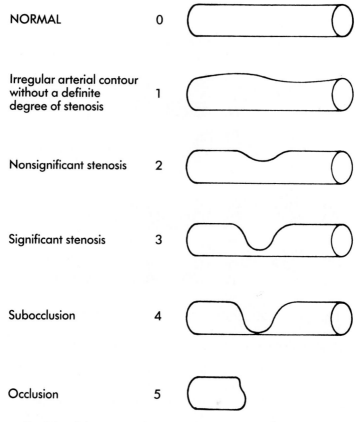

NORMAL	0	
Irregular arterial contour without a definite degree of stenosis	1	
Nonsignificant stenosis	2	
Significant stenosis	3	
Subocclusion	4	
Occlusion	5	

Fig. 5-8. Coronary stenosis grading. (From Pujadas G: *Coronary angiography: in the medical and surgical treatment of ischemic heart disease,* New York, 1980, McGraw-Hill.)

3. Poor distal runoff
4. Absence of distal runoff

Collateral circulation. The reopacification of a totally or subtotally (99%) occluded vessel is considered. The collateral circulation is graded as follows:

Grade	Collateral appearance
0	No collateral circulation
1	Very weakly (ghostlike) reopacification
2	Reopacified segment, less dense than the feeding vessel and filling slowly

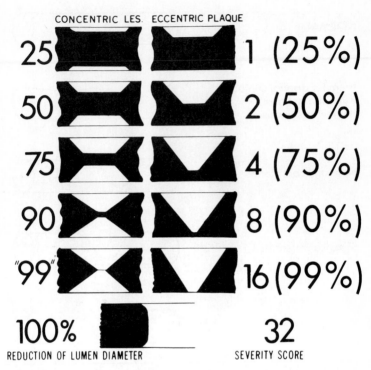

Fig. 5-9.   The angiographic appearance of concentric and eccentric plaques with, respectively, 25%, 50%, 75%, 90%, and
99% obstruction as well as complete occlusion (100%). Les,
lesion. (From Gensini GG: *Coronary arteriography*, Mount
Kisco, NY, 1975, Futura.)

3   Reopacified segment as dense as the feeding vessel
          and filling rapidly

It is useful to establish the size of the recipient vessel
exactly. Determine if the collateral circulation is ipsi (e.g.,
proximal RCA to distal RCA collateral supply) or contralateral (e.g., CFX to distal RCA collateral supply). Identify exactly which region is affected by collateral supply and lesions
in the feeding artery. Note whether the reopacification is
forward (anterograde) or backward (retrograde). This evaluation is important for making decisions on which vessels
might be protected or lost during coronary angioplasty.

PROBLEMS AND SOLUTIONS IN THE INTERPRETATION OF CORONARY ANGIOGRAMS

Vessel Overlap

Because coronary angioplasty requires a clear view of the target vessel that may be overlapped, multiple angles are required to reveal locations of lesions not previously considered important.

Poor Opacification

Poor contrast opacification of the vessel may falsely lead to an impression of an angiographically significant lesion or lucency that could be considered a clot. Inadequate mixing of contrast and blood would present itself as a luminal irregularity. A satisfactory bolus injection of contrast must be delivered if adequate opacification is to be achieved and the angiogram interpreted correctly. Enhanced contrast delivery can be achieved by using a larger-size catheter, injecting during Valsalva maneuver phase III, or using a power injector.

Total Occlusion

Total occlusion of a vessel may be erroneously suspected if a catheter is subselective in its location or an anomalous origin and course of a vessel is not recognized. A short left main coronary artery may lead to opacification of only the LAD and a presumption of a circumflex occlusion or anomalous position may result. If this is thought to be the case, an aortic cusp "flush" injection of contrast may reveal the second vessel. Subselective injections into each vessel separately may be necessary if the left main artery is too short to opacify both vessels simultaneously. This problem may also occur for subselective injection into a large RCA conus branch not adequately visualizing the main RCA.

Spasm

Catheter-induced spasm may appear as a fixed stenotic lesion. This has been observed in both right and left (and left main) coronary arteries and must be considered when an organic lesion is the only suspected anomaly. Nitroglycerin will reverse coronary spasm and should be administered in such cases where a question of catheter-induced spasm exists. Catheter-induced spasm may occur not only at the tip of the catheter touching the artery but also more distally. Repositioning of the catheter and administration of nitroglycerin (100 to 200 μg through the catheter) may clarify if the presumed lesion is structural and not spastic. Often a change to a smaller diameter (6 or 5 French) catheter or catheters that do not seat deeply may help.

Special Problems

LMCA stenosis.   A commonly encountered and potentially critical problem is the safe coronary angiography of patients having LMCA stenosis. The approach to the patient with LMCA stenosis remains one of the few critical situations in which the operator and his team may affect the life and death of the patient directly.

LMCA stenosis is encountered in two clinical presentations:

1. Patients with *suspected* disease have suspicious clinical history (e.g., resting angina pectoris) or evidence of significant low work load ischemia or hypotension during exercise treadmill testing. Unstable angina may be due to LMCA stenosis in about 10% of patients.
2. Patients with *unsuspected left main* stenosis may present with either typical or atypical angina. The clinical history, resting, or stress ECG may not be helpful, and often patients with resting or atypical chest pain syndromes may not have previous exercise test data.

TECHNICAL NOTES FOR THE ANGIOGRAPHY OF THE LEFT MAIN STENOSIS:

1. Either the Judkins femoral technique or the Sones brachial approach can be used safely. This decision should be based on whichever is the operator's best working method.
2. Coronary arteriography for identification of the suspected LMCA lesion before left ventriculography is recommended to obtain the most important information first, should a complication occur.
3. Careful slow advancement and seating of the Judkins left coronary catheter will prevent this preshaped catheter from jumping into the ostia. This maneuver is very important for an ostial narrowing.
4. If the catheter can be positioned beneath the ostia, a "cusp" flush of contrast in the aortic sinus in an AP or

shallow RAO projection may identify an ostial LMCA stenosis.

5. After catheter engagement, look for aortic pressure wave deformation (damping). If pressure damping occurs, a limited contrast flush (1 to 2 ml) and rapid catheter withdrawal ("hit and run") during cineangiography should be performed to obtain a first look (Fig. 5-10). Rarely, aortic pressure damping may occur without LMCA narrowing because the coronary catheter is seated deeply and subselectively. Gradual withdrawal and repositioning of the catheter may eliminate pressure damping. No reflux of contrast media into the aortic root on coronary injection is associated with an ostial LMCA stenosis.

6. Limit the number of coronary views. Distal coronary artery anatomy suitable for bypass grafting will be assessed from the few views (usually two or three) that are available. Additional views should be kept to a minimum. Two projections, an LAO (cranial angulation) projection (Fig. 5-11**A**) and a steeper RAO with caudal angulation (Fig. 5-11**B**), are usually sufficient. LAO/caudal for ostial is sometimes better. In less critical left main stenosis with 40% to 60% narrowing, more views may be obtained. Frequent catheter engagement of the LMCA segment and contrast jet stimulation of the lesion may precipitate coronary spasm or occlusion. The number of angiographic shots should be limited.

7. Use nonionic or low osmolar contrast agents. When using standard ionic contrast agents (meglumine diatrizoate),

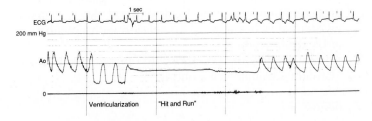

Fig. 5-10. Damping of aortic (*Ao*) pressure in the left main coronary artery with ventricularization in which immediate angiography was performed with removal of the catheter in a "hit and run" maneuver, rapidly restoring flow and perfusion after contrast injection.

lethal complications of hypotension or bradycardia may occur with reduced coronary perfusion. For the most part, hypotension and bradycardia have been eliminated with nonionic low-osmolar contrast agents.

8. After the left coronary views are completed, right coronary angiography is performed.

Left ventriculography. In patients with LMCA stenosis one may substitute noninvasive techniques (two-dimensional and Doppler echocardiography, radionuclide angiography) to determine LV function and mitral regurgitation. Safe contrast ventriculography can be performed using low-volume (<30 ml) nonionic contrast, facilitating a rapid "one-test" surgical decision. Digital ventriculography with low-volume contrast is acceptable. Nonionic or low-osmolar contrast agents are preferred over the standard ionic contrast media in these patients. Caution during catheter manipulation, including the pigtail catheter (especially in patients with LMCA stenosis and unstable angina) must be used to prevent a benign, transient arrhythmia from becoming a catastrophe. Left ventriculography should be considered only in those patients in whom the clinical presentation and severity of the lesion have a low risk/benefit ratio.

There are several important points to remember in post-catheterization care of the patients with LMCA stenosis:

1. Prevention of hypotension is paramount. If one assumes a left main stenosis pressure gradient of 40 mm Hg, aortic diastolic blood pressure of 80 mm Hg and LV end diastolic pressure of 10 mm Hg, the coronary perfusion pressure can be approximated as $80 - (40 + 10) = 30$ mm Hg. If diastolic blood pressure drops to 60 mm Hg, the perfusion pressure can fall as low as 10 mm Hg and may exacerbate myocardial ischemia and hypotension with potentiation of LV dysfunction.

2. Administer adequate volume with intravenous fluids.

3. Maintain adequate urine output.

4. Attend to any signs of ischemia in the postcatheterization period.

5. Change status from routine elective admittance to one requiring monitoring (such as in an intensive care unit).

6. Should a problem develop, immediate contact with the cardiologist or surgeon makes a critical difference in preventing the downward spiral of ischemia in patients with

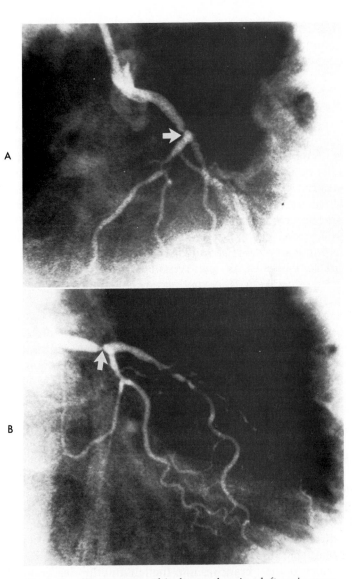

Fig. 5-11. Cineangiographic frame showing left main coronary stenosis (*arrow*). **A,** Left anterior oblique projection. **B,** Right anterior oblique projection. See text for details.

LMCA stenosis. Early insertion of intraaortic balloon pump should be considered in case of unstable hemodynamics.
7. Early review of the developed cineangiographic films with the cardiothoracic surgeon will determine timing of (emergency) coronary bypass.

Approach to common coronary anomalies.   Misdiagnosis of unsuspected anomalous origin of the coronary arteries is a potential problem in a busy catheterization laboratory. As the natural history of a patient with an anomalous origin of a coronary artery is dependent on the initial course of the anomalous vessel, it is the angiographer's responsibility to define accurately the origin and course as well as the severity of the coronary atherosclerosis in such vessels. It is an error to assume a vessel is occluded when in fact it has not been visualized because of an anomalous origin. It has often proved difficult even for experienced angiographers to delineate the true course of the anomalous vessel.

A simple "dot and eye" method for determining the proximal course of anomalous coronary arteries from an RAO ventriculogram, an RAO aortogram, or selective injection of the anomalous coronary artery in an RAO projection is described as follows. The RAO view best separates the normally positioned aorta and pulmonary artery. Placement of right-sided catheters or injection of contrast in the pulmonary artery is unnecessary and often misleading.

Anomalous origin of the left main coronary artery from right sinus of Valsalva.   This is the most clinically important anomalous artery. When the left main coronary artery arises from the right sinus of Valsalva or the proximal RCA, it may follow one of four pathways:
1. *Septal course.* The LMCA runs an intramuscular course through the septum along the floor of the RV outflow tract (Fig. 5-12). It then surfaces in the midseptum, at which point it branches into the left anterior descending and the left circumflex artery. Because the artery divides in the midseptum the initial portion of the circumflex courses toward the aorta (the normal position of the proximal LAD) and the LAD is thus relatively short (i.e., mid and distal LAD only are present). During RAO ventriculography, aortography, or coronary arteriography, the left main and the CFX coronary arteries will form an ellipse

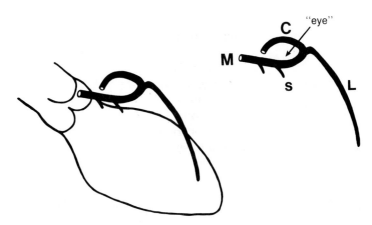

Fig. 5-12. Diagram of septal course of anomalous left coronary artery. *M,* Left main; *S,* septals; *C,* circumflex; *L,* left anterior descending artery.

(similar to the shape of an "eye") to the left of the aorta. The LM forms the inferior portion and the CFX forms the superior portion. Septal perforating arteries will be evident off the LMCA.

NOTE: This variant is considered benign and is not associated with myocardial ischemia.

2. *Anterior free wall course.* The LMCA crosses the anterior free wall of the right ventricle and then divides at the midseptum into the LAD and circumflex (Fig. 5-13). Because the artery divides at the midseptum the initial portion of the CFX courses toward the aorta (the normal position of the proximal LAD) and the LAD is thus relatively short (i.e., mid and distal LAD only are present). During RAO ventriculography, aortography, or coronary arteriography the LM and the CFX will form an ellipse ("eye") to the left of the aorta with the LM forming the superior portion and the CFX forming the inferior portion.

NOTE: This variant has not been associated with myocardial ischemia.

3. *Retroaortic course.* The LMCA passes posteriorly around the aortic root to its normal position on the anterior surface of the heart (Fig. 5-14). It divides into the LAD and CFX at the normal point and thus gives rise to LAD and CFX coronary arteries of normal length and course. Dur-

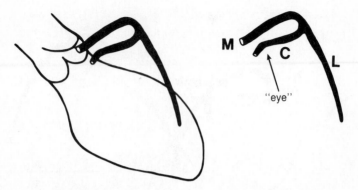

Fig. 5-13. Diagram of anterior course of anomalous left coronary artery. (See abbreviations in Fig. 5-12.)

ing RAO ventriculography, aortography, or coronary angiography the LM will be seen "on end," posterior to the aorta, and appear as a radiopaque dot. This retroaortic dot is diagnostic of a posteriorly coursing anomalous vessel.

NOTE: This variant is considered benign with evidence of myocardial ischemia being reported in only a few individuals.

4. *Interarterial course.* The LMCA courses between the aorta and pulmonary artery to its normal position on the anterior surface of the heart (Fig. 5-15). It divides into the LAD and CFX at the normal point and thus gives rise to

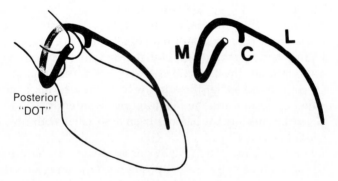

Fig. 5-14. Diagram of retroaortic course of anomalous left coronary artery. (See abbreviations in Fig. 5-12.)

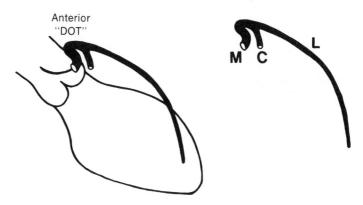

Fig. 5-15. Diagram of interarterial course of left main coronary artery. (See abbreviations in Fig. 5-12.)

LAD and CFX coronary arteries of normal length and course. During RAO ventriculography, aortography, or coronary arteriography, the LMCA will be "on end," anterior to the aorta, and appear as a radiopaque dot to the left of the aortic root.

The interarterial course of the LMCA originating from the right sinus of Valsalva has been demonstrated to be associated with exertional angina, syncope, and sudden death at a young age. Therefore, its identification is imperative. The mechanism by which myocardial ischemia is caused is unclear, but it may be caused by dynamic compression of the obliquely arising LMCA at the ostium or as it courses between the aortic root and the root of the pulmonary trunk. Once identified, coronary revascularization or translocation is indicated in young patients with symptoms of myocardial ischemia. The need for revascularization in older patients with this anomaly is less clear. However, a decision for revascularization should be based on the severity of concomitant obstructive coronary disease.

Anomalous origin of the CFX coronary artery from right sinus of Valsalva. When the CFX coronary artery arises from the right coronary cusp or the proximal right coronary artery it invariably follows a retroaortic course with the CFX coronary artery passing posteriorly around the aortic root to its normal position (Fig. 5-16). During RAO ventriculography, aortog-

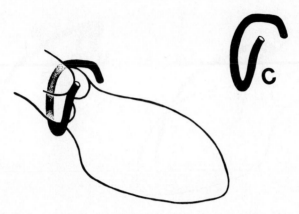

Fig. 5-16.   Diagram of retroaortic course of circumflex (C) from the left coronary cusp.

raphy, or coronary angiography, the CFX will be on end, posterior to the aorta, and appear as a radiopaque dot.

Anomalous circumflex artery. The most common coronary anomaly is the circumflex artery arising from the proximal RCA. This feature is often suggested during left coronary angiography by seeing a very long LMCA segment with a very small or trivial circumflex branch. The circumflex may also be thought to be occluded. This variant is benign.

Anomalous origin of the RCA from the left sinus of Valsalva. When the RCA arises from the left coronary cusp or the proximal LMCA it generally follows only one path, although other courses are theoretically possible (Fig. 5-17). The RCA courses between the aorta and pulmonary artery to its normal position. During RAO ventriculography, aortography, or coronary arteriography, the RCA will be on end, anterior to the aorta, and appear as a radiopaque dot. This coronary anomaly has been associated with symptoms of myocardial ischemia, particularly when the RCA is dominant. Therefore, coronary revascularization should be considered when associated with symptoms of myocardial ischemia.

Anomalous origin of the LAD coronary artery from the right sinus of Valsalva. When the LAD arises from the right aortic

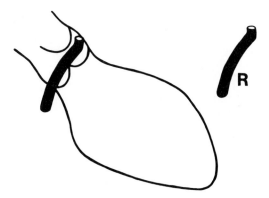

Fig. 5-17.   Diagram of anterior course of right coronary artery (*R*) from the left coronary cusp.

cusp or the proximal RCA, it generally follows one of two pathways, although other courses are possible (Fig. 5-18).

1. *Anterior free wall course.* The LAD coronary artery crosses the anterior free wall of the right ventricle and then at the midseptum turns toward the apex. During RAO ventriculography, aortography, or coronary arteriography, the LAD will pass to the left and upward before turning toward the apex. This coronary anomaly is benign.

2. *Septal course.* The LAD coronary artery runs an intramuscular course through the septum, along the floor of the RV outflow tract (Fig. 5-19). It then surfaces in the midseptum and turns toward the apex. During RAO ventriculography, aortography or coronary arteriography, the LAD will pass to the left and downward before turning toward the apex. This anomaly is benign.

LAD and CFX coronary arteries from separate ostium in the left aortic sinus. When the LAD and CFX coronary arteries arise from separate ostium in the left coronary cusp the normal proximal course is followed.

Rare anomalies of aortic coronary origin.   There have been rare reports of anomalous origin of the LMCA, RCA, or CFX from the posterior sinus of Valsalva, although most of these are necropsy reports. Angiographic identification of these anomalies is so infrequent that delineation of angiographic hallmarks is difficult. The clinical significance of these anomalies is uncertain.

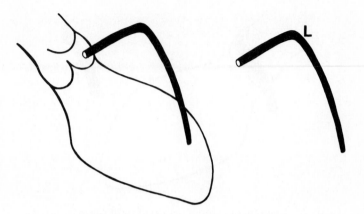

Fig. 5-18.   Diagram of anterior course of left coronary artery (*L*).

The four types of anomalous courses of the LMCA are summarized in Table 5-2.

VENTRICULOGRAPHY (Fig. 5-20)

Contrast ventriculography produces images of the LV or RV chambers. The left ventriculogram is an integral part of every coronary arteriographic study. The motion of the wall of the heart can be observed and quantitated. Abnormal wall motion indicates the presence of coronary disease, infarction, aneurysm, or hypertrophy. Left ventriculography also provides quantitative information such as the volume

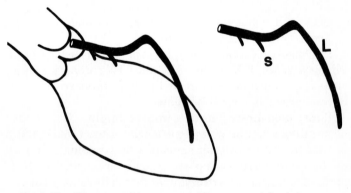

Fig. 5-19.   Diagram of intraseptal (*S*) course of the left coronary artery (*L*).

TABLE 5-2. Radiographic appearance of anomalous origin of the left main coronary artery from the right sinus of Valsalva

Course of anomalous left main coronary	RAO aortography or ventriculography		LAD length	Septals arising from LMCA
	Dot	Eye		
Septal	−	+ (upper CFX) (lower LMCA)	Short	Yes
Anterior	−	+ (upper LMCA) (lower CFX)	Short	No
Retroaortic	+ (posterior)	−	Normal	No
Interarterial	+ (anterior)	−	Normal	No

+, present; −, absent. Posterior and anterior are in reference to the aorta root. LAD, left anterior descending coronary artery; LMCA, left main coronary artery; CFX, circumflex coronary artery.

of the ventricle during systole, diastole, the ejection fraction, the rate of ejection, the quality of contractility, the presence of hypertrophic myopathy, and valvular regurgitation. Ventricular function predicts the long-term outcome of patients with coronary artery disease.

Ventriculography may be performed before or after coronary arteriography. Many laboratories routinely perform coronary arteriography first because ventricular function can be obtained through noninvasive methods in case of complications that terminate the study prematurely. In patients with LMCA stenosis, left ventriculography has often been omitted due to the potential postventriculography hypotension that occurs when ionic contrast media is used. Low-volume nonionic or low-osmolar contrast ventriculograms can be performed with little or no hypotension for these patients. These same concerns apply to patients with critical aortic stenosis in whom hypotension after left ventriculography may cause heart failure from LV ischemic dysfunction.

Indications for Left Ventriculography

1. Identify LV function for patients with coronary artery disease, myopathy, or valvular heart disease.
2. Quantitate degree of mitral regurgitation.
3. Identify ventricular septal defect.
4. Quantitate mass of myocardium for regression of hypertrophy or other similar research studies.

Diastole

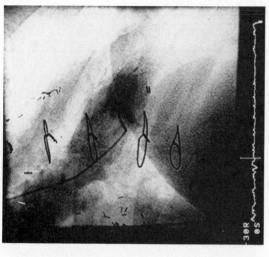

Systole

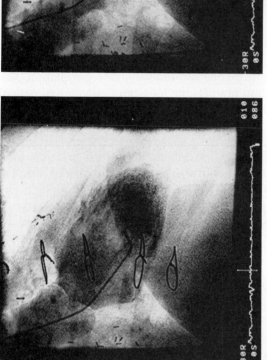

Fig. 5-20. Left ventriculography with a halo catheter.

Indications for Right Ventriculography
1. Documentation of tricuspid regurgitation
2. RV dysplasia for arrhythmias
3. Pulmonary stenosis
4. Abnormalities of pulmonary outflow tract
5. Right-to-left atrial or ventricular shunts

Technical Notes for Ventriculographic Setup

Contrast volume.   Adequate visualization and opacification of the ventricle chambers is accomplished by delivery of a large amount (30 to 60 ml) of x-ray contrast media over a short period of time (1 to 3 seconds), always using the power injector. Typical power injector settings for an average adult would be total volume 45 ml at 15 ml/sec. The rate of rise to maximal pressure is also a variable that can be set for smoother contrast delivery. Typically a 0.5-second rise time is chosen. With the catheter in the far apical position, a lower rate and volume can be used (e.g., 10 ml/sec or 30 to 35 ml total).

Catheter position.   The optimal catheter position for left ventriculography is one that avoids contact with the papillary muscles or positioning too close to the mitral valve, allowing contrast injection to artifactually produce mitral regurgitation. A midcavity position appears to be the best because adequate contrast is delivered to the majority of the LV chamber and apex and does not interfere with mitral valve function. In addition, most catheter side holes are well below the aortic valve, improving opacification of the ventricular chamber. Angled (145°) catheters and helical tip designs (halo) may provide better-quality ventriculography by reduced mitral regurgitation and ectopy.

The "pigtail" loop of the catheter may be coiled upward or downward in front of the mitral valve in the RAO plane so long as it does not interfere with mitral valve apparatus. Twisting of the pigtail loop with each beat indicates interference with the mitral valve apparatus.

Before performing the cineangiography a test injection of 5 to 8 ml of contrast will confirm proper catheter position (i.e., not entrapped in the valve structures or trabeculae) and identify problems with the power injector settings. For right ventriculography, a 7 or 8 French Berman balloon-tipped catheter produces excellent opacification. The angle of right ventriculography is not standardized. An AP or lateral projection is commonly used.

Ventricular ectopy. Ventricular ectopy during powerful contrast injection is common and generally does not require lidocaine. A stable rhythm should be maintained before contrast injection. Ventricular ectopy is produced more commonly by end hole catheters (Sones, multipurpose) than the pigtail shape.

Pressure injectors. Pressure injectors always are used to deliver a preset contrast volume over a brief period of time. In general there is no advantage to an ECG-synchronized pressure injection of contrast into the ventricle. Injection pressure and flow rates are chosen based on the catheter type (end hole or pigtail) and size (8 vs 5 French), size of ventricular chamber, cardiac output, valvular regurgitation, and prestudy hemodynamics. The range of ventricular injections may be as low as 8 to 10 ml/sec or as large as 20 to 25 ml/sec for total volumes from 25 to 60 ml. The choice and method are often those of laboratory routine based on patient size and conditions mentioned previously. Critical controls of the contrast injector are as follows:

1. Flow rate control
2. Volume termination control
3. Pressure limit control
4. Injection cutoff switch
5. Contrast media heater

Air bubbles should be expelled from the pressure injection transparent syringe and tubing before any injection. This is the mandatory feature of the setup of which all physicians and nurses should be especially conscious. There is no excuse for injection of air during contrast ventriculography.

Left ventriculography in patients with LV dysfunction. In patients with LV dysfunction and/or elevated LV end-diastolic pressure (i.e., >25 mm Hg) a reduction in the LV pressure may be required before contrast ventriculography. Use of sublingual, IV, or intraventricular nitroglycerin (100- to 200-μg boluses) is a safe and rapid method to produce the desired results. As a rule, LV systolic pressure should be <180 mm Hg before contrast injection. Extreme caution should be used in compromised patients not responding to conventional medical treatment for heart failure (i.e., left ventricular end-diastolic pressure >35 mm Hg). Ionic contrast media are not recommended for patients with LV dysfunction because of the adverse hemodynamic effects of these drugs.

Operator technique.   The physician performing the ventriculogram should be holding the catheter and the sheath, observing the monitor, and looking for problems (using the fluoroscope) during contrast injection. Myocardial contrast staining, ventricular tachycardia, or other adverse events may occur. Rapid catheter withdrawal may be required. The distance the catheter must be pulled includes 10 to 15 cm to take out the slack around the aorta before the end of the catheter moves out of the ventricle. Use of small-diameter (e.g., 5 French) catheters require high pressures. Injector connections to the manifold or direct connection to the catheter must be secured so that inadvertent separation does not spray the operator, patient, and laboratory with contrast.

Instructions to the patient before the injection will avoid surprises and help to insure comfort and ease of performance. Telling the patient that the "warm sensation" (of contrast vasodilation) will last for 30 to 60 seconds and will pass without incident is usually satisfactory.

Ventriculography views.   When available, biplane ventriculography is preferred (a two [pictures] for one [contrast injection] situation). Standard left ventriculographic views are: (1) a 30° RAO that visualizes the high lateral, anterior, apical, and inferior LV walls and (2) a 60° LAO, 20° cranial angulation that best identifies the lateral and septal LV walls.

The LAO with cranial angulation provides a view of the interventricular septum, projected on edge and tilted downward to give the best view of ventricular septal defects and septal wall motion. Biplane ventriculography may be unavailable in some catheterization laboratories. It involves increased radiation and more time spent positioning equipment. These considerations are offset by providing more information with less contrast media, which is often important. If no biplane system is available, all patients with coronary disease affecting the lateral wall should have a second left ventriculogram in 60° LAO, 20° cranial view. Almost every such patient can tolerate an additional 40 ml of contrast. In some patients the lateral view may be useful for assessment of mitral regurgitation.

Film rates should be 30 to 60 frames/sec depending on

TABLE 5-3. Recommended sites of injection and filming projections in angiocardiographic evaluation of valvular regurgitation and shunts

	Filming projections	Site of injection
Type of valvular regurgitation		
Aortic	LAO, RAO	Aortic root
Mitral	RAO, cranial LAO (lateral)	Left ventricle
Tricuspid	RAO (shallow, lateral)	Right ventricle
Pulmonic	RAO, LAO, AP	Main PA
Type of cardiac shunt		
ASD	LAO, cranial	PA
VSD	LAO, cranial	Left ventricle
PDA	AP, cranial	Aorta

LAO, left anterior oblique; RAO, right anterior oblique; PA, pulmonary artery; AP, anterior posterior; ASD, atrial septal defect; VSD, ventricular septal defect; PDA, patent ductus arteriosus.

heart rate (30 frames/sec for rates of <95 bpm). A 9-inch image intensifier is routine. Recommended views for valvular regurgitation are shown in Table 5-3.

Employ image intensifier collimator "shutters" to limit radiation scatter. The angiographic quantitation of valvular regurgitation is shown on Table 5-4.

Complications of ventriculography

1. Cardiac arrhythmias, especially ventricular tachycardia and ventricular fibrillation, require immediate cardioversion. All arrhythmias are more common with end hole catheters.
2. Intramyocardial "staining" or injection of contrast into the myocardium is generally transient and of no clinical importance unless it is deep or perforating (emergency pericardiocentesis may be required).
3. Embolism from thrombi or air may occur. These events are minimized with careful catheter preparation, flushing, and systemic heparinization.
4. Contrast-related complications noted previously may occur during this procedure. Transient hypotension (<15 to 30 seconds) is common with ionic contrast media.

Regional LV wall motion.   The normal pattern of LV contraction has been defined as a uniform, almost concentric, inward motion of all points along the ventricular inner sur-

TABLE 5-4. Angiographic quantitation of valvular regurgitation

Mitral regurgitation	Aortic regurgitation
+ Mild LA opacification; clears rapidly, often jet-like	+ Small regurgitant jet only; LV ejects contrast each systole
++ Moderate LA opacification, <LV	++ Regurgitant jet faintly opacifies LV cavity; not cleared each systole
+++ Diffuse contrast regurgitation; LA opacification = LV; LA significantly enlarged*	+++ Persistent LV opacification = aortic root density; LV enlargement*
++++ LA opacification >LV, persistent; systolic pulmonary vein opacification may occur; often marked LV enlargement*	++++ Persistent LV opacification > aortic root concentration; often marked LV enlargement*

LA, left atrium; LV, left ventricle.
* Chronic regurgitation.

face during systole. Uniform wall motion is dependent upon the cooperative and sequential contraction of the heart muscle, producing maximal effective work at minimal energy costs. This coordinated contraction has been called *synergy*. Local disturbances (from ischemia, infarction, or myopathy) in the pattern of wall motion contraction is termed asynergy and results in a disrupted and uncoordinated ventricular contraction. This pattern is particularly obvious in patients with severe coronary artery disease or cardiomyopathy.

There are three distinct types of asynergy (Fig. 5-21):
1. *Hypokinesia*—a diminished, but not absent, motion of one part of the LV wall (i.e., weak or poor contraction).
2. *Akinesia*—total lack of motion of a portion of the LV wall (no contraction).
3. *Dyskinesia*—paradoxical systolic motion or expansion of one part of the LV wall (i.e., an abnormal bulging out during systole).

Also, there are several methods by which the LV wall motion can be analyzed semiquantitatively. A point system based on the regional severity of abnormal wall motion is used to produce a wall motion score from the Coronary Artery Surgery Study (CASS) reflecting overall LV function.

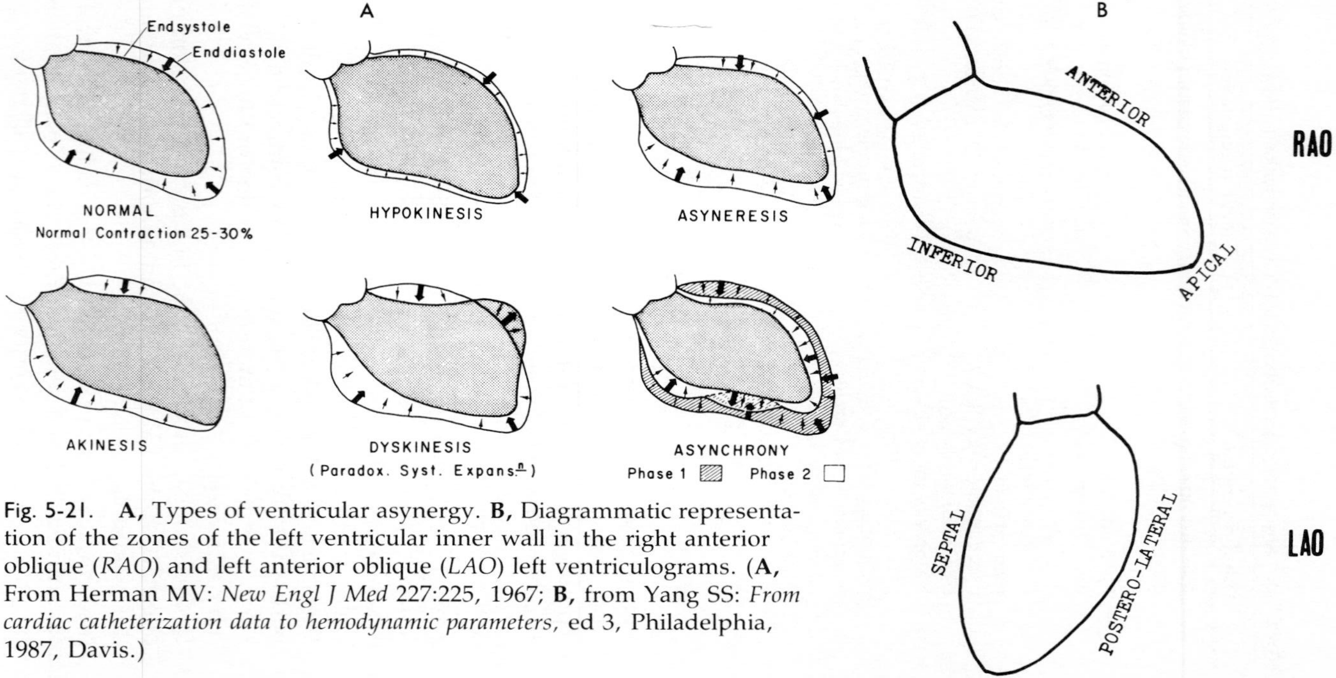

RAO

ANTERIOR

APICAL

INFERIOR

B

LAO

POSTERO-LATERAL

SEPTAL

NORMAL
Normal Contraction 25-30%

End systole

End diastole

AKINESIS

HYPOKINESIS

DYSKINESIS
(Paradox. Syst. Expans.ᴰ)

ASYNERESIS

ASYNCHRONY
Phase 1 ▨ Phase 2 ☐

A

Fig. 5-21. **A,** Types of ventricular asynergy. **B,** Diagrammatic representation of the zones of the left ventricular inner wall in the right anterior oblique (*RAO*) and left anterior oblique (*LAO*) left ventriculograms. (**A,** From Herman MV: *New Engl J Med* 227:225, 1967; **B,** from Yang SS: *From cardiac catheterization data to hemodynamic parameters*, ed 3, Philadelphia, 1987, Davis.)

The RAO and LAO left ventriculograms are divided into five segments. Points are assigned as follows:

1 = normal contraction
2 = moderate hypokinesis
3 = severe hypokinesis
4 = akinesis
5 = aneurysm-dyskinesis

Quantitation of regional wall motion.   Cineventriculography is the only established diagnostic procedure to evaluate LV wall motion quantitatively. Analysis of regional wall motion is described in Chapter 6 and Appendix II.

LV volume determination.   LV volumes can be calculated with biplane and single-plane methods (see Appendix VI), but these methods generally lead to overestimations of true ventricular volume because (1) a portion of the LV chamber is occupied by papillary muscles and trabeculae and is incorporated into the ventricular area measurement, and (2) there are the inadequacies of using an elliptical shape for the ventricular volume calculation when the ventricle is actually an irregular shape with variable margins.

Technique of Quantitative Ventriculography

The measurement of ventricular volume is derived from images obtained using high-speed cineangiography (Fig. 5-22). The volume of the left ventricle is computed by a formula previously calibrated against an image of known volume, such as a cast of a ventricle from an animal or postmortem specimen. The ventricular volume regression equation must be determined specifically for the laboratory in use. LV area is computed by the area-length method or the Simpson's rule formula. The ventricular area is converted into a volume, assuming that the ventricle has an ellipsoid shape rotated around its long axis. Image distortion and magnification should be taken into consideration. Methods for determination of ventricular volume by biplane ventriculography are described in Appendix VI. Precise imaging of the ventricle in an isocentered* projection is necessary for quantitation and calibration. Regression equations for precise ventricular volumes have been established by a number of laboratories

---

* The heart is directly in the center of the x-ray beam between the image intensifier and the x-ray tube in both angiographic planes.

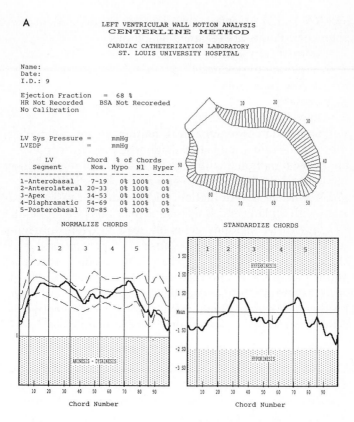

Fig. 5-22. **A,** Centerline method of regional wall motion analysis. End-diastolic and end-systolic left ventricular (*LV*) endocardial contours are traced manually and centerline constructed by the computer midway between the two contours. Motion is measured along 100 chords constructed perpendicular to the centerline. Motion at each chord is normalized by the end-diastolic perimeter to yield a shortening fraction. Motion along each chord is plotted for the patient (*dark line*). The mean motion in the normal ventriculogram group (*thin line*) and 1 standard deviation above and below the mean (*dotted line*) are shown for comparison. Wall motion is also plotted as the difference in units of standard deviations from the normal mean (*right panel*). The normal ventriculogram group mean is represented by the horizontal zero line. HR, heart rate; BSA, body surface area; LVEDP, left ventricular end diastolic pressure. *Continued on page 315.*

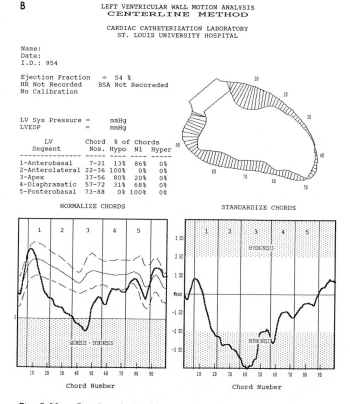

Fig. 5-22. *Continued.* **B,** Abnormal regional wall motion by centerline method. (Courtesy of St. Louis University Hospital.)

(Appendix VI). Adult values differ from those used in children.

Setup

1. Position ventricle in the isocenter of the fluoroscopic system.
2. Record the position of the center of the left ventricle (from catheter location) on lateral plane, so that the calibration grids can be positioned at this point. The image intensifier position should be marked so that it can be reproduced for grid filming. Do not move the image intensifier when filming the ventriculogram. Use a speed of 60 frames/

sec for the most precise image quality and ventricular volumes. Each frame of the cineangiogram may be analyzed.

For determination of quantitative regional wall motion abnormalities three methods are employed (see Appendix VI):

1. *Long axis method.* Determination of the major long axis and division of the long axis into equal segments with perpendicular lines.

2. *Center point method.* Midpoint of the major axis and division of the lines radiating out from the center point.

3. *Centerline method.* A centerline is established between the end-diastolic and end-systolic borders, 100 perpendicular chords are drawn and shortening of these chords determines wall motion abnormalities. Results are corrected using a normal motion value for each chord length. This is the preferred method for wall motion analysis.

Some of these methods of determining regional wall motion abnormality use computer planimetry available currently on most advanced x-ray systems. These methods have been widely employed and validated for studies involving identification of induction of angina by pacing tachycardia, drugs, coronary angioplasty, and other types of detailed study. Using regional wall motion abnormality the functional significance of coronary stenoses can be assessed.

Measurements of left ventricular contractility

Ejection fraction (EF, %)

$$\frac{EDV - ESV}{EDV} = \frac{SV}{EDV}$$

where EDV is end-diastolic volume, ESV is end-systolic volume, and SV is stroke volume. Velocity of circumferential fiber shortening (VCF, cm/sec)

$$\frac{\dfrac{D_{ed} - D_{es}}{D_{ed}}}{LVET}$$

where D_{ed} is diameter end diastole, D_{es} is diameter end systole, and LVET is LV ejection time (msec).

Regurgitant fraction (RF) for patients with valvular regurgitation

$$RF = \frac{\text{regurgitant flow}}{\text{total flow}}$$
$$= \frac{\text{CO from angiogram } - \text{ CO from Fick/thermodilution}}{\text{CO from angiogram}}$$

Semiquantitation of severity of regurgitation is determined as follows (Figs. 5-23 and 5-24):

RF < 40%	Mild
RF = 40% to 60%	Moderate
RF > 60%	Severe

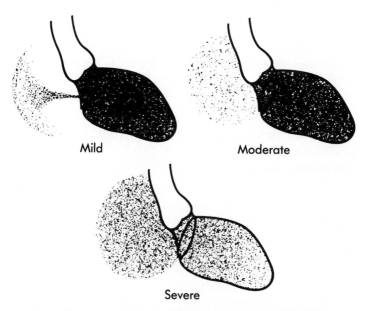

Fig. 5-23. Angiographic evaluation of mitral regurgitation. (From Pujadas G: *Coronary angiography: in the medical and surgical treatment of ischemic heart disease,* New York, 1980, McGraw-Hill.)

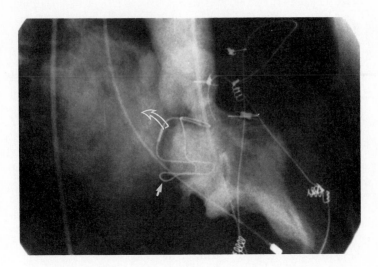

Fig. 5-24. Mitral regurgitation during left ventriculography. The bioprosthetic mitral (*small arrow*) valve has degenerated, permitting extensive opacification of the left atrium (*curved open arrow*) during contrast left ventricular injection. (From Kern MJ: *Hemodynamic rounds: interpretation of cardiac pathophysiology from pressure waveform analysis,* St. Louis, 1993, Wiley-Liss.)

SECTION II: OTHER CARDIOVASCULAR ANGIOGRAPHIC STUDIES
ASCENDING AORTOGRAPHY

Indications for aortography include the following:
1. Aortic aneurysm/aortic dissection
2. Aortic insufficiency
3. Nonselective coronary or bypass graft arteriography
4. Supravalvular aortic stenosis
5. Brachiocephalic or arch vessel disease
6. Coarctation of the aorta
7. Aortic to pulmonary artery communication
8. Aortic or periaortic neoplastic disease
9. Arterial thromboembolic disease
10. Arterial inflammatory disease

Contraindications for aortography are the following:
1. Contrast media reaction

2. Injection into false lumen of aortic dissection
3. End-hole catheter malposition
4. Inability to tolerate additional radiographic
   contrast media

Although cut film is an established radiologic method, for cardiac catheterization laboratories cineangiography is more suitable in patients with suspected dissection of the aorta.

Radiographic Projections for Aortography

LAO or lateral projection. This view is excellent for identifying dissection of the ascending aorta extending up to the neck vessels, optimally delineating the aortic arch, opening the curvature, and providing clear views of the innominate artery, common carotid, and left subclavian arteries. The coronary arteries at the root of the aorta are displayed in a semilateral projection.

RAO projection. The descending thoracic aorta, the ascending and descending aorta may be superimposed across the arch in the AP or LAO projection. The RAO view is more helpful in delineating the effect of dissection on intercostal arteries.

There are no advantages to cranial or caudal tilts for viewing of the aorta. In nonselective coronary arteriography in which aortic root angiography may help identify a vein graft takeoff the cranial and caudal angulation may provide some increased detail.

Angiographic Technique

Injection rates. Aortography can be performed using a minimum flow rate of 20 to 25 ml/sec for a total volume of 40 to 60 ml. High flow catheters are required with standard power injectors. Film rates of 30 frames/sec are satisfactory.

Catheter selection and position. Use of catheters without end holes reduces the risk of extending or inducing a dissection during contrast injection. The catheter should be positioned just above the aortic valve, but not close enough to interfere with valve opening or closing (Fig. 5-25). For descending aortic dissection, position the catheter above the suspected proximal tear. Extreme caution should be used with guidewires during catheter placement. Aortic regurgitation is estimated semiquantitatively as $1+$, $2+$, $3+$, or $4+$

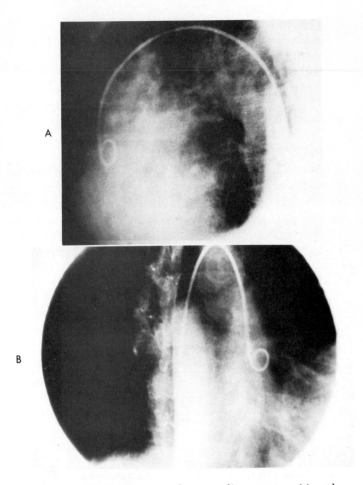

Fig. 5-25.   Pigtail catheter in the ascending aorta positioned for aortography. **A,** Left anterior oblique projection; **B,** right anterior oblique projection.

(Fig. 5-26), depending on the opacity of the ventricle after the third cycle following contrast injection. Care should be taken to avoid entrapping the catheter in a false lumen of a suspected aortic dissection. Check position with contrast test before full volume injection.

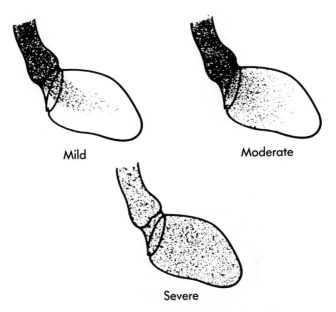

Mild

Moderate

Severe

Fig. 5-26. Angiographic evaluation of aortic regurgitation, right anterior oblique view. When the left anterior oblique view is utilized, overestimation of the aortic regurgitation occurs. (From Pujadas G: *Coronary angiography: in the medical and surgical treatment of ischemic heart disease,* New York, 1980, McGraw-Hill.)

PULMONARY ANGIOGRAPHY

Pulmonary angiography, the visualization of vascular abnormalities (e.g., intraluminal defects representing pulmonary emboli, shunts, AV malformation, and anomalous connections), should be preceded by the measurement of right heart pressures.

Indications for pulmonary angiography include the following:

1. Pulmonary embolism
2. Peripheral pulmonic stenosis or pulmonary AV fistula
3. Anomalous pulmonary venous drainage
4. Follow-through for left atrial opacification (suspected atrial mxyoma, large thrombi)

Contraindications and precautions for pulmonary angiography are the following:

1. Allergy to contrast agent
2. Pulmonary hypertension with PA systolic pressure (>60 mm Hg); use extreme caution (e.g., with primary pulmonary hypertension)
3. Acute right ventricular volume overload (after contrast media, increased volume may product RV failure, low output state, shock, or death)

Angiographic Technique

1. Venous entry
   a. Use brachial vein (percutaneous or cutdown technique), not cephalic vein.
   b. Percutaneous femoral vein approach may dislodge iliofemoral clot. Precede with brief contrast flush of IVC. Noninvasive Doppler studies may also indicate thrombus. If it is present, use the brachial approach.
2. Monitor systemic arterial pressure. Patients are often critically ill. A small arterial catheter in the femoral or brachial artery for pressure monitoring does not complicate the procedure.
3. Selection of angiographic catheters
   a. Large-diameter 7 or 8 French will reduce catheter recoil from PA to RV location. Recoil is common with high flow rates. Balloon-tipped flotation (Berman) catheters are easy to position. Ventriculographic catheters (Grollman, Eppendorf, or NIH) are stiffer and recoil less than balloon-tipped ones.
   b. CAUTION: A pacing catheter may be needed for patients with left bundle branch block. Right bundle branch block induced by passing stiff catheters through right heart would result in asystole or complete heart block in these patients.
4. Complications of pulmonary angiography
   a. Problems and complications of right heart catheterization (see Chapter 3): cardiac perforation and arrhythmia
   b. Angiography related complications: bronchospasm, anaphylaxis, hypotension, and cardiogenic shock

5. Right heart hemodynamic measurements
   a. Measurement of RA, RV, and PA pressures before angiography
   b. Measurement of CO before angiography
6. Angiographic views
   a. Position catheter in proximal portion of right PA (or where lung scan defect evident) (Fig. 5-27).
   b. Injection rate depends on hemodynamics.
      (1) If resting PA pressures are normal, use 30 to 40 ml at 20 ml/sec. Main PA injection is performed (30 frames/sec), in AP projection panning to site of presumed ventilation/perfusion (i.e., lung scan) defect.
      (2) If pulmonary hypertension (PA systolic >60 mm Hg) or RV failure (RV diastolic or RA mean pressure >10 mm Hg), reduce contrast volume and flow rate for selective PA branch injection of 15 to 20 ml at 10 ml/sec.
      (3) Selective PA branch injections by hand syringe (10 ml) may visualize a filling defect of pulmonary embolisms.
   c. For subselective injection, position catheter proximal to lobar artery in question.
   d. Do not inject if catheter is in PCW position.
   e. Pressure tracing should not be damped (do not use end-hole catheter to avoid accidental PCW injection).
   f. Angiographic views should be oblique (RAO or LAO) and AP.
7. Filming rate
   a. Cineangiography rate of 30 frames/sec is adequate. (Because pulmonary arteries are not moving quickly, slower rate is acceptable).
   b. If using cut films, capture peak arterial phase for 3 to 4 seconds. Two films per second are used to capture late levophase films as well.
8. Interpretation of the data
   a. Hemodynamics. With acute pulmonary embolism (PE), previously normal RV will fail at 40 to 60 mm Hg peak systolic pressure. The hemodynamic conse-

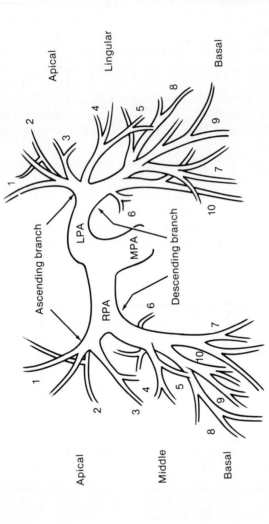

Fig. 5-27. Normal pulmonary arterial tree (anterioposterior projection). *MPA*, main pulmonary artery; *LPA*, left pulmonary artery; *RPA*, right pulmonary artery. (From Tilkian AG, Daily EK: *Cardiovascular procedures: diagnostic techniques and therapeutic procedures,* St Louis, 1986, Mosby.)

quences of pulmonary embolization may be summarized as follows:

Obstruction of the pulmonary vasculature	Mean RA pressure
Moderate <25%	<10 mm Hg
Severe 25% to 50%	10 mm Hg
Massive >50%	>10 mm Hg

Hypoxia increases CO. Only with massive PE and RV failure will CO decrease. Systemic hypotension is a late-occurring premorbid event with PE.

  b. Angiographic findings (Fig. 5-28)
    (1) Criteria for positive angiogram
      (a) Intraluminal filling defects—not explicable by superimposed adjacent structures
      (b) Abrupt arterial cutoffs—when embolus completely occludes an artery
    (2) Associated, suggestive, but not definitive findings (both findings are common in patients with severe lung disease)
      (a) Oligemia—underperfused areas of lung
      (b) Asymmetry of flow—delayed filling both common with chronic obstructive pulmonary disease

PERIPHERAL VASCULAR ANGIOGRAPHY

Once the techniques of coronary angiography have been mastered, peripheral vascular angiography is not difficult. Similar techniques are used for percutaneous entry of the superficial and deep arteries of the leg.

Digital subtraction angiography is the method of choice for identifying peripheral vascular disease. However, cineangiography can provide satisfactory information if the filming time, frame rates, and contrast dosages are properly established.

Renal Arteriography

Selective renal arteriography or arteriography obtained from aortic flush is used to evaluate the renal artery origins and vasculature. REMEMBER: For renal artery identification during aortography, the artery origins usually arise at L_1 vertebrate

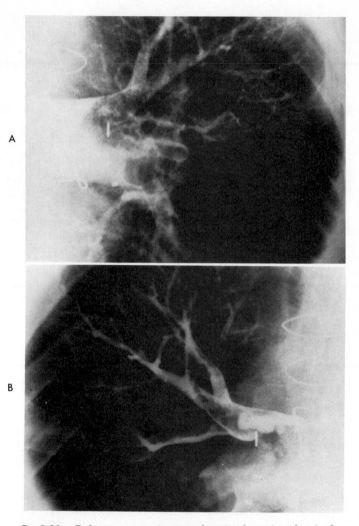

Fig. 5-28.   Pulmonary arteriogram showing large intraluminal filling defects of pulmonary embolus within pulmonary arteries. **A,** Left upper lobe; **B,** Right middle and upper lobe.

[just below the T_{12} ribs].) Selective renal arterial injections provide the most detail. The LAO projection often provides the best view of the renal artery ostia in a majority of patients. Acutely angled takeoffs of the renal artery may require specially shaped catheters or a brachial arterial approach from above. Atherosclerotic disease of the renal artery usually involves the proximal one-third of the renal artery and is seldom present without abdominal atherosclerotic plaques. A renal artery stenosis alone is rarely the sole determinant for surgery or angioplasty. Refractory hypertension and determination of the renin-angiotensin levels are usually the indicators for an interventional (angioplasty) procedure. Renal artery fibromuscular dysplasia may occur and appear as atherosclerotic disease. This finding is often present in middle-age women with other vessels involved, most commonly cerebral or visceral arteries. The proximal one-third of the main renal artery is usually free of disease with distal involvement, unlike that of atherosclerotic narrowing.

Angiography of the Thoracic and Abdominal Aorta

Aortography is indicated for suspected aneurysms or dissections, by clinical, historical, or procedural signs. Injection techniques are the same as for ascending aortography. Evaluation of peripherial lower extremity disease requires identification of iliac bifuration and common femoral artery patency before subselective injections.

Angiography of Lower Extremities (Figs. 5-29 to 5-31)

Based on clinical signs and symptoms of arterial insufficiency to the legs, suspected obstructions of vessel are screened with echo-Doppler before angiography is performed. Small-diameter (5 French) catheters are satisfactory. Reduced volumes of contrast (10 to 20 ml over 1 to 2 seconds) are injected during filming with panning down the artery, following the course to the most distal locations. Angulated views may be necessary to open bifurcations and overlying vessels that obscure the vessel origin. When possible, angiographic filming should extend, at least to the ankle. Long cut-films that cover the entire lower extremity on a moving table are available in radiologic suites. In cardiac catheterization laboratories, cineangiographic filming with prolonged filming and panning down to the ankle must be tested before obtaining final views. Digital subtraction techniques are available commonly in many modern laboratories. Nonionic contrast agents are less painful for peripheral vascular angiography as compared to ionic contrast agents.

The area most frequently involved in peripheral athero-

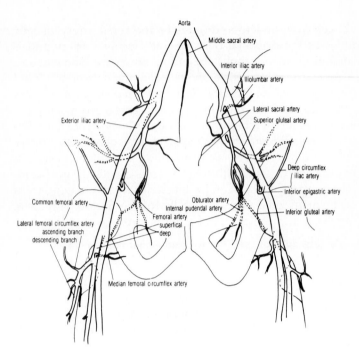

Fig. 5-29. Pelvic and proximal femoral arterial branches. (From Johnsrude IS, Jackson DC, Dunnick NR: *A practical approach to angiography*, ed 2, Boston, 1987, Little, Brown.)

sclerotic disease involves the distal superficial femoral artery at the abductor canal (Fig. 5-32). One major challenge encountered with femoral-iliac angiography is the contralateral (opposite leg) approach over the aortic bifurcation of the iliac vessels. To enter the opposite iliac artery, often a right Judkins or internal mammary artery graft catheter (see Chapter 2) is selected and advanced with a guidewire over the bifurcation and down into the opposite femoral artery. The wire is passed down into the selected artery. The catheter may be advanced and exchanged (over a long 300-cm wire) for an appropriate angiographic or balloon dilatation catheter, as required. The calf, tibial, and knee (popliteal) arteries are the next most commonly involved vessels after the superficial femoral artery. Disease in the deep femoral artery (femoral profunda) is rare. Pathways of collateralization are often rich and varied in patients with chronic distal femoral artery

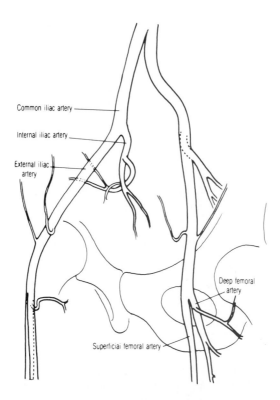

Common iliac artery

Internal iliac artery

External iliac artery

Deep femoral artery

Superficial femoral artery

Fig. 5-30. The right common iliac and left common femoral bifurcation are better seen in the right posterior oblique projection. The origin of the left deep femoral artery branch (profunda femoris) may be hidden on the anterioposterior projection. (From Johnsrude IS, Jackson DC, Dunnick NR: *A practical approach to angiography*, ed 2, Boston, 1987, Little, Brown.)

disease, especially in total occlusions of the superficial femoral artery that reconstitutes at or below the knee, close to the branching trifurcation of the tibial and deep peroneal arteries.

SECTION III: THE X-RAY IMAGE
GENERATION OF THE X-RAY IMAGE

Cardiac angiography uses a complex interaction of radiographic x-ray elements, transforming energy into a visual image. The x-ray image generation chain can be simplified

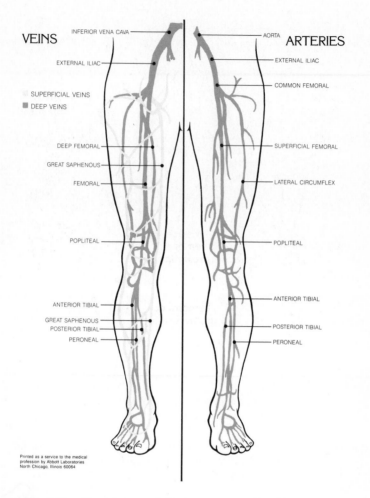

Fig. 5-31.   Vasculature of the lower extremity. (Courtesy of Abbott Laboratories, North Chicago, IL.)

into three major components: (1) the x-ray generator; (2) the x-ray tube; and (3) the image intensifier (Fig. 5-33). The details of x-ray equipment should be familiar to all personnel working in the catheterization laboratory.

X-Ray Generator

The generator provides the power source necessary to accelerate the electrons through the x-ray tube. The duration of x-ray exposure is similar to the shutter speed on a regular

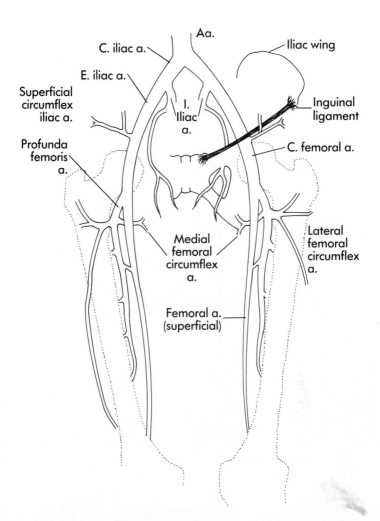

Fig. 5-32. Normal anatomy of the femoral artery, its branches, the distal runoff arteries, and the potential collateral vessels. Aa, aorta; a, artery; I, internal; C, common; E, external.

camera. During the cardiac "photographic" examination the exposure usually is set fast enough to stop blurring as a result of heart movement. During selective coronary arteriography, the shorter the exposure time, the better the image. Exposure times of 3 to 6 ms reduce "movement blur." Most modern generators are capable of delivering adequate power while

THE CINE RADIOGRAPHIC SYSTEM

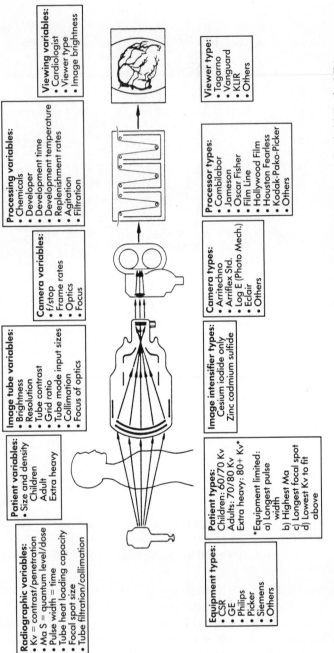

Radiographic variables:
- Kv = contrast/penetration
- Ma S = quantum level/dose
- Pulse width = time
- Tube heat loading capacity
- Focal spot size
- Tube filtration/collimation

Patient variables:
- Size and density
  - Children
  - Adult
  - Extra heavy

Image tube variables:
- Brightness
- Resolution
- Tube contrast
- Grid ratio
- Tube mode input sizes
- Collimation
- Focus of optics

Camera variables:
- f/stop
- Frame rates
- Optics
- Focus

Processing variables:
- Chemicals
- Developer
- Development time
- Development temperature
- Replenishment rates
- Agitation
- Filtration

Viewing variables:
- Cardiologist
- Viewer type
- Image brightness

Equipment types:
- CSR
- GE
- Philips
- Picker
- Siemens
- Others

Patient types:
- Children: 60/70 Kv
- Adults: 70/80 Kv
- Extra heavy: 80+ Kv*

*Equipment limited:
  a) Longest pulse width
  b) Highest Ma
  c) Longest focal spot
  d) Lowest Kv to fit above

Image intensifier types:
- Cesium iodide only
- Zinc cadmium sulfide

Camera types:
- Arritechno
- Arriflex Std.
- Log E (Photo Mech.)
- Eclair
- Others

Processor types:
- Combilabor
- Jameson
- Oscar Fisher
- Film Line
- Hollywood Film
- Houston Fearless
- Kodak-Pako-Picker
- Others

Viewer type:
- Tagarno
- Vanguard
- KLIR
- Others

Fig. 5-33. Schematic diagram of an x-ray system. (Courtesy of Cinerex, Inc., Ridgefield Park, NJ.)

providing precise and automatically adjusted exposure timing. Current generators are equipped with either multiple phase (alternating on/off) or short/long pulse widths that are automatically adjusted for correct exposure. Manual settings, which are operator selected, are limited to film frame rates (e.g., 30 to 60 frames/sec).

X-Ray Tubes

The function of the x-ray tube is to convert electrical energy, provided from the generator, to an x-ray beam. Electrons emitted from a heated filament (cathode) are accelerated toward a rapidly rotating disc (anode) and at contact undergo conversion to x-radiation (Fig. 5-34). This process generates extreme heat. The heat capacity of an x-ray tube is a major limiting factor in the design of x-ray tubes. Only 0.2% to

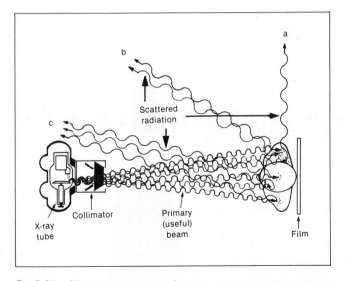

Fig. 5-34.   X-ray generation and scatter radiation. The radiographer receives the least amount of scattered radiation by standing at right angles to the scattering object (the patient), in position *a*. The most scattered radiation is recieved at point *c* because of backscatter coming from the patient. (From Statkiewicz MA, Ritenour ER: *Radiation protection for student radiographers,* Denver, 1983, Multi-Media Publishing, p 170.)

0.6% of the electric energy provided to the tube eventually is converted to x-rays.

In addition to the exposure times (controlled by the generator system) and the size of the imaging field (controlled by the x-ray tube), two other factors of the x-ray determine the quality of x-ray for proper image exposures:

1. *Electrical current (mA)*—(Fig. 5-35) the number of photons (electrical particles) generated per unit of time. The greater the electrical current the greater the number of photons, resulting in improved image resolution. If the photon volume is marginal the resulting image may be "mottled" or have a spotty appearance. Increasing the milliamperage will improve this result, but the level of milliamperage is limited by the heat capacity of the x-

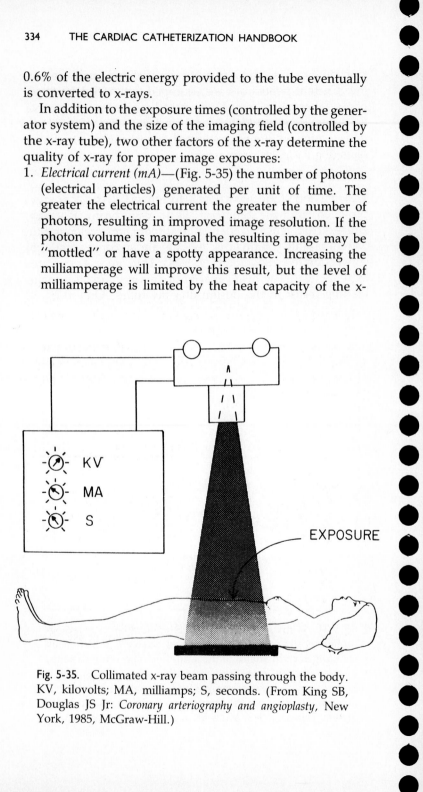

Fig. 5-35.   Collimated x-ray beam passing through the body. KV, kilovolts; MA, milliamps; S, seconds. (From King SB, Douglas JS Jr: *Coronary arteriography and angioplasty*, New York, 1985, McGraw-Hill.)

ray tubes. Also, increasing the number of milliamperes markedly increases radiation exposure and scatter to patient and catheterization personnel.

2. *The level of kilovoltage (kV)*—the energy spectrum (wavelengths) of the x-ray beam. The higher the level of kilovoltage the shorter the wavelength of radiation and the greater the ability of x-rays to penetrate target tissue. Increased kilovoltage is especially important in obese patients. In order to obtain better images through more tissue, a higher kilovolt level is required. Unfortunately, a high kilovolt level also will produce lower resolution because of wide scatter. There is also greater radiation exposure to patients and laboratory personnel. Modern radiographic equipment currently allows for variability of the amperage and voltage to attain optimal quality radiographic images. Results of using high kilovoltage are shown in the box above.

An automatic exposure control system sets exposure times by utilizing computers to incorporate changes in voltage, amperage, and exposure times, providing the desired images at the best exposures possible.

Results of High Kilovolt Exposure

THE OPTIMUM RADIOGRAPHIC TECHNIQUE

Lowest kilovoltage for penetration
Highest milliamperage for lowest tube heat

HIGH KILOVOLTAGE YIELDS

Low dose to patient
More mottle
More scatter
More contrast
More operator dose
REMEMBER: Kilovolts plus milliamperes vary inversely
Kilovoltage has greater effect on contrast than milliamperage
Tube heat is less with higher kilovoltage techniques
FOR EXAMPLE:

70 kV @	Settings of	80 kV @
400 mA =	equal density =	200 mA
× 5 sec	on film	× 5 sec
140 heat units		80 heat units

> EFFECT OF KILOVOLTS ON CINEANGIOGRAPHIC IMAGE:
>
> Increased kilovolts, high energy, short wavelength, uniform penetration—all images tend to become gray at high kilovoltage
> Decreased kilovoltage, discriminates among densities, provides contrast

Image Intensifier (Fig. 5-36)

After the x-rays have penetrated the body the partially absorbed beams are cast in a shadow fashion on the input screen of the image intensifier. The image intensifier converts the invisible x-ray image into a visual image. Image intensifiers are equipped with different-sized image fields that alter the image resolution. In general, the smaller the input screen diameter, the smaller the image field size and the sharper the resolution. Smaller input screen diameters (5- to 7-inch screens) are better suited for selective coronary cineangiography because of their enhanced resolution. For more detailed work, such as percutaneous transluminal coronary angioplasty, even smaller input diameter (4-inch) screens are particularly useful. In contrast, large-screen (or field) examinations (i.e., left ventriculography, aortography, or peripheral angiography) use input screen diameters of 9 to 11 inches. The trade-off, of course, is that detailed resolution is impaired.

Image Distortion

Magnification (Fig. 5-37). The x-ray image casts an x-ray shadow onto the input screen of the image intensifier. The distance of the object from the screen produces an image that may be either sharp or indistinct, depending on the distance. Fig. 5-37 displays the effect of the object-screen distance on image quality. When an object is held close to the surface on which the shadow falls, the image is sharp. The farther the object moves away from this surface, the larger and more indistinct the image becomes. When the image intensifier is closest to the chest wall and the heart, the image obtained is sharp. When the heart lies far away from the image intensifier, and closer to the x-ray source, the image is magnified, but poorly defined. Increasing the distance of the heart to the image intensifier also requires more kilovoltage, thereby further reducing image quality.

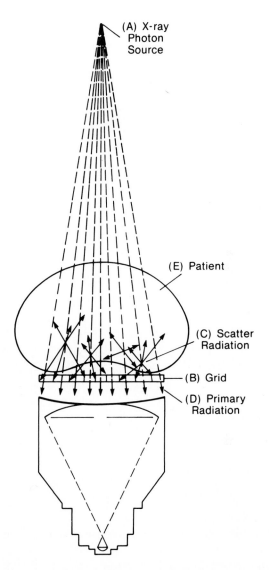

Fig. 5-36. The grid on the image intensifier aligns the beams. **A,** X-ray photon source; **B,** grid; **C,** scatter radiation; **D,** primary radiation; **E,** patient. Scatter radiation is reduced by grid in front of image intensifier. (From King SB, Douglas JS Jr: *Coronary arteriography and angioplasty*, New York, 1985.)

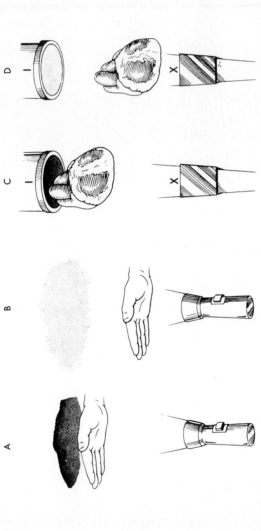

Fig. 5-37. Image magnification. **A,** When a hand is held close to the surface on which the shadow falls, the image is sharp. **B,** The farther the hand moves from this surface, the larger and "fuzzier" the image becomes. **C,** When the image intensifier (I) is close to the chest wall and the heart, the image obtained is sharp. **D,** When the heart lies farther from the image intensifier and close to the x-ray source (X), the image is magnified but poorly defined and hazy. Increased x-ray source-to-image distances require more kilovoltage, also degrading the image. (From King SB, Douglas JS Jr: *Coronary arteriography and angioplasty,* New York, 1985, McGraw-Hill.)

Foreshortening.   Distortion of the object's perspective is called *foreshortening*. Fig. 5-38 displays the effects of the shadow cast by an object such as a pencil that has a concentric narrowing (like an artery stenosis) in the middle portion. The foreshortening (change of true length) of the pencil changes

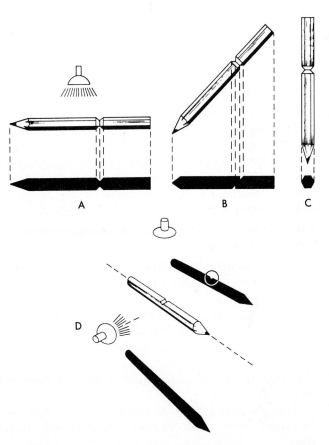

Fig. 5-38.   **A–C,** Foreshortening of the shadow of an object is not parallel with the filming plane. **D,** In order to evaluate accurately a slitlike lesion, it is necessary to use a view perpendicular to the longitudinal axis of the vessel but parallel to the longest diameter of the lesion. (From Pujadas G: *Coronary angiography in the medical and surgical treatment of ischemic heart disease,* New York, 1980, McGraw-Hill.)

depending on the axis in relation to the beam of the x-ray. When the pencil's long axis is perpendicular to the film plane (parallel to the x-ray beam), all contour details are lost and the shadow is seen as a dot. When the longitudinal axis is seen at an oblique angle, there is foreshortening of the length shadow, and when it is perpendicular to the x-ray beam (parallel to the film plane), there is a full and true image of the length and contour details. Because of foreshortening, arterial lesions that may appear severe in one projection may not appear at all or seem significantly less severe in other projections. For this reason multiple projections are used to identify the severity of lesions within the coronary tree.

Videotape Monitors and Recorders

A videotape recorder is used in combination with the angiographic system monitors to record the fluoroscopic images so that they can be rapidly reviewed and information will not be lost should something happen to the cineangiographic film. These video recorders commonly use $\frac{1}{2}$- to 1-inch tape. Newer laboratories also will use digital cardiac imaging to review angiographic data before a case is finished.

X-Ray System Preparations by the Angiographic Nurse/ Technician/Assistant

The cineangiography preparations include establishing a checklist sequence of steps from x-ray generation to film viewing.

A daily check of the x-ray unit should be performed by a staff member first thing each morning. The following is a list of parameters that need to be checked before the start of a case:

1. Unit powers up and makes fluoroscopic and cineangiographic exposures.
2. A short cineangiographic test strip of a resolution phantom should be run to check resolution of known mm line pairs.
3. TV monitor screens are cleaned. Contrast and brightness controls are adjusted to optimum.
4. Fluoroscopic timers are reset to zero.
5. Proper exposure station is selected for first case.
6. Kilovoltage and milliamperage levels (minimums and maximums) are set if the unit allows.

7. Before the start of each case, an adequate amount of film should be in the camera.

TECHNICAL NOTES: During the case the angiographic technician may be responsible for the angulation of the image intensifier and panning. In some institutions the physician may perform this function. The staff should be aware of the following principles in order to obtain optimum cineangiograms:

1. A patient name plate picture should be taken at the start of each case. The name plate should contain the patient's name, ID number, date, institution, and catheterization room number. The catheterization room number helps identify the room should the images look less than optimum or a repeat study with the same equipment be needed (for research). The name plate should be shot before the arterial puncture, thus assuring that the cineangiographic unit is working properly.

2. The image intensifier should be as close to the patient's chest as possible. This optimizes the image and decreases scatter radiation.

3. The patient should be instructed to take a deep breath before the start of the cineangiographic camera. This pulls the diaphragm downward, out of the field of view. During a deep breath the x-ray exposure changes automatically (automatic brightness control). The presence of the dense diaphragmatic image in the field can cause poor quality images. It is helpful if a staff member practices breath holding technique with the patient before the start of the case.

4. All electrocardiographic electrodes, metal snaps on patient's gown, electrocardiographic lead wires, etc., should be out of the field of view before the start of the procedure. Keeping the lines from hanging down under the table will prevent the x-ray tube from pulling out a lead or IV tube.

5. Use of the collimator (shutters) should be mandatory. Focus on the exact area of interest to be photographed. This technique will eliminate unwanted lung field brightness and will help optimize exposure parameters of the automatic brightness control system in the x-ray system.

6. During the cineangiograms, the staff member responsible for data recording should note the following information:
   a. Time of each contrast injection.
   b. The projection angulation of the cineangiographic unit (right or left obliques and the degree of cranial/caudal angulation). Most x-ray units have a digital readout for these angulations. A log sheet such as the one shown in Appendix I will aid in the recording of these projections.
   c. The type and French size of the catheter used for each angiogram.
   d. Record the names and dosages of any drugs that are given during the procedure. If drugs that affect coronary dilatation or constriction are given during the angiogram procedure, this should be recorded on the film with a lead letter marker.
   e. If an LV angiographic volume is to be calculated, a grid* is filmed to calculate a correction factor for ventricular volume analysis. The nurse/technician must record certain data during the ventriculogram that is necessary for grid and image intensifier placement. These data include (1) the position of the image intensifier in relation to the x-ray table top at the time of the left ventriculogram; (2) measurement of the patient's AP diameter so that grid placement can approximate the position of the left ventricle during the angiogram; and (3) if a dual or trimode (4-, 6-, or 9-inch) image intensifier is used, the image intensifier magnification for each angiogram.

Film Processing

In many laboratories film processing is done by the radiologic technologist or the laboratory technicians. Some laboratories cross-train all staff members (RNs or LPNs) to process film. Film processing is a precise procedure that requires attention to details to obtain an optimum result. Film transport speed, chemistry, temperature, and processor cleanliness all must be monitored and maintained in order to assure quality im-

---

* A grid is a series of 1-cm squares imbedded in plastic, which is used to calibrate an area on a cineangiogram.

ages. The most expensive, finely tuned x-ray equipment cannot produce good images if poor technique is used in film processing. Therefore, all persons processing film need a basic understanding of the film processor, while at least one staff member must be well versed in all aspects of photographic principles. The following steps should be performed in order to process high-quality cineangiograms.

Establish quality control.   The film should be sensitized by use of a sensitometer at the start of each day. The film should then be processed using the same parameters that have been established by the laboratory. These parameters are film transport speed, developer/fixer temperature, and replenishment rates. The densities of the processed test strip are then read and plotted on a graph that is compared to the previous day's readings. Certain standards for film speed, contrast, and base plus fog should be established for each laboratory. If the densities are outside the acceptable window, the processing parameters must be reexamined.

Troubleshoot quality control to identify factors that may adversely affect processing the factors include the following:

1. Inadequate chemical replenishment, causing *light* underdeveloped films
2. Overreplenishment of chemicals causing *dark* overdeveloped films
3. Low temperature of developing solution causing *light* underdeveloped films
4. High temperature of developing solution, causing *dark* overdeveloped films
5. Film transport speed out of calibration
6. Dirty solution tanks/dirty transport rollers causing fogged or scratched film

Imaging equipment preventive maintenance.   The x-ray unit should be placed on a scheduled preventive maintenance program performed by trained service technicians. This should be done at least biannually, with quarterly checks preferred. Maintenance and cleaning schedules should be monitored by the staff so that equipment can be scheduled for routine maintenance (see the boxes on p. 344).

Cineangiographic film projector.   Differences among projectors rarely affect image quality, but a difficult or malfunctioning machine makes film evaluation unpleasant for staff physicians and families.

Optimizing Cineangiographic Techniques

1. Cleaning image chain is important (at least every 1 to 2 months):
   a. Clean cineangiographic camera mirror and lenses
   b. Clean projector lenses, mirrors (every 2 months)
2. Check the following cineangiographic optic chain:
   a. Cineangiographic lens focus tight
   b. f-stop correct (no role in resolution because flat plane)
   c. Focus image on plane of image intensifier
   d. Film magazines secured tightly
3. Cineangiographic film: correct for changing technique if new angiographic equipment installed
4. Processor: fast enough for rapid processing for interventional (PTCA) procedures when problems need angiographic review
5. Dark room operator: cross trained for back-up staffing
6. Photographic chemistry: corrected for film and techniques
7. Quality control:
   a. Daily, weekly, monthly
   b. Single technician job for high level of reproducibility

Preventive Maintenance Scheduling for Imaging Equipment

DAILY

Clean TV monitor screen.
Clean projector screens.
Monitor densitometer results.
Run a daily cineangiographic of resolution phantom and check line pairs visible.

WEEKLY

Clean lenses on cineangiographic projectors.
Clean film debris from cineangiographic camera.
Check lens on cineangiographic camera and clean as needed.
Clean film processor.
Change tapes on videotape decks.
Clean heads on videotape decks.

There are two types of cineangiographic projectors:
1. Intermittent claw-driven or belt-driven type (Vanguard)
   a. Sharpest images
   b. Good light source for distant projection
   c. Variable speeds (mostly 1 or 2)

 d. Noisy motor (consideration for conferences)
 e. Hard to thread
2. Rotating prism type (CAP 12, General Electric, Siemens, Tagarno)
 a. Dust accumulation that dulls image—needs periodic cleaning
 b. Low light collection
 c. Highly variable speed
 d. Quiet operation
 e. Easy to load

DIGITAL ANGIOGRAPHY (Fig. 5-39)

The objective of digital angiography is to convert the x-ray image into a quantitative format for storage on a computer. Digital angiography stores x-ray images on magnetic tapes, disks, or other electronic media rather than on x-ray film.

Advantages

It is possible to acquire useful arterial images with much smaller amounts of contrast than with film angiography and to store and analyze images in a more quantitative fashion. In addition, the digital approach allows the performance of a number of manipulations on the stored images. The contrast image can be amplified or enhanced. One image can be subtracted from another and then that image can be subtracted from a third image. Digital image manipulations allow many views that are not possible with film radiograms.

Disadvantages

Digital angiography systems may not provide the exquisite detail found in radiographic films. Moreover, the digital subtraction procedure is very sensitive to motion. It often requires a patient who is alert and aware of what is going on and who can cooperate during the procedure.

Digital (Subtraction) Angiography System (Fig. 5-40)

There are two types of digital subtraction angiography systems.

Pulsed system. The pulsed system acquires images relatively infrequently. One image per second with a 512×512 digital matrix is a typical acquisition rate. Some systems may indicate that five to ten images per second can be acquired.

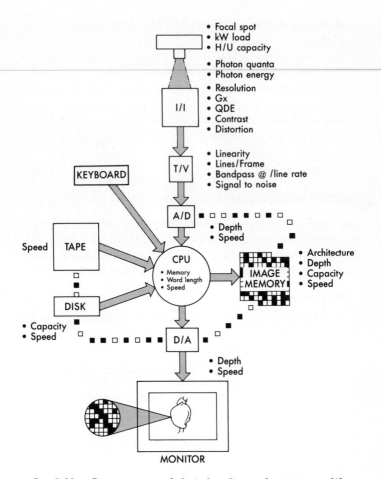

Fig. 5-39. Components of digital radiography system. *I/I,* image intensifier; *T/V,* television converter; *A/D,* analog-to-digital signal converter; *CPU,* central processing unit; *D/A,* digital-to-analog signal converter.

(Cineangiographic filming acquisition rates are >30 frames/ sec.)

Pulsed systems require special TV cameras. Pulsing requires high-powered, three-phase, 12-pulse x-ray generators. They operate by pulsing the generator at high-milliamperage currents, which provides a heavy burst of x-ray energy to the image intensifier, in an attempt to obtain

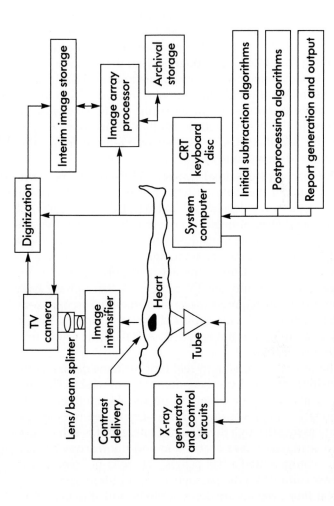

Fig. 5-40. Components required for digital subtraction angiography. CRT, cathode ray tube. (From Schroeder JS: *Invasive cardiology*, Philadelphia, 1985, Davis.)

sharp images. A single image is scanned by the TV camera, which overcomes the blurring of the x-ray image. Images are stored until after the run is complete.

Once the run is complete the operator retrieves these images and subtracts them from each other. Image acquisition runs must begin several seconds before the contrast media is due to arrive at the anatomical region of interest and must continue long enough so that the operator can be certain that a person with slow circulation has passed all the contrast media through the region of interest. The unopacified image (mask) is subtracted from the images with the contrast in the vessels with a resultant image remaining of only the opacified vessel without interference from other structures such as bones.

Fluoroscopic (real-time) system.   The second type of system is called a real-time system. These systems operate at fluoroscopic x-ray levels and normal TV frame rates (30 frames/sec). They normally do not require a special TV camera, and fluoroscopic milliamperage levels from 5 to 20 mA produce quite satisfactory imaging. The milliamperage required will depend upon the age and performance of the image intensifier and the TV camera. A three-phase x-ray generator is not required. Because of the fluoroscopic x-ray requirements, and unlike pulsed systems, special heavy-duty x-ray tubes are not required. A 300,000 heat unit tube is quite satisfactory.

The image processing in real-time systems occurs as the acquisition run (and the examination) progresses. The subtracted image can be observed on the TV monitor as the examination is proceeding. This ability to see the contrast agent passing through the region of interest allows the operator to terminate image acquisition and fluoroscopy as soon as the contrast media has passed. There is no need to run on past contrast media passage as with pulsed systems.

Real-time systems are designed to be added to most fluoroscopic x-ray generators. Real-time systems have the ability to do subtraction angiography with IV injection for primary and secondary arteries (peripheral vessels only). To visualize tertiary and very small vessels, intraarterial catheterization often is required.

Other Digital Angiographic System Capabilities (Figs. 5-41 and 5-42)

Vascular tracing.   A procedure called *vascular tracing,* or *road mapping,* often is provided in digital angiographic systems. After arterial injection of small amounts of contrast material the vascular tracing function will "remember" the path of the contrast media as it travels through the arteries. As the contrast media travels down the artery, it traces out the path of the entire arterial system in that area. Once the digital trace is complete a "hardcopy" (photograph or print) can be made, or it can be subtracted from an image with no contrast media in it. The major value of this technique for relatively stationary vascular anatomy is in "runoff" studies for detecting blood clots or blockages in the legs or arms.

Digital fluoroscopy aids.   Many digital angiographic systems utilize functions of the image processor during fluoroscopy, when subtraction angiography is not being performed. One of these functions is image noise reduction during fluoroscopy by integrating several successive frames. Another is "last image hold," which allows the operator to retain the last image displayed on the monitor each time the fluoroscopic foot switch is released.

Another capability is *electronic radiogaphy.* This turns the x-rays on just long enough for the system to acquire and freeze an image and then automatically turns the x-rays off again. This is similar to spot-filming with the fluoroscope. One other function that can be provided during normal fluoroscopy is contrast enhancement.

Quantitative Coronary Angiography

The degree of coronary stenosis is quantitated from the cineangiogram and, in clincial practice, is usually a visual estimation of the percentage of diameter narrowing using the presumed proximal normal arterial segment and the ratio of normal diameters to stenosis diameters. This technique is widely applicable in clinical practice but is inadequate for the quantitative methodology done in most research studies. The intraobserver variability may range between 40% and 80%, and there is frequently as wide as 20% range on interobserver differences. Quantitative methodology uses digital

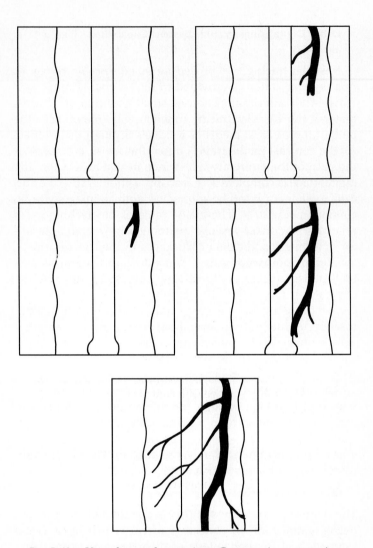

Fig. 5-41. Vascular road mapping. Contrast is progressing through arteries in the thigh. The computer using digital angiography "remembers" the path traveled, even after dye has passed.

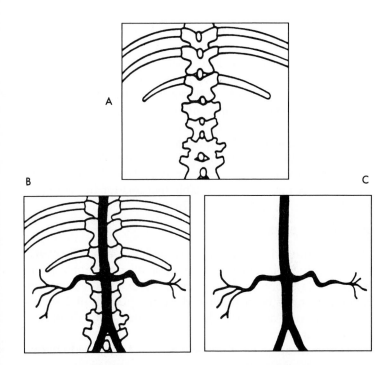

Fig. 5-42. Subtraction imaging. **A,** Image prior to arrival of contrast in artery. **B,** Image with contrast in artery. **C,** Image **A** subtracted from image **B.**

calipers or automated or manual edge detection systems. Densitometric analysis with digital angiography also provides quantitative lesion measurements.

COMPARISON OF CONVENTIONAL ANGIOGRAPHY AND SUBTRACTION

Because contrast media tend to dilute rapidly after their injection, conventional angiography normally places small amounts of contrast material in a specific problematic circulatory region. A large number of x-ray pictures are taken in a short period of time.

Because the human body contains bones and other dense structures, it is sometimes difficult to observe blood vessels even when they are filled with contrast agents.

Conventional angiographers have therefore found it useful to compare radiographs taken before blood carrying a contrast agent arrives at a given point and after contrast-carrying blood arrives in that vessel.

Techniques were developed to subtract the earlier (non–contrast-enhanced) radiograph from the later (containing contrast) radiograph and thereby obtain a composite picture showing only the contrast-filled blood vessels or structures in question. These subtacting procedures are now widely available and have proved to be valuable in diagnosing many disorders of the circulatory system. A comparison of advantages and other available features for three angiographic imaging techniques is shown in Table 5-5.

RADIATION SAFETY

Radiation protection equipment should be available in every cardiac catheterization laboratory for all personnel. Standards for radiation protection in the cardiac catheterization laboratory have been published by the Society of Cardiac Angiography. Four principles in radiation safety should be self-evident:

1. The less exposure, the less chance of absorbed-energy biologic interaction.
2. No known level of ionizing radiation is a permissible dose or absolutely safe.

TABLE 5-5. Comparison of angiographic imaging techniques

	Cut-film changer	35-mm cineangiography	Digital subtraction
Resolution	++++	++	+++
Field of view	++++	++	++
Magnification	+++	+	++
Ease of use	+	+++	++
Flexibility for intervention	−	+++	+++
Panning	−	+++	−
Video replay	−	++	++
Contrast volume used	+++	++	+/−
Postprocessing facility	−	−	++
High-density resolution	++	+	+++
Radiation	+++	++	+

+, Present and comparative value; ++++, highest value or easiest to use; −, feature not present.

3. Radiation exposure is cumulative. There is no washout phenomenon.
4. All participants in the cardiac catheterization laboratory have voluntarily accepted some degree of radiation exposure, but they are obliged to minimize and reduce risks to other personnel and themselves.

The source of radiation in the cardiac catheterization laboratory is the primary x-ray beam emanating from the undertable tube upward and outward toward the image intensifier. Scatter of this beam exposes all subjects to radiation in a dose geometrically inverse to the distance from the source. Radiation scatter is increased when the angle of the tube is set obliquely. A high degree of angulation with large obliquities increases the amount of radiation scatter (Fig. 5-43). Acrylic lead shields and lead table mounted aprons should be used to reduce the amount of scatter.

Fluoroscopy generates x-ray approximately one-fifth that of cineangiography. The increased use of cineangiography for complex catheterization procedures has increased the total exposure to radiation and should be a consideration in procedures requiring extensive intracardiac manipulation such as angioplasty or valvuloplasty.

Personal Radiation Protection (see Chapter 1)

Personal protection from radiation should include eye protection. Physicians performing caridac angiography with U-arm systems should be protected by room-installed radiation shields. The exposure with a shield resulting from performing 25 examinations per week on a continuous basis will be within the recommendations of the National Commission on Radiologic Protection and Units.

Radiation exposure is greater during angioplasty than during diagnostic catheterization. If the protective shields are employed carefully the radiation exposure for single- and double-vessel angioplasty as compared to diagnostic catheterization may be comparable. However, it should be understood that radiation exposures are generally higher for these procedures, especially when biplane angiography is performed.

During angiographic studies, 90% of the x-ray energy entering the body is absorbed. It has been shown that a single

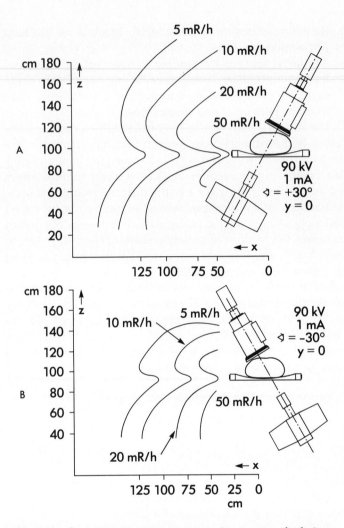

Fig. 5-43.   Isoexposure curves representing ranges of relative exposure in the position usually occupied by the operator performing an angiographic procedure from the right arm. **A,** 30° left anterior oblique. **B,** 30° right anterior oblique. (From Balter S, Sones FM, Brancato R: Radiation exposure to the operator preforming cardiac angiography with U-arm systems, *Circulation* 58(5):925, 1978.)

exposure of 200 R can produce cataract formation in humans. Thyroid cancers and other carcinomas are associated with x-rays. Ironically, techniques often used to improve image quality (i.e., increased mA, kV, LAO views, and the like) have resulted in increased exposure.

Radiation During Catheterization

RADIATION TO PATIENT

From the primary x-ray beam
Affects thyroid, eyes, gonads, bone marrow, or tract
Highest exposure of any diagnostic test

RADIATION TO STAFF

Chronic low dose from scatter, tube leakage
Affects thyroid and eyes
Accepted occupational exposure

LIMIT DOSE BY

Maintain equipment safeguards
Optimize milliamperage and kilovoltage
Minimize exposure time
Minimize scatter with shielding and techniques
Employ all protective measures

A summary of radiation safety for the cardiac catheterization laboratory is provided in the box on page 355 and reviewed in Chapter 1 in the "Radiation Safety" section, beginning on page 36.

SECTION IV: ANGIOGRAPHIC EQUIPMENT AND SUPPLIES
INJECTORS AND CONTRAST MATERIALS (Fig. 5-44)

The angiographic power injector allows the angiographer to administer a precise volume (bolus) of contrast at a rapid preset flow rate.

High-quality power injectors are necessary for performing either conventional or digital angiography. The injector accepts a large syringe for radiographic contrast media. The power injector settings are selected and upon receiving an electronic signal an accurately calibrated motor discharges

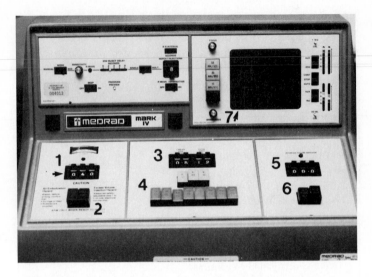

Fig. 5-44. Close-up of contrast power injector. *1*, Setting for total volume injected. *2*, Setting for arming the device. *3*, Rate of rise setting and flow rate. *4*, Pressure setting. *5*, Interface. *6*, Single or multiple injections. *7*, The synchronizing system for electrocardiographic injection.

the contrast material at the predetermined rate through a connecting tube and into the catheter. The quantity and type of contrast material, concentration or dilution, and rate of injection are selected by the operator-physician. Normally, the signal to the injector to begin contrast injection is received from a technician.

Bolus contrast injections for visualization of the left ventricle, PA, aorta, or other heart chamber require from 30 to 60 ml of contrast to be delivered at flow rates of 15 to 30 ml/sec. The power injector is capable of pushing the contrast through the catheter at rapid flow rates under varying degrees of pressure.

Responsibilities of the Nurse/Technician

1. Load the syringe with contrast media.
2. Set the volume, flow rate, and rate of pressure rise parameters as instructed by the physician.
3. Press the inject button that triggers the injection.

Power injection. The staff member must be aware of the following points in order to provide technical assistance in angiographic procedures requiring power injection.

Clear air bubbles. All air must be expelled from the contrast-filled syringe prior to making the injector available to the physician for the catheter connection. Under no circumstances should the head of the power injector be tilted toward the catheterization table or made available for the physician if air is in the syringe.

There are several techniques used to establish an air-free system when connecting the catheter to the syringe. A "running connection" is a technique where the injector operator squirts a small amount of contrast out of the syringe while the catheter is being connected to the syringe. Merging of the streams of blood from the catheter and the forward flow of contrast from the syringe prevents any air bubbles from entering the system upon connection. After connection the injector operator always will aspirate fluid into the syringe to assure that there are no air bubbles present. If air is present, expel the air and start the clearing procedure over.

One must be careful when aspirating blood into the contrast syringe for two reasons: (1) a large blood volume in the syringe will dilute the contrast; and (2) more important, the blood may cause clot formation in the injector syringe. There have been rare reports of clot formation when nonionic contrast is used.

Test injection in ventricle. Once the system is free of air, the injector operator and the physician should be sure that the catheter is cleared of blood if an aspiration technique has been used. To accomplish this, the injector operator should squirt a small amount of contrast out the tip of the catheter under x-ray visualization. This small test injection of contrast also helps the physician ascertain proper catheter position.

Confirm injector settings. The physician should verbally confirm the power injector settings for the contrast volume and delivery rate desired. The injector operator should *repeat* the injection parameters back to the physician to eliminate any chance of error in injector set up.

Depending on the type of injector being used the flow rate may be determined by setting an amount in milliliters per second or by setting the pressure. Regardless of the system the staff member must make sure that the catheter being used can accept the flow rate that has been dialed into the injector.

Safety features.   Once the physician has initiated a cine-angiographic run the injector operator must listen for the physician's command to start the injection. The nurse/technician should be prepared to stop the injection (by hitting or releasing the correct button) at any time as directed by the physician or his own discretion (e.g., when the catheter is pulled back).

NOTE: All personnel should be watching the power injection setup and injections looking for small bubbles or other problems. Six eyes are better than four for seeing catheterization laboratory problems.

Power injectors have many safety features that must be known by the staff of the cardiac catheterization laboratory. Understanding all aspects of the operation of the power injector and the built-in safeguards is required to ensure patient safety during angiography.

Contrast Media

The nurse/technician provides the technical support with regard to contrast media during angiography in the following areas.

The setup for administration of contrast media during angiography is the responsibility of the staff of the catheterization laboratory.

Contrast agents should be warmed to body temperature before administration. Commerical warmers are available from the companies that manufacture contrast. A warm water bath is sometimes used to warm contrast, but temperature control is difficult to regulate.

The nurse/technician preparing the patient for angiography should (again) ask the patient if he is aware of any known contrast allergy. Iodine gives contrast its radiopaque qualities and is a known allergen. If there is a history of iodine or seafood allergy (iodine is found in certain seafoods, especially shellfish), the physician should be notified. The physician may wish to give corticosteroids and/or antihistamines before performing angiography (see Chapter 1).

Before the administration of contrast agents the patient should be prepared as to what sensations are associated with contrast administration. Some patients experience nausea and vomiting. Therefore the patient should not have ingested food or water before angiography. If vomiting occurs, the staff member should be quick to respond; the patient's head should be turned down and to the side to prevent aspiration. This is particularly important in patients that have been sedated heavily for the procedure. The newer low-osmolality and nonionic contrast agents produce less nausea and vomiting.

Patients should also be instructed that they may experience a hot flushing sensation (caused by artery vasodilation) during bolus injections of contrast media. Again, this sensation has been reduced with the use of nonionic contrast agents. Direct injection of ionic contrast into peripheral vessels produces a painful burning and cramping sensation of the injected area. The nonionic/low-osmolar agents are highly recommended for peripheral vascular angiography.

During angiography, it is important for the nurse to document the type and amount of contrast delivered. The patient should be observed for any signs of allergy such as hives, flushed skin, bronchospasm, or laryngeal edema (hoarseness). Appropriate medications for treatment of anaphylaxis such as epinephrine should be readily available. An airway always should be available and easily accessible when administering contrast agents.

Because hypotension, bradycardia, and arrhythmia commonly are associated with iodinated contrast administration, the ECG and arterial pressure should be monitored continuously by a laboratory staff member specifically given this responsibility. Atropine, vasopressors, and antiarrhythmic agents should be available for prompt administration.

Immediately following the injection of contrast into the coronary artery, transient bradycardia and/or hypotension may occur. The physician may want the patient to cough after the injection. The staff should instruct the patient before the coronary arteriograms when and how to cough (one or two deep, rapid coughs). Coughing maintains arterial pressure and cerebral blood flow and influences vagal tone as well. Coughing does not increase coronary blood flow.

Increased use of nonionic and low-osmolality contrast agents has greatly reduced the incidence of bradycardia, arrhythmia, hypotension, and the need for coughing during coronary arteriography.

After angiography, the nurse/technician should monitor urine output. It is normal for the urine output to increase postcontrast administration. A decrease in urine output postcontrast administration should be documented and the physician notified. Because of increased diuresis caused by the hypertonicity of contast agents, the patient should be instructed to increase fluid intake after catheterization in order to replace body fluids lost from contrast administration. It is common practice to administer 1 to 2 L of D5½ normal saline or normal saline over 12 to 24 hours intravenously after the catheterization.

Selection of Radiographic Contrast Media

The contast material is selected from commercially available liquid solutions appropriate for the specific examination to be conducted. All contrast materials are x-ray "dense" (as a result of iodine) as compared to anatomical structures that are x-ray "lucent" and absorb x-rays in order to provide different gray shades in x-ray images. The quantity and concentration of contrast materials used are specific medical decisions. Factors included in these decisions are the patient's age, size, general health, and allergies.

All contrast agents contain iodine, an effective absorber of x-rays. Although all agents are derivatives of benzoic acid the number of iodine molecules and ionic and osmolar compostion will vary (Fig. 5-45). Osmolarity, viscosity, sodium content, and other additives and properties are different among these agents. Table 5-6 provides a summary of commonly used contrast agents for coronary and left ventricular angiographic studies. Selection of a contrast agent for the particular laboratory is, to a large extent, a matter of personal preferences. Major differences between the contrast agents include cost, induction of bradycardia and hypotension, and impairment of left ventricular function. Thousands of studies have been performed safely with conventional high-osmolar/ionic agents and pose no major risks. However, considerable data exist to suggest that the newer low-

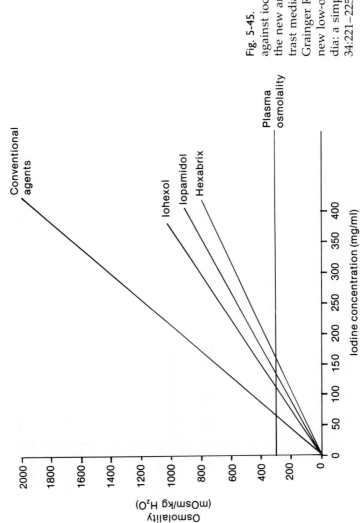

Fig. 5-45. A plot of osmolality against iodine concentration for the new and conventional contrast media. (From Dawson P, Grainger RG, Pitfield J: The new low-osmolar contrast media: a simple guide, *Clin Radiol* 34:221–225, 1983.)

TABLE 5-6. Commonly used contrast media

Composition	U.S. proprietary name	Source	Sodium content* (mEq/L)	Osmolarity†	Iodine content (mg/ml)
Ionic media					
Sodium and meglumine diatrizoate	Renografin-76‡	Squibb	190	1700	370
	Urografin	Schering	1-1050	Variable	270–370
	Hypaque	Winthrop		1400–2400	
	Angiovist	Berlex			
Sodium and meglumine iothalamate	Conray	Mallinckrodt	1-1050	Same as above	270–370
Sodium meglumine, and calcium metrizoate	Isopaque	Winthrop	1-1050	Same as above	270–370
	Triosil	Glaxo			
Nonionic, low-osmolar contrast media					
Metrizamide (nonionic)	Amipaque	Winthrop	0	580	390

Generic (type)	Brand	Manufacturer	Sodium		
Sodium and meglumine ioxaglate (ionic), low osmolar	Hexabrix	Mallinckrodt	0	485	300
			0	600	320
Iopamidol (nonionic)	Isovue	Squibb	0	796	370
Iohexol (nonionic)	Omnipaque	Winthrop-Breon	0	844	350
			0	672	300
Iopromide (nonionic)		Schering (Germany)	0	670	320
Iotasul (nonionic)		Schering	0	300	400
Iotol (nonionic)	Iotrolan	Berlex	0	360	300
Ioversol (nonionic)	Optiray	Mallinckrodt	0	360	320

From Tilkian AG, Daily EK: *Cardiovascular procedures: diagnostic techniques and therapeutic procedures*, St Louis, 1986, Mosby.

* Most preparations for coronary arteriography have a sodium content of 150 to 190 mEq/L to reduce the risk of ventricular fibrillation.

† Osmolarity of blood is approximately 300 mOsm/kg at 37°C.

‡ Renografin-76 (10% sodium diatrizoate, 66% meglumine diatrizoate, 0.04 mg/ml sodium EDTA, 0.32 mg/ml sodium citrate) is an example.

osmolar/nonionic agents may be safer and provide satisfactory diagnostic quality, especially for high-risk patients. Indications for low-osmolar/nonionic contrast agents include unstable ischemic syndromes, congestive heart failure, diabetes, renal insufficiency, hypotension, severe bradycardia, history of contrast allergy, severe valvular heart disease, and use for internal mammary artery injection.

Ionic contrast media produces hypotension by peripheral arterial vasodilation, transient myocardial dysfunction, and decreasing circulating volume and blood pressure after osmotic diuresis (initially contrast media increases circulating fluid volume by osmotically shifting fluid into vascular space).

ANGIOGRAPHIC CATHETERS (See Chapter 2)

There are numerous shapes and sizes of catheters available to the angiographer. Basic routine catheters that are pre-shaped for normal anatomy are available for both the brachial and femoral approaches. There is an array of shapes and sizes to aid the angiographer when abnormal anatomy is present. The nurse/technician is responsible for knowing the different types of catheters that are available and the indications for their use. The experienced staff member becomes familiar with the different types of difficult anatomy and anticipates what type of catheter may be necessary to achieve proper catheter placement. Anticipation of the physician's needs for special equipment during difficult procedures is not only the mark of a good support staff but also greatly reduces procedure length and improves patient safety and comfort.

MEDICATIONS USED IN CORONARY ANGIOGRAPHY

The box on pp. 365–366 lists medications used commonly during cardiac catheterization.

Coronary Vasodilators

Nitroglycerin.   Nitroglycerin is the most commonly used drug during coronary arteriography and ventriculography. Nitroglycerin dilates peripheral arteries, venous beds, and coronary arteries. Nitroglycerin is a very safe and short-acting drug. It can be given through the sublingual, IV, intracoronary, or intraventricular route. Sublingual (or oral spray) nitroglycerin (0.4 mg) is almost always given before coronary arteriography. Exceptions include patients in whom coronary spasm may be suspected and those with hypotension (<90 mm Hg systolic pressure). In patients with documented coronary spasm, sublingual or intracoronary nitroglycerin is given to eliminate coronary spasm. In patients with unstable angina, IV infusions of nitroglycerin of up to 250 μg/min with a systolic blood pressure of 90 mm Hg is permissible. In patients with elevated LV end-diastolic pressure in the catheterization laboratory from ischemia or from congestive heart failure, intraventricular or IV boluses of 200 μg of nitroglycerin will reduce LV end-diastolic pressure and are appropriate if not required before or after ventriculography. Nitroglycerin increases coronary blood flow without a marked reduction in pressure in doses of 50, 100, and 200 μg (intracoronary). In doses of more than 250 μg, hypotension without further increases in coronary blood flow may be evident.

Medications Used in the Cardiac Catheterization Laboratory*

INOTROPICS

Digitalis, 0.125 to 0.25 mg IV >4 hours apart
Dobutamine, 2 to 10 μg/kg/min IV drip
Dopamine, 2 to 10 μg/kg/min IV drip
Epinephrine, 1 : 10,000 IV
Isoproterenol, 1 mg/min IV drip

ANTIARRHYTHMICS, ANTICHOLINERGICS, BETA BLOCKERS, CALCIUM BLOCKERS

Adenosine, 5 to 12 mg IV bolus
Atropine, 0.6 to 1.2 mg IV
Bretylium, 100 to 300 mg IV bolus
Diltiazem, 10 mg IV
Esmolol, 4 to 24 mg/kg IV drip (beta blocker)
Lidocaine, 50 to 100 mg IV bolus; 2 to 4 mg/min IV drip
Procainamide, 50 to 100 mg IV
Propranolol, 1 mg bolus; 0.1 mg/kg in three divided doses (beta blocker)
Verapamil, 2 to 5 mg IV, may repeat dose to 10 mg (calcium channel blocker)

ANALGESICS, SEDATIVES

Diazepam, 2 to 5 mg IV
Diphenhydramine, 25 to 50 mg IV
Meperidine, 12.5 to 50 mg IV
Morphine sulfate, 2.5 mg IV
Naloxone, 0.5 mg IV

ANTICOAGULANTS

Heparin 2000 to 5000 U IV; 1000 U/hr IV drip; 10,000-U bolus for
   PTCA

VASODILATORS

Nitroglycerin 1/150 sublingual, 100 to 300 μg IC
Nitroprusside, 5 to 50 μg/kg/min IV

VASOCONSTRICTORS

Aramine, 10 mg in 100 mL Saline, 1 mL IV
Ergonovine, 0.4 mg IV in divided doses
Norepinephrine 1:10,000 IV, 1 mL doses IV

DIURETIC

Furosemide, 20 to 100 mg IV

METABOLIC BUFFERS

Calcium chloride and/or gluconate, 10 mEq
Sodium bicarbonate, 50 mEq

MISCELLANEOUS

Protamine, 15 to 50 mg IV
Succinylcholine, 1 to 4 mg IV

* The list is meant to be neither all inclusive nor exclusive of emergency life support techniques or standards.

Calcium channel blockers.   Calcium channel blockers dilate vascular smooth muscle and reduce heart muscle contractility, and some agents block AV nodal conduction. Calcium channel blockers are used to reduce peripheral vascular
resistance, reduce blood pressure, and increase coronary
blood flow. These agents are given orally before the performance of angioplasty and are in use chronically by patients
with ischemic heart disease. Acute use in the cardiac catheterization laboratory is indicated for hypertension and ongo-

ing myocardial ischemia with increased blood pressure or sudden recurrent supraventricular tachycardia (verapamil, diltiazem). Doses for calcium channel blockers are as follows:

1. Nifedipine; 10 to 20 mg pO
2. Diltiazem; 30 to 60 mg pO, 10 mg IV
3. Verapamil; 120 mg pO, 2.5 to 5 mg IV

Coronary Vasodilators for Research

Papaverine. Papaverine is a potent arterial vasodilator used in the investigation of coronary vasodilatory reserve. Intracoronary papaverine causes a marked increase in blood flow in the RCA in doses from 4 to 8 mg and in the LCA in doses of from 8 to 12 mg. Doses exceeding these recommended levels do not appear to provide an increase over the maximal blood flow. Rare cases of papaverine-induced torsade de pointe have been reported, and antiarrhythmic preparations for this unusual event should be in place before administraion of intracoronary papaverine.

Adenosine. Adenosine is used for breaking SVT and is the drug of choice for intracoronary induction of maximal hyperemia for coronary vasodilator reserve. For the RCA IC Adenosine in 6 to 8 μg and for the LCA 12 to 18 μg produces optimal results. Adenosine, 0.14 μg/kg/min IV, infusions produce sustained hyperemia. Adenosine hyperemia lasts <60 seconds after drug administration is ended.

Acetylcholine. Acetylcholine dilates normal coronary arteries and constricts diseased vessels. Intracoronary doses of 20, 50, and 100 μg have been used to induce coronary spasm in patients in Japan. The drug is very short-acting and rapidly reversed, making it excellent for catheterization laboratory use. Marked bradycardia and heart block have been reported with the use of acetylcholine. Temporary pacing is required during its administration. Continuous infusions of 0.02 to 2.2 μg/min/kg (10^{-8}, 10^{-7}, 10^{-6} M) have been used to identify normal endothelial function of coronary vessels (vasodilation).

Coronary Vasoconstrictor (for Provocation of Coronary Spasm Only)

Ergonovine. Ergonovine is used to produce coronary vasospasm in patients with chest pain syndromes and normal or nearly normal coronary arteriograms. The regimens for the administration of ergonovine are varied. One commonly used regimen is sequential dosing with 0.02, 0.18, and 0.2 mg intravenously at 3-minute intervals, obtaining ECGs at the end of each dose for total dose of 0.4 mg. If the patient develops typical symptoms an ECG is obtained and arteriograms performed immediately on both the left and right coronary arteries. Ergonovine-induced diffuse coronary vasoconstriction is a physiologic response. Ergonovine-induced focal coronary constriction (relieved with nitroglycerin) is a positive response for coronary spasm. These angiographic changes should be associated with electrocardiographic or symptomatic alterations. Ergonovine-induced coronary vasospasm or physiologic narrowing can be reversed immediately with intracoronary nitroglycerin.

Anticholinergics for Vagal Reactions

Atropine.   Atropine is used to block vagally induced slowing of the heart rate and hypotension. Doses of 0.6 to 1.2 mg IV given immediately will reverse bradycardia and hypotension within 2 minutes. It is important to remember that in elderly patients heart rate may not slow during vagal episodes in which the only manifestation is that of low blood pressure. This low blood pressure can be alleviated by the administration of IV atropine and normal saline. In the rare patient in whom IV access is not immediately available, intraarterial atropine (in the aorta) can be administered.

Antiarrhythmic Drugs

Lidocaine.   Lidocaine is an antiarrhythmic drug used to block or reduce the number of ventricular extrasystoles. Lidocaine can be administered as a bolus of 50 to 100 mg intravenously before ventriculography if a stable and quiet catheter position within the left ventricle cannot be obtained. In patients in whom myocardial iscehmia is developing during cardiac catheterization or angioplasty, lidocaine for frequent ventricular ectopy is indicated. A bolus of 50 to 100 mg intravenously followed by 1 to 2 mg/min infusion is usually satisfactory.

Cardiac Agonists

Isoproterenol.   Isoproterenol (Isuprel) is a pure beta agonist that increases heart rate and causes peripheral vasodilatation. It is indicated during cardiac arrest with refractory bradycardia. Isuprel has been used for provocation of heart stress (increase heart rate) in patients with valvular heart disease or hypertrophic cardiomyopathy.

Dopamine.   Dopamine is a potent vasoconstrictor. In low doses it causes renal vasodilatation. In high doses it causes peripheral vasoconstriction, elevating the blood pressure and increasing myocardial contractility. Dopamine from 2 to 15 μg/min will act to cause vasoconstriction, elevating the blood pressure for problems resulting in severe hypotension.

Dobutamine.   Dobutamine is a potent inotropic agent with no peripheral vasoconstrictor effects. It increases cardiac contractility (inotropy) and so is especially useful in patients with congestive heart failure. It may be used in conjunction with a potent vasodilator such as nitroprusside in those patients with markedly elevated filling pressures and poor cardiac output.

Epinephrine.   Epinephrine (1 : 10,000) is a naturally occurring catecholamine that stimulates cardiac function. It is administered only during cardiac emergencies. This medicine will increase heart rate and blood pressure immediately, sometimes to excessive levels. This should be reserved for cases in which cardiac resuscitation is required or in which refractory hypotension is present and not responding to peripheral vasoconstrictors. Transthoracic administration of epinephrine through a long needle is not required during cardiac catheterization in which IV or intraarterial access already is obtained. One milliliter of 1 : 10,000 dilution given intravenously can increase systemic pressure during hypotension to a safe level until IV vasopressors have been prepared. This dose has a duration of action between 5 and 10 minutes.

Arterial Vasodilator

Nitroprusside.   Nitroprusside is a potent short-acting intravenous arterial vasodilator used in the treatment of aortic insufficiency, mitral regurgitation, hypertensive crisis, and congestive heart failure. Doses administered range from 10 to 100 μg/min and must be monitored by direct arterial pressure measurement.

Recording Medications on Cinefilm During Angiography

If drugs are given during the course of the catheterization that may affect the angiograms in any way, the medication may be marked on the film with a cineangiographic exposure of the radiopaque drug marker to identify the drug and indicate that a change in the subsequent arteriograms may be present. Examples of such drugs are sublingual or intracoronary nitroglycerin, ergonovine, and drugs used during thrombolytic therapy (e.g., streptokinase). A radiographic clock marker also may be used to indicate the time of such events.

PACEMAKERS

Cardiac pacing is a low-risk means of providing emergency cardiac rhythm, especially in cases of symptomatic bradycardia or asystole. Since the introduction of low-osmolar or nonionic contrast media, significant bradycardia and asystole during coronary angiography has decreased, obviating the need for prophylactic pacing in this setting. Cardiac pacemakers may be used prophylactically during cardiac catheterization to reduce hemodynamic compromise of heart block and have been used to rescue patients after development of conduction abnormalities requiring atrial or ventricular pacing.

The use of pacemakers for routine coronary arteriography and ventriculography and a majority of coronary angioplasty procedures is not required.

Indications

1. Previously demonstrated high degree conduction block
2. Symptomatic bradycardia (after contrast or angiography of RCA)
3. Left bundle branch block for anticipated right heart studies

4. Acetylcholine studies
5. Acute myocardial ischemia studies

In patients with left bundle branch block, passage of catheters through the right heart should be accomplished with great care because the induction of right heart block will lead to complete heart block, requiring a pacemaker in some patients. Atropine may be used to prevent bradycardia, but a pacemaker should be on standby for patients who experience severe bradycardia during coronary injections.

Technique

Venous access from either the femoral or brachial approach may be used. The easiest access is usually the vein next to the arterial entry site. Temporary transvenous pacemaker placement can be achieved through the internal jugular, subclavian, brachial, or femoral vein route.

RV pacing is accomplished with standard pacing catheters. End-hole or balloon-tipped pacing catheters are available. A pulmonary artery (Zucker) catheter in which pacing electrodes lie along the catheter as it passes through the right ventricle before passing into the PA has been used during coronary angioplasty (see Catheters, Chapter 2). Among the safest catheters is a 5 French balloon-tipped pacing catheter.

Setting the Pacemaker (Fig. 5-46)

The pacemaker is set either in the "demand" or "fixed" mode. *Demand* mode means the pacemaker will pace when the heart rate drops below the level set by the demand rate (e.g., demand set at 50 bpm). This would be useful when a patient has a vasovagal reaction or heart block with a heart rate of 40 bpm. Pacing would start when pacer detected a rate of less than 50 bpm. *Fixed* rate mode means that the pacer is working all the time at the rate set.

Milliamperes are a measure of the amount of current delivered through the pacing wire to the heart muscle. This setting should be three times the threshold value (see Determining Pacemaker Threshold below). A well-positioned pacemaker wire has milliamperage set around 2 to 3 mA. A poorly positioned wire may not pace even with milliamperage as high as 6 to 7 mA. Repositioning is then required.

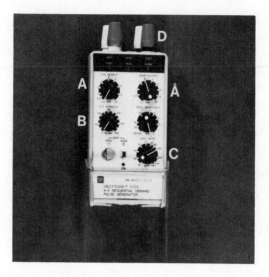

Fig. 5-46. A close-up of pacemaker controls. *A*, *Å*, Output setting in milliamps for atrial and ventricular channels. *B*, The AV interval. Opposite *B* is the sensitivity control, which on full counterclockwise to asynchronism is a fixed mode and can be set clockwise to demand rates (see text for details). *C*, The ventricular pacing rate. *D*, Connectors to pacemaker cable.

Determining Pacemaker Threshold

The *threshold* value is the lowest milliamperage at which the pacemaker will pace. After the wire is positioned:

Step 1: Set milliamperage at 5 mA.

Step 2: Turn pacer mode fixed at rate higher than patient's rate.

Step 3: Turn the milliamperage down in 1-mA increments until the pacing fails. This level is the threshold.

Step 4: For use during studies set the milliamperage at three to four times the threshold on demand mode.

Complications

Complications related to the placement of pacemakers are principally those related to the site of venous access. The complications and problems with these access sites have been discussed in Chapter 2 (Fig. 5-47). Direct transthoracic pacing should be avoided. Complications of transthoracic placement of a pacemaker into the heart include pneumothorax, hemopericardium, coronary sinus laceration, cardiac

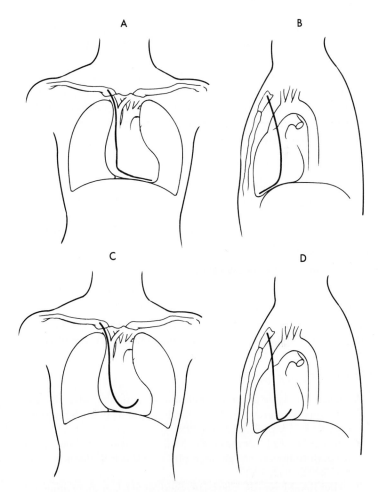

Fig. 5-47.   Normal pacemaker position in the right ventricle on (**A**) anterioposterior and (**B**) lateral chest films as compared to coronary sinus position in the same views (**C** and **D**). (From Tilkian AG, Daily EK: *Cardiovascular procedures: diagnostic techniques and therapeutic procedures,* St Louis, 1986, Mosby.)

tamponade, and major organ or vessel injury. Additional injuries reported include inferior vena cava puncture, right atrial puncture, pulmonary artery puncture, lung or liver puncture, internal mammary artery puncture, and right or left coronary artery laceration.

RV pacing is complicated by RV perforation with tamponade in a small percentage of patients. This may be a significant limitation to the use of pacemakers in patients who are anticoagulated (on heparin). This is especially problematic in patients who are undergoing angioplasty and for whom large doses of heparin are required. Carefully select patients for prophylactic pacemakers. Perforation of the right ventricle, although uncommon, will complicate an otherwise benign yet important procedure for patients with atherosclerotic coronary artery disease.

Other Pacemaker Uses

Pacemakers are also used for:
1. Provocative testing for ischemia through rapid atrial pacing
2. Electrocardiographic signal input and sampling for EPSs (see Chapter 4).

Alternatives to Invasive Pacing

External noninvasive cardiac stimulation can be performed with wide patch electrodes placed over the anterior and posterior chest. Although these pacemakers leads may produce some discomfort in the awake patient, they will create a temporary rhythm when needed.

SUGGESTED READINGS

Arvidson H: Angiographic observations in mitral valve disease, with special reference to the volume variations in the left atrium, *Acta Radiol* (Suppl 158):1–40, 1958.

Balter S, Sones M Jr, Brancato RL: Radiation exposure to the operator performing cardiac angiography with U-arm systems, *Circulation* 58:925–932, 1978.

Boucher RA, Myler RK, Clark DA, Stertzer SH: Coronary angiography and angioplasty, *Cathet Cardiovasc Diagn* 14:269–285, 1988.

Dillon JC: Inexpensive radiation protective glasses, *Cathet Cardiovasc Diagn* 5:203–208, 1979.

Dodge HT, Sandler H, Ballew DW, Lord JD Jr: The use of biplane angiocardiography for the measurment of left ventricular volume in man. *Am Heart J* 60:762–776, 1960.

Finci L, Meier B, Steffenino G, Roy P, Rutishauser W: Radiation exposure during diagnostic catheterization and single- and double-vessel percutaneous transluminal coronary angioplasty, *Am J Cardiol* 60:1401–1403, 1987.

Gertz EW, Wisneski JA, Gould RG, Akin JR: Improved radiation protection for physicians performing cardiac catheterization, *Am J Cardiol* 50:1283–1286, 1982.

James TN, Bruschke AVG, Bothig S, Dodu SRA, Gil JF, Kawamura K, Paulin SJ, Piessens J: *Report of WHO/ISFC task force on nomenclature of coronary arteriograms*, American Heart Association, 451A–455A.

Judkins MP: Guidelines for radiation protection in the cardiac catheterization laboratory, *Cathet Cardiovasc Diagn* 10:87–92, 1984.

Levin DC, Dunham LR, Stueve R: Causes of cine image quality deterioration in cardiac catheterization laboratories, *Am J Cardiol* 52:881–886, 1983.

Miller SW, Castronovo FP Jr: Radiation exposure and protection in cardiac catheterization laboratories, *Am J Cardiol* 55:171–176, 1985.

Rackley CE, Dodge HT, Coble YD Jr, and others: A method for determining left ventricular mass in man, *Circulation* 29:666–671, 1964.

Sandler H, Dodge HT: The use of single plane angiocardiograms for the calculation of left ventricular volume in man, *Am Heart J* 75:325–334, 1968.

Wynne J, Green LH, Mann T, and others: Estimation of left ventricular volumes in man for biplane cineangiograms filmed in oblique projections, *Am J Cardiol* 41:726–732, 1978.

6

RESEARCH TECHNIQUES

Morton J. Kern and Thomas J. Donohue

Research techniques commonly are performed in catheterization laboratories where cardiology fellows train and have been of great value in understanding common problems in cardiology. This chapter is an overview of commonly used research procedures in the cardiac catheterization laboratory. Many of our clinical methods were once research techniques that have been incorporated into the routine of diagnostic cardiac catheterization. Tables 6-1 and 6-2 show the most commonly used research techniques and their functions.

In the cardiac catheterization laboratory the support staff may view research as unnecessary, unimportant, or dangerous to the patient. These commonly held misconceptions should be alleviated by the physician who should explain the utility and safety of the procedure. Only skilled physicians with directed goals apply these research techniques. The information has been invaluable in identifying new therapies and advancing the frontiers of treatment for cardiac disease. It is most helpful for nurses and catheterization laboratory physicians to appreciate these problems and convey a sense of confidence and enthusiasm to the patient. The most common research catheterization techniques described below may be used alone or combined with others:

TABLE 6-I.   Research techniques

Objective	Method
I. Ventricular function	
1. Systolic function	Ventricular pressure-volume (P-V) relationship (simultaneous LV pressure with LV volume by echocardiogram, contrast angiogram, nuclear angiogram or impedance catheter)
	Variables derived: end-systolic P-V slope, intercept; contractility ($+dP/dt$)
2. Diastolic function	Ventricular pressure-volume relationship (as above)
	Variables derived: end-diastolic P-V slope, intercept; relaxation ($-dP/dt$, Tau, K)
3. Exercise studies	
4. Combined hemodynamic and echocardiographic studies	
II. Myocardial blood flow (coronary vasodilatory reserve, effects of drugs, etc.)	Indicator dilution; inert gas (xenon, nitrogen); thermodilution
	Doppler flow velocity
	Digital radiographic studies
III. Electrical function (abnormal conduction, excitation)	Electrophysiologic studies
	His bundle
	Atrial and ventricular refractory periods
	Conduction abnormalities
	Inducible ventricular ectopy
	Bypass tracts

LV, Left ventricular; P-V, pressure-volume.

1. High-fidelity pressure measurements
2. Quantitative angiographic analysis
3. Myocardial blood flow determination
4. Myocardial metabolism measurement
5. Combined hemodynamic-echocardiographic methodologies
6. Angioscopic and two-dimensional ultrasound imaging techniques

TABLE 6-2. Additional research techniques in the catheterization laboratory

LV function	Methods
Pressure-volume relationships	High-fidelity pressure
End systole	LV volume
End diastole	LV-gram (cineangiographic, digital)
	RV-gram
	Two-dimensional echocardiogram
	Impedance catheter
Wall stress	
LV mass	Quantitative ventriculography
Diastolic function	High-fidelity pressure
	Doppler mitral inflow
Ventricular interaction	RV/LV high-fidelity pressures
Aortic impedance	Aortic flow velocity, high-fidelity pressure
Coronary physiology	
Coronary blood flow, coronary reserve, coronary vasodilation (response to drugs)	Pharmacologic studies with papaverine and adenosine, acetylcholine
	Physiologic flow responses during interventional procedures such as angioplasty or hemodynamic studies
Ischemia testing	
Induced tachycardia	Electrical pacing
Isoproterenol, dopamine	Pharmacologic infusion
Transient coronary occlusion	Coronary angioplasty

LV, left ventricular; RV, right ventricular.

HIGH-FIDELITY MICROMANOMETER-TIP PRESSURE MEASUREMENTS
Indications

Indications for high-fidelity transducer-tipped pressure measurements include those studies requiring precise determination of the pressure waveform for analysis of highly accurate and small changes in absolute pressure as well as upstroke and downstroke slopes for assessment of contractility. High-fidelity pressure measurements are useful for studies of conditions affecting cardiac contractility, afterload reduction, or improved myocardial metabolism (e.g., drugs). In addition, high-fidelity pressures combined with quantitative volume measurements are used to determine myocardial functional curves. The most precise hemodynamic studies utilize this technique.

Assessment of Ventricular Function from High-Fidelity Pressure Catheters

Contractility is the force or rate of myocardial muscle activity and often is measured by the electronically derived rate of rise (the first derivative dP/dt: i.e., change in pressure, dP, divided by change in time, dt) of pressure in the left ventricle. (Fig. 6-1). This measurement is obtained with a micromanometer-tipped (high-fidelity) catheter because of its precise and instantaneous pressure transmission. The frequency responses of fluid-filled systems are too slow for research data. Various other isovolumetric measurements are also derived from the dP/dt taken at different pressure levels (e.g., pressure at 40 mm Hg or at end diastole).

High-Fidelity Catheter Setup

High-fidelity micromanometer-tip catheters are available from several different manufacturers. The Millar Instruments catheter has a small silicon piezo crystal that often requires warming of the micromanometer-tip transducer to blood temperature before insertion. A sterile cable connects the catheter to the recorder. This connector cable has a calibration box used to set the baseline (zero) and range of the pressure signal. Patch cables transmit the pressure signal from the pressure amplifier to the differentiation module on the physiologic recorder. After the catheter is inserted, matching the high-fidelity pressure to the fluid-filled pressure may verify the correct setup before the study. The pigtail catheter configuration is used from the femoral approach, but an 0.032-inch guidewire is generally the largest wire that can be accommodated.

QUANTITATIVE VENTRICULOGRAPHY AND WALL MOTION

These techniques are sophisticated approaches to routine ventriculographic techniques described earlier. The precise

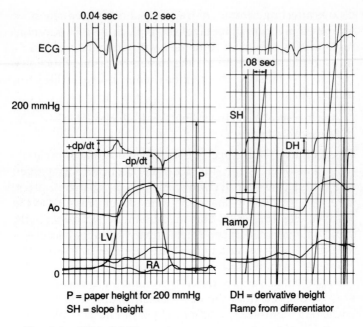

Fig. 6-1. High-fidelity, micromanometer-tipped hemodynamic tracings of aortic and left ventricular pressures with
differentiated dP/dt signal demonstrating method of calculation of dP/dt. See text for details. *SH,* Slope height; *DH,*
Derivative height; *P,* paper height for 200 mm Hg full-scale
deflection. To compute dP/dt:

1. SH: mm deflection from *ramp* over 80 m
2. DH: mm deflection of *square* box of derivative
3. Compute K : K = (12.5 × SH)/DH
4. Scale factor P = mm paper deflection of 200 mm Hg
5. Compute dP/dt:

$$dP/dt = \frac{200 \text{ mm Hg}}{P} (K)$$

Peak dP/dt positive or negative deflection; normal value
range: 1500 to 1800 mm Hg/sec

angiographic setup and later computer analysis facilitates
quantitative measurements (Fig. 6-2). Further details are
given in Chapter 5 and Appendix VI.

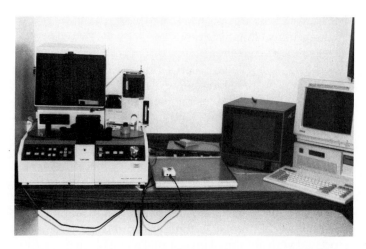

Fig. 6-2.   Equipment used for analysis of ventriculography. A desk-top computer and tracing tablet convert the ventriculogram from the film projector to digital data and provide quantitative analysis of regional wall motion.

MYOCARDIAL BLOOD FLOW

Techniques for determination of myocardial blood flow include coronary sinus thermodilution, intracoronary Doppler velocity measurement, digital coronary angiographic blood flow velocity, and older, less facile techniques of injected gas washout (xenon-133 [radioactive] or nitrogen [inert]). These techniques, for the most part, need to be applied during well-defined research protocols with approval of human subject research committees.

Indications

1. Coronary blood flow velocity assessment of coronary stenoses (Doppler guidewire technique)
2. Coronary vasodilatory reserve
3. Effects of drugs or interventions on myocardial blood flow and/or metabolism
4. Identification of syndrome X (chest pain with normal coronary arteries)
5. Coronary endothelial function

6. Coronary flow during mechanical interventions; PTCA, atherectomy, Rotablator, etc.

7. Detection of collateral flow

Coronary vasodilator reserve (maximal coronary blood flow/resting coronary blood flow) can be measured by coronary sinus blood flow using continuous thermodilution technique or, most recently and more precisely, with intracoronary arterial flow velocity using miniaturized Doppler-tipped coronary catheters or guidewires. This methodology involves measurement of coronary blood flow at rest and again during stimulation with rapid atrial pacing, intracoronary nitroglycerin, contrast media, papaverine, dipyridamole (IV), or adenosine (IC or IV). When the methodologies indicate abnormal coronary vasodilatory responses associated with abnormal myocardial metabolism in patients with chest pain syndromes, the diagnosis of syndrome X is made. Coronary reserve may be affected by both epicardial and microvascular circulatory abnormalities (Fig. 6-3).

The measurement of absolute changes in coronary blood flow, indicating the response of the heart to various drugs, should be combined with measurement of transmyocardial oxygen (arterial and coronary sinus blood) to identify whether increases in blood flow are caused by increased myocardial oxygen demand (secondary to autoregulation) or by primary coronary action without changes in myocardial demand (primary vasodilation/constriction). The coronary sinus thermodilution catheter is ideally suited for these studies. Coronary flow velocity measurements provide relative, but not absolute, flow values and a second catheter needs to be placed in the coronary sinus to measure transmyocardial oxygen extraction. Alternatively, coronary blood flow velocity can be combined with quantitative cineangiography to provide a calculated absolute blood flow.

MYOCARDIAL METABOLISM
Measurement of Specialized Blood Products

Transmyocardial (arterial and coronary vein blood) determinations of myocardial metabolism can be obtained by measuring pyruvate, lactate, and oxygen extraction. The transmyocardial extraction of drugs after systemic delivery can also be determined. Most commonly, lactate and oxygen are

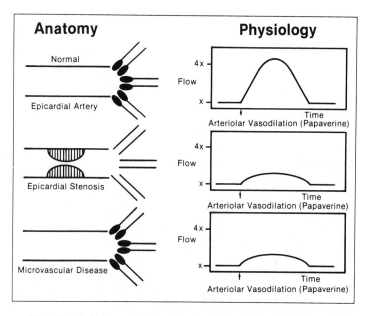

Fig. 6-3. A diagram of normal epicardial coronary artery and microvascular bed. Coronary vasodilatory reserve is normal. Coronary vasodilator reserve can be abnormal due to either epicardial artery narrowing or microvascular disease. (From White CW, Wilson RF: Assessment of the human coronary circulation using a Doppler catheter. *Am J Cardiol* 67:44D–56D, 1991).

measured for studies involving ischemic myocardial metabolism. Specialized collection tubes for lactate and heparinized syringes for paired serial oxygen blood samples from both the arterial and coronary sinus should be prepared in advance. In addition, myocardial catecholamines (norepinephrine, epinephrine) and other specialized prostaglandin products can be obtained with this technique. Specialized heparin-coated catheters may facilitate sampling of platelet products without platelet activation on withdrawal through the catheter lumen.

In the setup for any measurement of specialized blood products, advanced preparation of the sampling tubes should be made so that the physician can quickly pass the drawn blood to the technicians for insertion into the collecting tubes. In addition to sample tube preparation, ice, a centrifuge in the laboratory, or a series of dilutional tubes may be required. These techniques are not complicated, but advanced preparation with correct labeling and anticipation of which samples will be obtained at which point in the procedure facilitate measurements without error or prolongation of the study.

CORONARY SINUS CATHETERIZATION
Technique

Coronary sinus (CS) catheterization is generally performed from the left brachial venous approach or through the right internal jugular vein. The ostium of the CS is located inferiorly and posterior to the tricuspid valve.

The 8 French relatively stiff Dacron catheter is inserted by cutdown or through a percutaneously placed 8 French venous sheath. After carefully entering the heart, the catheter is directed toward the tricuspid valve and in a posterior direction. Gentle medial advancement with a 1- to 2-ml flush of contrast will enable the physician to know when the catheter has entered the CS. If ventricular ectopy is noted (contact with RV wall or septum), the catheter is withdrawn and readvanced after slight rotation.

The CS catheter is usually positioned in the AP view with the catheter seen passing upward across the tricuspid valve and spine. In the LAO position it appears to be coming directly in plane toward the observer. In the RAO position, it should pass away from the ventricular apex (i.e., not into the right ventricle).

This technique is particularly difficult from the IVC, and this approach probably should be avoided unless specifically shaped catheters are available.

Care should be taken not to cannulate the inferior cardiac vein and to avoid perforation of the CS, right ventricle, or atrium. Once positioned, the catheter must be secured to the vein so that movement of the temperature thermistors on the distal catheter tip will not produce artifactual signals. If a brachial approach is utilized, the patient's arm also should remain fixed during the study.

Catheter Setup

After the catheter position is secured, the electrical connections from the catheter to the CS Wheatstone bridge (temperature-sensing device) are made and connections from the Wheatstone bridge to the physiologic recorder calibrated. Thermistor signals (i.e., patient's body temperature) are then set to the baseline (zero) position.

The indicator solution (D_5W at room temperature) is injected through the catheter at a rate of 25 to 50 ml/min using a Harvard pump or Medrad injector. Typical data records are shown in Figs. 6-4 and 6-5.

DOPPLER CORONARY FLOW VELOCITY TECHNIQUES

The Doppler coronary flow velocity techniques allow measurement of quantitative characteristics of coronary flow by sending out a pulsed sound waves (12 to 20 mHz) and measuring the return times bouncing off moving red cells (Fig. 6-6). Measurement of the physiologic response of the coronary circulation to various drugs and the significance of coronary obstructive lesions are examples of useful applications.

Types of Doppler Catheters

There are four commercially available Doppler catheters with two types of velocimeters for measuring blood flow velocity in the coronary arteries (Fig. 6-7): (1) the nonselective Judkins Doppler catheter (Cordis Corp., Miami, Florida), (2) the 3 French subselective end-mounted catheter (Millar Instruments, Houston, Texas), (3) the side-mounted ultrasonic crystal catheter (NuMed, Inc., Hopkinton, New York), and (4) the FloWire/FloMap System (Cardiometrics, Inc., Mountain View, California). The two velocimeters are the zero-crossing type (Millar Instruments and Triton Medical, San Diego, California), compatible with the three Doppler catheters, and the spectral velocity analyzer, compatible only with the Doppler FloWire. The 3 French subselective Doppler catheters have been used to assess the hemodynamic significance of coronary lesions and interventions but have not been put into routine practice for several reasons. These include a relatively large catheter size, limitation of measurements to the proximal vessel before any lesions, the need

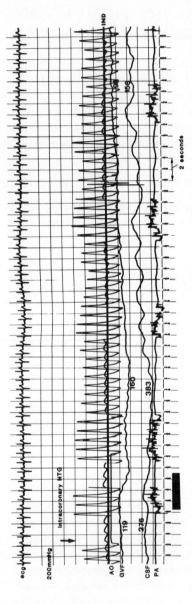

Fig. 6-4. Data record from a patient during measurement of coronary sinus blood flow by thermodilution technique receiving intracoronary nitroglycerin. At the arrow, 200 μg intracoronary nitroglycerin is given and great vein flow increases. (Higher flow is toward the bottom of the tracing.) The solid line (*IND*) is the indicator temperature of the thermodilution signal. *AO*, Aorta, mean and phasic; *GVF*, great vein flow; *CSF*, coronary sinus flow; *PA*, pulmonary artery pressure. (From Kern MJ, Eilen SD, O'Rourke RA: Coronary vasomotion in rest angina and effect of nitroglycerin on coronary blood flow. *Am J Cardiol* 56:484–485, 1985.)

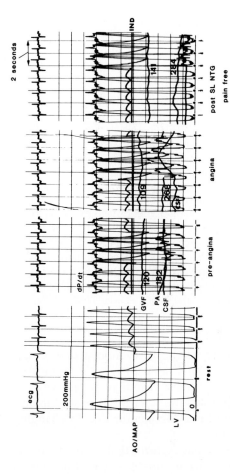

Fig. 6-5. Coronary sinus thermodilution measurements in a patient with severe coronary artery disease before and during angina and immediately after receiving sublingual nitroglycerin demonstrating the changes in hemodynamics and coronary sinus blood flow. During preanginal period, ST segment depression is noted. Baseline great vein flow (*GVF*) and coronary sinus flow (*CSF*) are 120 and 182 ml/min, respectively, with pulmonary artery (*PA*) mean pressure of 25 mm Hg. During angina, mean pulmonary pressure increases slightly. Great cardiac vein flow decreases to 109 ml/min while coronary sinus flow increases (268 ml/min). After the administration of sublingual nitroglycerin, both great vein flow and coronary sinus flow increase and pulmonary pressure drops to a mean of 18 mm Hg. ST segment changes have resolved demonstrating the effect of ischemia on coronary sinus blood flow before and after nitroglycerin. (From Kern MJ, Eilen SD, O'Rourke RA: Coronary vasomotion in rest angina and effect of nitroglycerin on coronary blood flow. *Am J Cardiol* 56:484–485, 1985.)

387

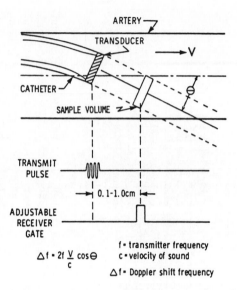

Fig. 6-6. A diagram of coronary Doppler principles. The catheter or guidewire emits high-frequency sound from the tip-mounted crystal, which reflects off moving red cells passing through the sample volume. The velocity of the blood flow is calculated using the Doppler shift formula. (From Hartley CJ, Cole JS: An ultrasonic pulsed Doppler system for measuring blood flow in small vessels. *J Appl Physiol* 37:626, 1974.)

to exchange catheters to insert the interventional device, and difficulty ascertaining optimal signals with the zero-cross technique. In addition, coronary vasodilatory reserve (i.e., the hyperemic-to-basal flow ratio [CVR]) has proved to be a poor indicator of procedural completion due to changing basal and hyperemic flows.

The Doppler guidewire has features that overcome many of these limitations, making it suitable for routine clinical use. Some of the clinical uses are listed on Table 6-3. The FloWire is small enough (0.014 to 0.018 inch in diameter) to assess coronary flow velocity proximal and distal to any coronary stenosis. It can also determine whether normal blood flow velocity has been restored following angioplasty and monitor flow changes related to procedural complications. During diagnostic angiography, the FloWire can detect

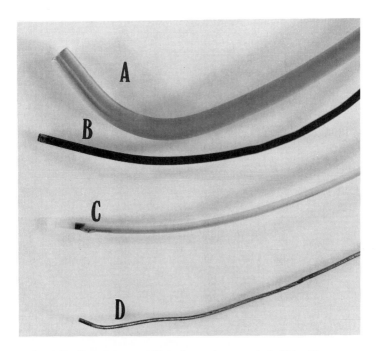

Fig. 6-7. Intracoronary Doppler catheters. *A*, Judkins Doppler (Cordis Corp., Miami, FL); *B*, Millar 3 French end-mounted crystal Doppler (Millar Instruments, Houston, Tex.); *C*, NuMed 3 French side-mounted catheter (NuMed, Hopkinton, NY); and *D*, FloWire 0.018-inch Doppler-tipped angioplasty guidewire (Cardiometrics, Inc., Mountain View, CA). (From Ofili EO, Kern MJ, Labovitz AJ, St. Vrain JA, Segal J, Aguirre F, Castello R: Analysis of coronary blood flow velocity dynamics in angiographically normal and stenosed arteries before and after endolumen enlargement by angioplasty. *J Am Coll Cardiol* 21:308–316, 1993.)

flow velocity impairment caused by an intermediately severe angiographic lesion and can then help direct mechanical intervention.

Setup for Measurement

1. Arterial access is easiest from femoral approach with 6-8 French sheath.
2. A 5 or 6 French diagnostic or larger angioplasty guiding catheter is positioned in coronary ostium.

TABLE 6-3.   Clinical uses of the Doppler FloWire

Angioplasty
End points
Complications
Additional lesions
Collateral flow
Stent placement
Atherectomy

Intermediate (40% to 70%) lesion assessment

Coronary vasodilatory reserve assessment
Syndrome X
Transplant coronary arteriopathy
Saphenous vein graft, internal mammary artery

Coronary research
Pharmacologic studies
Intraaortic balloon pumping
Coronary physiology of vascular disease
Thallium correlation

---

3. A 5000-unit IV heparin bolus dose is given.
4. Through an angioplasty Y connector on guiding catheter, Doppler guidewire is inserted. If using a Doppler catheter, it is inserted over a 0.014-inch angioplasty guidewire.
5. The Doppler guidewire or catheter is advanced to the proximal part of the vessel, beyond major branch bifurcations.
   a. For catheters only, the electrical Doppler lead is connected to the velocimeter.
   b. Velocimeter range gate (2 to 4 mm) is adjusted for optimal diastolic phasic waveform.
   c. After baseline flow is measured, a vasodilatory drug is instilled through the guiding catheter. *Alternatively* the guidewire in the Doppler catheter is withdrawn and the vasodilatory agent is injected through Doppler catheter.
   d. Commonly used coronary vasodilators include 50 to 200 μg nitroglycerin, 2 to 8 ml contrast media, 6 to 12 mg papaverine, and 8 to 18 μg adenosine.

Characteristics and Methods of Use of the Doppler FloWire

The 12-mHz crystal on the tip of the guidewire sends and receives ultrasound waves. The timing allows the FloWire to measure blood flow velocities from moving red cells in a sample area 5 mm from the tip of the wire (and 2 mm deep), far enough away that the blood velocity is not affected by the wake of the wire. The returning signal is transmitted in real time to the display console. The gray-scale spectral scrolling display shows the velocities of all the red blood cells within the sample volume. The key parameters are derived from the automatically tracked peak blood velocities, making them less position sensitive (Fig. 6-8).

The Doppler angioplasty guidewire has a forward-directed ultrasound beam that diverges in a 27° arc from the long axis (measured in the -6 dB roundtrip points of the ultrasound beam pattern). The pulse repetition frequency of >40 Hz, pulse duration of $+0.83$ second, and sampling delay of 6.5 seconds are standard for clinical use. The system is coupled to a real-time spectrum analyzer, videocassette recorder, and video page printer. The quadrature-Doppler audio signals are processed by the spectrum analyzer using on-line fast-Fourier transformation (Fig. 6-8). Simultaneous electrocardiographic and arterial pressure data are also input to the video display. During in vivo testing, the Doppler guidewire measured velocity demonstrated excellent correlation with electromagnetic measurements of flow velocity and volumetric flow.

Prior to placing the Doppler guidewire into an artery, the patient should be treated with 3000 to 5000 units of IV heparin. Pressure and velocity signals should be recorded continuously at slow paper speed (10 cm/sec), and brief runs should be made at fast paper speed (100 cm/sec) for waveform analysis (Fig. 6-9).

Measurement of Translesional Velocity

After diagnostic angiography or during angioplasty, the Doppler guidewire is passed through a standard angioplasty Y connector attached to either a 6 French or 8 French guiding catheter. The guidewire is then advanced into the artery. Baseline flow velocity data are obtained at least 1 cm proximal

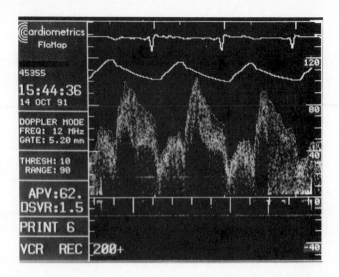

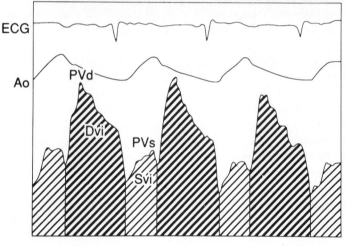

Fig. 6-8. Normal coronary flow velocity spectra demonstrating small systolic and large diastolic velocity components. The diagram of measurements in the lower panel shows a darkly hatched diastolic velocity integral (*Dvi*), a lightly hatched systolic velocity integral (*Svi*), and peak systolic (*PVs*) and peak diastolic (*PVd*) velocities. The means of both diastole and systole can be computed as well as total cycle variables. *Ao*, Aortic pressure; *DSVR*, diastolic-to-systolic velocity ratio; *ECG*, electrocardiogram; *APV*, average peak velocity (mean). (From Ofili EO, Kern MJ, Labovitz AJ, St. Vrain JA, Segal J, Aguirre F, Castello R: Analysis of coronary blood flow velocity dynamics in angiographically normal and stenosed arteries before and after endolumen enlargement by angioplasty. *J Am Coll Cardiol* 21:308–316, 1993.)

to the lesion. The wire is then advanced by a distance equivalent to at least five to ten times the arterial diameter (approximately 2 cm) beyond the stenosis. Placement in any side branches is avoided. Distal flow velocity data are then obtained.

Coronary Flow Reserve

Proximal and distal hyperemic measurements are obtained by intracoronary injections of adenosine (6 to 8 mg in the RCA and 12 to 18 mg in the left coronary artery). [Papaverine has rarely caused ventricular tachycardia/ventricular fibrillation (VT/VF).] Coronary flow reserve is computed as the quotient of hyperemic and basal mean flow velocities.

Setting up of the FloWire system usually takes less than 10 minutes. It is easily incorporated into routine angioplasty procedures and provides additional physiologic information on lesion severity and responses to balloon occlusions; it also monitors flow in the postprocedural period without the need for frequent contrast injections.

Methodologic Difficulties

Doppler coronary velocity only measures relative changes in velocity, not absolute blood flow. Measurements assume the following:

1. The cross-sectional area of the vessel being studied remains fixed.
2. The velocity profile across the vessel is not distorted by arterial disease.
3. The angle between the crystal and sample volume remains constant and less than 30° from the horizontal flow stream.

Intravascular Imaging

Additional intracoronary research techniques include high-frequency two-dimensional coronary ultrasound imaging and coronary angioscopy. Catheter-based coronary ultrasound imaging uses catheters ranging in size from 2.9 to 5.0 French with either mechanically or electronically rotating 20- to 30-MHz echo crystals, which produce a cross-sectional image of the artery (Fig. 6-12). The ultrasound image appearance of a normal coronary artery is homogenous. In even mildly diseased arteries, the more characteristic three-

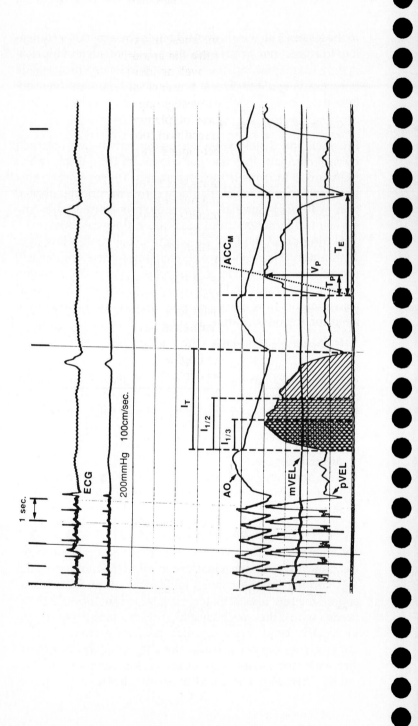

layered image is the norm. These images are more accurate than angiography to identify the amount of atherosclerotic material inside a vessel as well as identifying morphologic characteristics such as the presence of calcium. Research studies using this tool are investigating endothelial function, progression and regression of plaque, responses to new pharmacologic agents and results of coronary artery catheter-based interventional techniques (e.g., atherectomy or PTCA).

Ultrasound catheters that are currently available are introduced over guidewires in a monorail fashion. The proximal end of the catheter is connected through sterile drapes to the motor drive unit that rotates the crystal.

Angioscopy catheters utilize fiberoptic technology to provide a topographical, real-time image of the coronary artery. The glass fibers that transmit the light for imaging are managed in a bundle and collectively constitute the fiberoptic array. There is also a distal lens that serves to focus the transmitted light. These catheters have improved dramatically over the past decade with a reduction in size, increase in flexibility, and improved optics.

The catheter is introduced into the artery over a guidewire and a small, compliant balloon is inflated to the size of the vessel to block antegrade blood flow. A continuous flush system of warm saline is irrigated through the angioscope to clear the viewing field. This technique has allowed direct

---

Fig. 6-9. Coronary flow velocity signals with aortic (AO) pressure. The shaded area is the integral of diastolic flow velocity divided into first one half ($I_{1/2}$) and one third ($I_{1/3}$) of the diastolic flow velocity integral (I_T). $mVEL$, Mean velocity; $pVEL$, phasic velocity; T_p, time to peak; V_p, peak velocity; T_E, total extent or duration of diastolic flow. These measurements are useful in research analysis of flow velocity data. (From Kern MJ, Deligonul U, Vandormael M, Labovitz A, Gudipati CV, Gabliani G, Bodet J, Shah Y, Kennedy HL: Impaired coronary vasodilator reserve in the immediate postcoronary angioplasty period: analysis of coronary artery flow velocity indexes and regional cardiac venous efflux. *J Am Coll Cardiol* 13:860–872, 1989.)

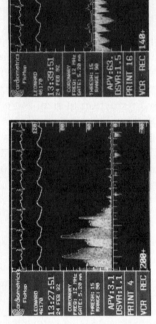

Fig. 6-10. Time sequence of flow velocity during coronary balloon occlusion in a patient with a left anterior descending (*LAD*) coronary artery filled with collaterals originating from the right coronary artery. Note the retrograde collateral flow velocity below the baseline in a phasic pattern appearing after 15 seconds of coronary occlusion. On release of balloon occlusion, immediate anterograde hyperemia can be observed in the distal bed with a loss of the retrograde flow pattern, corresponding with successful angioplasty. Abbreviations as in Fig. 6-8. (From Kern MJ, Donohue TJ, Bach RG, Aguirre FV, Caracciolo EA, Ofili EO: Quantitating coronary collateral flow velocity in patients during coronary angioplasty using a Doppler guidewire. *Am J Cardiol* 71(14):34D–40D, 1993.)

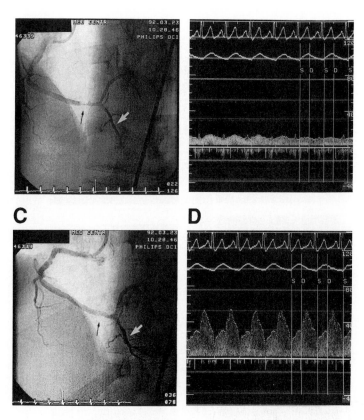

Fig. 6-11.   Distal coronary flow velocity before (**A**) and after (**C**) successful percutaneous transluminal coronary balloon angioplasty of the distal right coronary artery 90% stenosis. Distal pre-percutaneous transluminal coronary balloon angioplasty flow velocity is 12 cm/sec (**B**) with reduced phasic pattern. After percutaneous transluminal coronary balloon angioplasty (**D**), the mean flow velocity is 35 cm/sec with normal phasic pattern. The black arrows show percutaneous transluminal coronary balloon angioplasty sites, and white arrow shows Doppler guidewire sample volume location.

Normal LAD Transplant

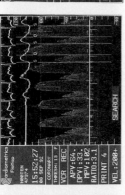

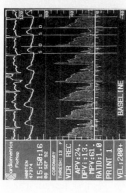

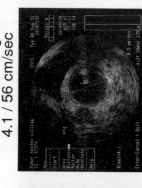

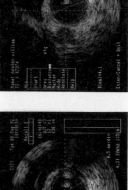

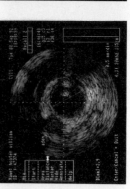

NTG, 200 mg
4.1 / 56 cm/sec

Adenosine, 12 µg
3.9 / 64 cm/sec

Base
3.9 / 24 cm/sec

visual identification of thrombus, arterial dissection, and plaque surface characteristics. Image quantitation remains a significant limitation.

ANGIOGRAPHIC BLOOD FLOW TECHNIQUES: VIDEODENSITOMETRY

Videodensitometry is based on determining the contrast media transit time from one point in the arterial tree to another. The time of transit of the wave front of contrast density is proportional to coronary blood flow. Digital angiographic computer software and hardware systems are required.

Technique

Videodensitometry measures of contrast time have been combined with subtraction digital angiography in which spatial resolution has been markedly improved by computer coding of the contrast rates. The transmural distribution of perfusion, as with other techniques in patients, cannot be assessed. Absolute flow cannot be determined because baseline flow is unknown. Intraarterial injection of contrast must be performed using standardized flow velocity and volume techniques (power injection of coronary arteries is needed). A further description of digital angiography can be found in Chapter 5.

Limitations

Accurate measurement of contrast transit time is seriously limited by the complex, geometric courses of the coronary arteries with their three-dimensional anatomy and multiple arterial branch points. Variables affecting the accuracy of digital videodensitometric coronary flow measurements include the technique of arterial contrast injection, the effect

---

Fig. 6-12. *Top,* Doppler guidewire flow velocity and 4.3 French two-dimensional coronary ultrasound images. *Bottom,* The cross-sectional artery images show a normal lumen with a diameter of 3.9 mm and minimal changes to adenosine or nitroglycerin (*NTG*). *LAD,* left anterior descending artery. APV, average peak velocity; DPVi, diastolic peak velocity integral; MPV, maximal peak velocity; Ratio, coronary reserve ratio; VEL, velocity scale.

of contrast on coronary hyperemia, the digital subtraction protocol employed, and the computer algorithms. Coronary flow reserve computed by digital subtraction angiography is approximately 2 (ratio of hyperemic/basal coronary flow), whereas assessments using other techniques in normal patients (e.g., intracoronary Doppler) generally demonstrate higher levels (three- to fivefold).

COMBINED HEMODYNAMIC AND ECHOCARDIOGRAPHIC METHODOLOGIES

Two-dimensional or M-mode echocardiography of LV wall motion provides detailed information of myocardial contractile responses, which can be recorded with simultaneous hemodynamic measurements. The echocardiogram is safe and provides a method of continuous observation of LV or valvular flow functions during cardiac catheterization without radiation. The recent introduction of transesophageal echocardiography for use during valvuloplasty in the catheterization laboratory has demonstrated that the echocardiogram provides a useful, novel method of guiding transseptal balloon placement and improving the results of such procedures.

Echocardiographic machines used in the cardiac catherization laboratory obviously must be modified to accept pressure and other signals from the hemodynamic studies (Figs. 6-13 to 6-15). Specialized input amplifiers for echocardiographic machines are available from several manufacturers, facilitating the recording of pressures simultaneously with echocardiographic parameters. Use of Doppler echocardiography and simultaneous hemodynamics has advanced the understanding of cardiac function and will provide a means of examining questions heretofore unanswered using other techniques.

PHYSIOLOGIC MANEUVERS IN THE CATHETERIZATION LABORATORY
Exercise During Cardiac Catheterization

Exercise evaluation of cardiac function is helpful to relate symptoms of fatigue or dyspnea to hemodynamic changes of cardiac dysfunction, especially for patients with valvular heart disease (e.g., mitral stenosis). Hemodynamics are measured at rest and during peak exercise using bicycle ergome-

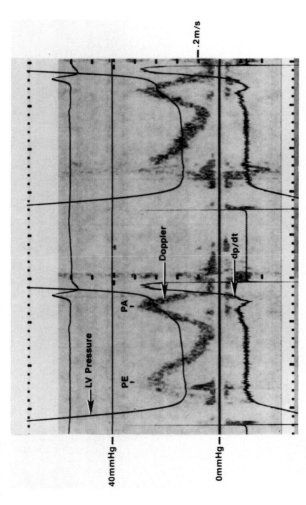

Fig. 6-13. Simultaneous high-fidelity left ventricular (*LV*) pressure (0 to 40 mm Hg scale) superimposed on Doppler echocardiogram showing peak early (*PE*) and peak atrial (*PA*) filling waves of the mitral valve inflow. Also superimposed is the dP/dt signal from the left ventricular pressure tracing and the electrocardiogram. These combined methodologies permit analysis of function not previously available by a single technique.

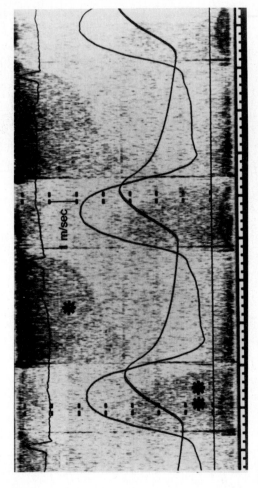

Fig. 6-14. Aortic (*Ao*) and left ventricular (*LV*) pressure superimposed on the Doppler aortic flow velocity demonstrating aortic stenosis and insufficiency characterized by the Doppler waveform. Aortic stenosis is superimposed on the systolic ejection gradient (**) and the aortic insufficiency can be observed over the diastolic period with the reversed diastolic velocity observed (*).

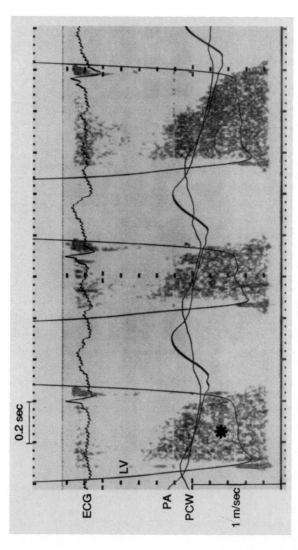

Fig. 6-15. Mitral stenosis as evidenced by simultaneous pulmonary capillary wedge (*PCW*), pulmonary artery (*PA*) pressure, and left ventricular (*LV*) pressure superimposed on the Doppler mitral inflow velocity showing a high prolonged initial flow velocity (*) characteristic of severe mitral stenosis.

403

try, repeated leg lift, and, occasionally, arm bicycle ergometry. Adequate response to exercise includes

1. Normal ventilatory responses (i.e., arterial oxygen extraction)
2. Normal heart rate increase in response to increases in cardiac output
3. Normal ventricular volume responses (decrease in filling pressures)
4. Adequate metabolic substrate utilization (i.e., appropriate use of glucose without lactate production)

Exercise may be *dynamic* or *isometric*. Measurement of each type demonstrates different features of left ventricular function.

Dynamic exercise.   Dynamic exercise measures the ability of the cardiovascular system to supply oxygen in keeping with the demands of the heart. Oxygen consumption and work load increases should be parallel until the maximal oxygen consumption for the patient's size is reached. Dynamic exercise in the cardiac catheterization laboratory requires simultaneous right and left heart pressure measurements during exercise (e.g., treadmill device mounted on the catheterization table). The patient's oxygen consumption also is measured and compared to the hemodynamic responses. Supine exercise in the catheterization laboratory differs from normal upright exercise in several ways:

1. Ventricular volumes are larger when the patient is supine rather than upright.
2. Heart rate and diastolic arterial pressure are higher when the patient is upright rather than supine.
3. Pulmonary and intracardiac filling pressures are lower when the patient is upright.
4. Stroke volume increases 100% with maximal exercise when the patient is upright and only 20% to 50% when the patient is supine.
5. Both upright exercise and supine exercise are normally associated with increases in LV end-diastolic volume and decreases in end-systolic volume with concomitant increase in ejection fraction. In patients with coronary artery disease, these findings may not occur.

Method.   The performance of a dynamic exercise test in the catheterization laboratory is a follows:

1. With the patient in a supine position, resting hemodynamic data are obtained.
2. Exercise begins. Heart rate and changes in hemodynamics are recorded during the 6 minutes of exercise at constant load with bicycle ergometry.
3. At minute 4, exercise hemodynamic data collection is begun.
4. At minute 5, peak cardiac output measurements are obtained.
5. Exercise is terminated at minute 6. Fick oxygen consumption is obtained over minutes 4 to 6.

Data are analyzed with respect to change in hemodynamics (valve gradients), cardiac output, and oxygen consumption. Patients may be unable to exercise because of leg weakness, depressed cardiac function, peripheral vascular disease, or severe deconditioning. These factors may preclude determination of accurate exercise results in the catheterization laboratory and should be considered before undertaking the study.

Measurements of response to exercise

1. CO (a useful measurement for studying practically all types of heart disease) predicts a normal response and allows categorization of a given patient's response.
   a. Dexter index: The predicted CI with exercise is equal to $2.99 + 0.0059 \times$ (measured O_2 consumption index with exercise). The measured CI is the CO divided by body surface area. The normal Dexter index equals the measured CI with exercise divided by the predicted CI, and should be greater than 1.
   b. Normal exercise factor: For every 100 ml/min increase in O_2 consumption with exercise, the CO should increase by at least 600 ml/min, thus normal exercise factor:

$$= \frac{\text{ml/min CO}}{\text{ml/min } O_2 \text{ consumption}} \geq 6$$

NOTE: Exercise factor is calculated directly from observed changes in CO and O_2 consumption; it is not indexed to BSA.

2. Appropriate increases in arterial blood pressure and heart rate should be noted.

3. Compute left ventricular volumes (useful in myopathic, coronary, and valvular disease). Changes in left LV end-diastolic volume of LV end-diastolic pressure (more commonly used) with exercise may be plotted against observed changes in some parameter of LV systolic function (stroke volume or stroke work) to define a modified LV function curve.

4. Changes in filling pressures or valvular gradients are useful in valvular, myopathic, and coronary disease.

Isometric exercise.   Isometric exercise consists of skeletal muscle contraction without shortening. In the cardiac catheterization laboratory, isometric exercise commonly is performed using a hand grip with a graded hand dynamometer. Measurements of hemodynamics and ventricular function are obtained during sustained hand grip at a predetermined range (15% to 50% of the maximal hand grip contraction) for a period of 3 to 4 minutes. The size of the involved muscle group is unimportant, provided that maximal voluntary contraction is maintained to increase oxygen demand during the isometric exercise period. Isometric exercise is easy to perform and easy to repeat and requires inexpensive equipment. It does not involve body motion that may interfere with hemodynamic measurements. An involuntary Valsalva maneuver during straining may occur during unsupervised isometric exercise. Careful monitoring, patient cooperation, and practice in use of the hand grip dynamometer will minimize false hemodynamic information. In patients with coronary artery disease, isometric exercise rarely precipitates ischemia but may induce new LV wall motion abnormalities, decrease in LV ejection fraction, and an increase in end-systolic volume with no change in diastolic volume. SV and CO may decline during isometric exercise. In patients with congestive heart failure, heart rate and systemic pressure may rise appropriately with a fall in SV and CO resulting in increase in LV end-diastolic volume and PA pressure.

Valsalva maneuver (Fig. 6-16).   This maneuver is performed by having the patient forcibly expire against a closed glotus and straining as if using the toilet. The magnitude of the Valsalva can be quantitated by measuring the pressure against which the patient must expire. The Valsalva maneuver can be performed safely and without complications by

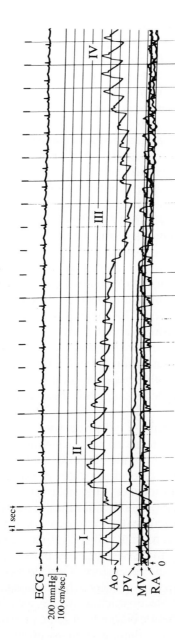

Fig. 6-16. Valsalva maneuver showing the effects on aortic (*Ao*) pressure, mean coronary velocity (*MV*), phasic coronary velocity (*PV*), and right atrial (*RA*) pressure. The four phases of the Valsalva maneuver (see text) are enumerated (*I, II, III,* and *IV*).

almost every type of patient. The four phases of the normal Valsalva maneuver (strain, hypotension, release, and pressure overshoot) may be absent in patients with specific cardiac diseases (congestive heart failure, coronary artery disease, and obstructive cardiomyopathy). In addition, the hemodynamics demonstrated for different types of valvular lesions may be more pronounced during the Valsalva maneuver because of changes in ventricular filling.

The Muller maneuver. The Muller maneuver is performed by inspiring against a closed glottis, and it is considered the inverse or opposite of the Valsalva maneuver. The subject inhales and the force of inhalation is measured with a manometer, usually -30 to -60 mm Hg for 30 seconds. Hemodynamic alterations of the Muller maneuver include increased RV filling, increased period of diminished filling as a result of the collapse of the vena cavae at thoracic inlets, increasing LV afterload with increase in LV end-diastolic and end-systolic volumes, diminished SV, reduced CO, and reduced ejection fraction. This maneuver is used to augment right-sided heart murmurs and to decrease the physical findings of obstructive cardiomyopathy by a reduction in LV outflow gradient. A reduction in the intensity of the systolic murmur in patients with echocardiographic evidence of anterior mitral valve leaflet motion can also be demonstrated with this maneuver.

Cold pressor testing. Cold pressor testing is an alpha-adrenergic stimulus, mediated by cold-induced pain in the forearm, hand, or forehead. Hemodynamic findings occurring with cold pressor testing include an increase in heart rate (5% to 15%), an increase in systolic and mean arterial pressure (15% to 20%), and a mild increase in CO. These responses usually occur within 2 minutes of application of the cold stimulus. In normal subjects, alpha stimulation by cold pressor testing increases coronary blood flow and reduces coronary vascular resistance. Cold pressor testing in patients with coronary artery disease has been demonstrated to cause coronary vasoconstriction, which may be potentiated by a beta-adrenergic blockade in some patients. Angina is rarely precipitated, although changes in left ventricular function have been identified. Coronary vasospasm has also been reported during cold pressor testing.

Hyperventilation.   Hyperventilation has been used to induce coronary spasm. Deep breathing (30 breaths/min for 5 minutes) is a commonly used method. Ischemia is rarely precipitated during hyperventilation but may commonly occur at the termination of rapid breathing. Heart rate, oxygen consumption, AV oxygen difference, and arterial pH increase during hyperventilation. Arterial pressure, PA pressure, and arterial Pco_2 fall. Peripheral vascular resistance, CO, and LV SV are unchanged with the increase in LV ejection fraction seen in normal patients. These abnormalities may not be observed in patients with stable or variant angina.

Pharmacologic stress.   Pharmacologic stresses are used to assess alterations of ventricular function. (See Chapter 5.)

Nitroglycerin.   Nitrates decrease systolic and mean arterial pressure and often produce a reflex increase in heart rate. Preload is markedly reduced with nitrates. There is no demonstrable effect on left ventricular performance, unless there is a profound decrease in systemic arterial pressure, resulting in a marked reflex stimulation. Nitroglycerin relieves coronary ischemia and coronary vasospasm and may improve LV function through this mechanism.

Amyl nitrate.   Amyl nitrate acts in a similar fashion to that of nitroglycerin. Its pronounced effects, quick onset, and rapid resolution make this drug an ideal agent for the study of brief but intense changes in preload.

Isoproterenol.   Isoproterenol is a pure beta agonist. It has been used as a pharmacologic replacement for exercise or for rapid atrial pacing, and it permits more precise hemodynamic monitoring than occurs during active exercise.

The hemodynamic effects of isoproterenol are similar to those of dynamic exercise, with increases in heart rate and CO. SV increases in young individuals and falls or is unchanged in older individuals where CO is more dependent on heart rate alone. Diastolic pressure falls and systolic pressure rises or remains unchanged resulting in a decline in mean arterial pressure. Both systemic and pulmonary vascular resistances are also reduced. Isoproterenol increases ejection fraction, maximum dP/dt, mean ejection rate, and LV work, demonstrating improved LV contractility. LV end-diastolic filling pressure is unchanged or falls while both

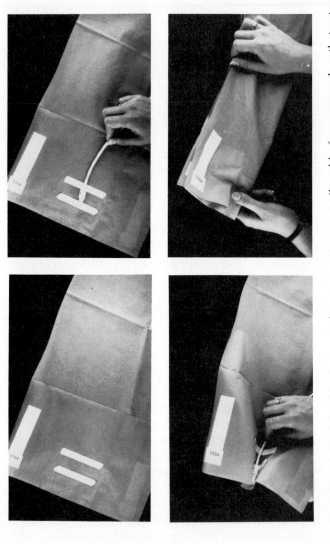

Fig. 6-17. Specialized "Roth" cable drape used to connect a nonsterile cable for a research catheter to a sterile connector in the catheter field. This drape is especially useful for the Doppler catheter and guidewire connections.

myocardial oxygen consumption and coronary blood flow markedly increase. In patients with coronary artery disease, the LV ejection fraction may fall, angina may be induced, and LV regional wall motion abnormalities may be provoked.

Dobutamine. Dobutamine is a synthetic catecholamine that increases contractility and reduces vascular resistance. IV infusions and two-dimensional echocardiographic examination of LV wall motion are used to screen for severe coronary artery narrowings.

Nurse/Technician Viewpoint

The nursing/technical staff should be presented with a clear, concise, project protocol. The protocol should include

1. Overview of the project with clearly delineated objectives
2. Patient safety
3. Special equipment if necessary
4. Additional staffing if required
5. Data sheets (prepared to facilitate study periods)

If additional sterile equipment is necessary, a "protocol pack" with all additional equipment will aid with setup.

Many research techniques require the use of special catheters that must be interfaced with various flow meters, CO computers, and the like. Personnel must be careful not to contaminate the sterile field when connecting the catheter to the inferface cable. There are two ways to approach this situation. One is to sterilize all interface cables. The other is to wrap the nonsterile cable in a sterile drape (Fig. 6-17). If the latter technique is used the physician must be careful not to pull the nonsterile cable into the sterile field.

If medications are involved, dose/calculation worksheets will aid the staff in drug preparation.

SUGGESTED READINGS

Braunwald E, Goldblatt A, Harrison DC, Mason DT: Studies on cardiac dimensions in intact, unanesthetized man. III. Effects of muscular exercise, *Circ Res* 13:460, 1963.

Chapman CB, editor: Physiology of muscular exercise, *Circ Res* 20(Suppl 1):I1–I255, 1967. (Also available as Monograph Fifteen from American Heart Association.)

Donald KW, Bishop JM, Cumming G, Wade OL: The effect of exercise on the cardiac output and circulatory dynamics of normal subjects, *Clin Sci* 14:37, 1955.

Donohue TJ, Kern MJ, Aguirre FV, et al.: Determination of the hemodynamic significance of angiographically intermediate coronary stenoses by intracoronary Doppler flow velocity (abstr), *J Am Coll Cardiol* 19:242A, 1992.

Donohue TJ, Kern MJ, Aguirre FV, et al.: Comparison of hemodynamic and pharmacologic perturbations of coronary collateral flow velocity in patients during angioplasty (abstr), *J Am Coll Cardiol* 19:383A, 1992.

Doucette JW, Corl PD, Payne HM, et al.: Validation of a Doppler guide wire for intravascular measurement of coronary artery flow velocity, *Circulation* 85:1899–1911, 1992.

Grines CL, Mancini GBJ, McGillem MJ, Gallagher KP, Vogel RA: Measurement of regional myocardial perfusion and mass by subselective hydrogen infusion and washout techniques: a validation study, *Circulation* 76:1373–1379, 1987.

Herman MV, Heinle RA, Klein MD, Gorlin R: Localized disorders in myocardial contraction: asynergy and its role in congestive heart failure, *N Engl J Med* 277:222–232, 1967.

Kass DA, Maughan WL: From 'Emax' to pressure-volume relations: a broader view, *Circulation* 77:1203–1212, 1988.

Kern MJ: Intracoronary flow velocity: current techniques and clinical applications of Doppler catheter methods. In Tobis JM, Yock PG, editors: *Intravascular ultrasound imaging,* New York, 1992, Churchill Livingstone, pp 93–111.

Kern MJ, Aguirre F, Bach R, et al.: Augmentation of coronary blood flow by intra-aortic balloon pumping in patients after coronary angioplasty, *Circulation* 87:500–511, 1993.

McLaurin LP, Grossman W: Dynamic and isometric exercise during cardiac catheterization. In Grossman W, editor: *Cardiac catheterization and angiography,* Philadelphia, 1974, Lea & Febiger, pp 159–167.

Mirsky I: Assessment of diastolic function: suggested methods and future considerations, *Circulation* 69:836–841, 1984.

Mitchell JH, Harris MD: Exercise and the heart: physiologic and clinical considerations. In Willerson JT, Sanders CA, editors: *Clinical cardiology,* New York, 1977, Grune & Stratton, pp 208–213.

Otili EO, Kern MJ, Labovitz AJ, et al.: Analysis of coronary blood flow velocity dynamics in angiographically normal and stenosed arteries before and after endoluminal enlargement by angioplasty, *J Am Coll Cardiol* 21:308–318, 1993.

Ross J Jr, Linhart JW, Braunwald E: Effects of changing heart rate in man by electrical stimulation of the right atrium: studies at rest, during exercise and with isoproterenol, *Circulation* 32:549–558, 1965.

Sagawa K, Suga H, Shoukas AA, Bakalar KM: End-systolic pressure-volume ratio: a new index of contractility, *Am J Cardiol* 40:748–753, 1979.

Segal J, Kern MJ, Scott NA, et al.: Alterations of phasic coronary artery flow velocity in man during percutaneous coronary angioplasty, *J Am Coll Cardiol* 20:276–286, 1992.

Sheehan FH, Schofer J, Mathey DG, Kellett MA, Smith H, Bolson EL, Dodge HT: Measurement of regional wall motion from biplane contrast ventriculograms: a comparison of the 30 degree right anterior oblique and 60 degree left anterior oblique projections in patients with acute myocardial infarction, *Circulation* 74:796–804, 1986.

Sonnenblick EH, Braunwald E, Williams JF Jr, Glick G: Effects of exercise on myocardial force-velocity relations in heart rate, sympathetic activity and ventricular dimensions, *J Clin Invest* 44:2051, 1965.

Suga H, Hayashi T, Shirahata M: Ventricular systolic pressure volume area as predictor of cardiac oxygen consumption, *Am J Physiol* 240 (*Heart Circ Physiol* 9):H39–H44, 1981.

Suga H, Sagawa K: Instantaneous pressure-volume relationships and their ratio in the excised, supported canine left ventricle, *Circ Res* 35:117–126, 1974.

Weiss JL, Frederiksen JW, Weisfeldt ML: Hemodynamic determinants of the time-course of fall in canine left ventricular pressure, *J Clin Invest* 58:751–760, 1976.

7

SPECIAL TECHNIQUES

Ubeydullah Deligonul, Richard G. Bach, Morton J. Kern, Michael S. Flynn, and Eugene A. Caracciolo

TRANSSEPTAL HEART CATHETERIZATION

Retrograde left heart catheterization for aortic stenosis or prosthetic aortic valve dysfunction may not be suitable in all patients. Transseptal access across the thin atrial septal membrane at the fossa ovalis into the left atrium and left ventricle is an established technique that should be performed only by experienced operators.

Indications (See the box on p. 415)

1. Conditions that require direct LA or LV measurement of pressure (such as mitral stenosis, pulmonary venous disease, left intraventricular gradient, aortic stenosis, or hypertrophic cardiomyopathy)
2. Access for mitral balloon-catheter valvuloplasty
3. Severe peripheral vascular disease that impairs retrograde catheter attempts at crossing the aortic valve
4. Prosthetic aortic or mitral heart valves

Crossing a tilting disc-type prosthetic valve in the aortic position has been performed with varying success using a retrograde catheter technique, although death in some patients from lodged catheters has been reported.

Contraindications

1. Patients who cannot lie flat or fully cooperate
2. Anticoagulant therapy or other hemostatic abnormalities (coumadin should be discontinued several days before transseptal puncture so that the prothrombin time is less than or equal to 14 seconds)
3. Left atrial thrombus
4. Atrial myxoma

Transseptal left heart catheterization should be considered carefully in patients with distorted cardiac anatomy secondary to congenital heart disease, dilated aortic root, marked atrial enlargement, or thoracic skeletal deformity.

Indications for Transseptal Left Heart Catheterization

MEASUREMENT OF LEFT ATRIAL OR LV HEMODYNAMICS

Mitral valve

PCWP in question
Doppler gradient in question
Prosthetic mitral valve
Previous mitral valve surgery
Exclude pulmonary veno occlusive disease

Aortic valve

Retrograde catheterization not possible
Tilting disc prosthetic valve
Echocardiographic data inconclusive
Question of hypertrophic obstructive cardiomyopathy

LEFT VENTRICULAR ANGIOGRAPHY

To assess mitral regurgitation when retrograde catheterization not possible

VALVULOPLASTY

Mitral approach

Antegrade aortic approach

Procedural Highlights

Crossing the interatrial septum is performed in the AP projection after correct positioning of the transseptal Brockenbrough catheter. Steps to performing transseptal catheterization are as follows:

1. A pigtail catheter is placed in the sinus of Valsalva of the aorta for anatomic reference. (A Swan-Ganz catheter positioned in a pulmonary artery via the left femoral vein may also serve as a useful marker of the tricuspid valve.)
2. The right femoral vein is used for access. The guidewire is advanced to the SVC.
3. The Brockenbrough catheter is advanced over guidewire to superior vena cava.
4. The wire is withdrawn and a transseptal needle is advanced through the catheter permitting free rotation of the needle. The needle is positioned in the SVC at the twelve o'clock position, keeping the needle within the catheter. The needle is connected to a pressure transducer with a three-way stopcock for continuous observation during atrial crossing.
5. The catheter and needle assembly are withdrawn into the right atrium with a clockwise rotation, with the needle angle indicator pointing posteriorly between three and five o'clock (Fig. 7-1).
6. On withdrawal downward into the right atrium, the catheter assembly will pass over the aortic knob, with a for-

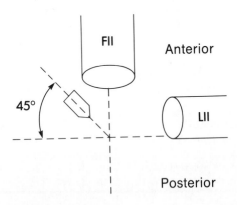

Fig. 7-1. Transseptal arrow is oriented approximately 45° posteriorly. *FII,* Frontal image intensifier; *LII,* lateral image intensifier. (From Weiner RI, Maranhao V: Development and application of transseptal left heart catheterization, *Cathet Cardiovasc Diagn* 15:112, 1988.)

ward motion, and on further withdrawal pass under the aortic indentation into the fossa ovale. Slight advancement until contact with the septum is performed at this point. Approximately 15% to 20% of patients will have a patent foramen ovale allowing unobstructed passage of the catheter assembly into the left atrium without puncture.

7. To localize precisely the point of puncture on the interatrial septum, the technique described by Croft et al. is used (Fig. 7-2). This consists of RAO angulation and identification of the pigtail catheter within the sinus of Valsalva in the aorta and RA posterior wall. A line is drawn from the lower end of the pigtail horizontally to the verti-

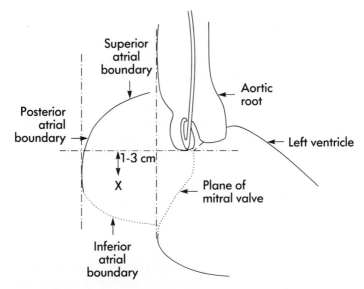

Fig. 7-2. X marks the optimal spot for transseptal puncture. Diagrammatic representation of the structures visualized in 40° right anterior oblique projection. The limits of the atria are depicted behind the aorta. The pigtail catheter positioned in the noncoronary aortic cusp defines the posterior boundary of the aortic root. The point of intended atrial septal puncture is delineated by X. (From Croft CH, Lipscomb K: Modified technique of transseptal left heart catheterization. *J Am Coll Cardiol* 5:904, 1985. Reprinted with permission of the American College of Cardiology.)

cal line of the RA border. Bisecting this line, the operator drops 1 cm below the line at the midpoint. This point usually is centered within the fossa ovale.

8. After contact with the interatrial septum is felt, firm pressure is maintained and the needle is advanced into the septum while pressure is continuously monitored. Some operators advocate "tagging" the atrial septum by injecting a small amount of contrast through the transeptal needle if it does not pass directly and fairly easily into the left atrium. This septal stain can aid in excluding inappropriate positioning and can serve as a landmark for further attempts. Entry into the left atrium is signified by observing LA pressure waveforms. If in doubt of the location of the needle tip, the operator may aspirate blood for determination of oxygen saturation (which should be arterial) and/or inject a small amount of contrast under fluoroscopy. After confirmation of proper positioning in the left atrium, the needle is advanced slightly and the catheter is then advanced over the needle with a counter-clockwise rotation of the needle permitting the Brockenbrough catheter to turn anteriorly into the mitral valve area. The needle is then withdrawn and the Brockenbrough catheter is carefully aspirated and connected to pressure. (Remember, left-sided injections of thrombus or bubbles will enter the systemic circulation.) After positioning the Brockenbrough catheter in the left atrium, a small amount of contrast may be injected to identify its position and so avoid advancing guidewires or catheters into pulmonary veins.

9. To enter the left ventricle, the guidewire (0.038-inch J) is inserted into the Brockenbrough catheter and advanced across the mitral valve and into the left ventricle. The catheter then follows this guidewire.

Preparatory notes

1. The Brockenbrough catheter must be measured against the transeptal needle to identify the position at which the needle extends outside the catheter (Fig. 7-3). This measurement is done before insertion of the catheter/ needle assembly. Placing the catheter over the needle and noting at what point the needle leaves the catheter end,

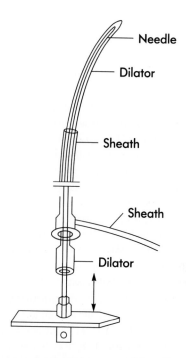

Fig. 7-3. Transseptal catheter assembly. The distance between the transseptal needle and the dilator hub (*arrow*) is
noted so that the needle lies just inside the dilator. (From
Weiner RI, Maranhao V: Development and application of
transseptal left heart catheterization, *Cathet Cardiovasc Diagn*
15:112, 1988.)

the operator marks this distance with the fingertips. Keeping the needle inside the catheter will protect the wall of
the atrium from inadvertent needle damage.

2. Note on passing the transseptal needle up through the
Brockenbrough catheter: There are three points along its
course in which a curve and turning of the needle will
occur. One is the iliac crest, the second is over the spine
near the renal vein, and the third is at the inferior junction
of the cardiac silhouette. The needle should rotate freely
over these three segments and slide smoothly and carefully up through the Brockenbrough catheter. Otherwise,
damage to the catheter and/or injury to the patient can
occur.

3. An alternative catheter system is that of the Mullins sheath and catheter that will provide a sheath positioned within the left atrium or ventricle suitable for inserting a pigtail or balloon-tipped ventriculographic (Berman) catheter.

4. Left ventriculography through the Brockenbrough catheter should be performed at low volume (30 to 40 ml) and moderate flow rates (10 to 12 ml/sec) because of its end-hole configuration. A small test injection should be performed to avoid catheter malposition. Rarely, perforation of the left ventricle with this catheter has been reported.

5. In the normal heart, the fossa ovalis is located in the middle third of the atrial septum and is concave toward the left atrium. Valvular disease may significantly alter the location of the fossa ovalis. In aortic valve disease, the dilated ascending aorta may displace the fossa superiorly and anteriorly. In mitral valve disease, the left atrium usually enlarges posteriorly and inferiorly, displacing the fossa ovalis inferiorly. In severe disease, the fossa may become everted and displaced into the lower third of the septum, becoming difficult to locate on catheter descent. Therefore, in severe valvular disease, the transseptal puncture site requires appropriate modification.

Risks Related to Transseptal Catheterization

Cardiac perforation of
   Right atrium
   Posterior left atrium
   Left atrial appendage
   Pulmonary vein
   Left ventricle
Puncture into the aortic root
Pericardial tamponade*
Embolus from the left atrium

* Almost all deaths related to transseptal catheterization are secondary to tamponade.

Risks of Transseptal Catheterization (See the box above)

Puncture of the aortic root, CS, or the posterior free wall of the atrium are potentially lethal problems. In patients who have not been given anticoagulants, the 21-gauge tip of the needle rarely causes a problem. However, if the large catheter is advanced into these spaces, cardiac tamponade may occur. If the operator is not satisfied with the position of the Brockenbrough catheter in the right atria, the catheter/needle combination should not be advanced. If the catheter assembly is not in the correct position, the procedure must start over again with removal of the transseptal needle, reinsertion of the guidewire to the SVC, repositioning of the catheter, and then repositioning of the needle with withdrawal and turning as indicated earlier.

DIRECT TRANSTHORACIC LV PUNCTURE

The development of retrograde arterial catheterization and transseptal catheterization has enabled clinicians to obtain hemodynamic data without direct transthoracic puncture techniques, except in very unusual situtations.

Indications

Transthoracic LV puncture is required to measure LV pressure or perform LV angiography when no other access is available. This occurs mainly in patients with combined mitral and aortic valve replacement with mechanical tilting disc prostheses. Although several investigators report techniques for crossing mechanical tilting discs, retrograde complications have been reported involving catheter entrapment and occlusion of the ball valves or tilting discs with disastrous results. When double valve replacement is the condition in which the ventricular pressure and angiography are required, direct puncture with echocardiographic guidance can be performed at relatively low risk.

Before the procedure, a two-dimensional echocardiography from the apical window is very helpful in locating the true LV apex and determining the direction of the long axis of the left ventricle. After placement of the arterial and right heart catheters, an 18-gauge, $4\frac{1}{4}$-inch-long needle with Teflon sheath connected to a pressure transducer is inserted at the apical area through the intercostal space close to the upper border of the lower rib in this space. It is directed posteriorly toward the right shoulder. The pressure tracing is monitored continuously while the needle is advanced. Following entry into the ventricle, the needle is removed, leaving the Teflon sheath in place through which pressure recordings and angiograms are performed. The hemodynamic data should be obtained quickly and the sheath should be removed.

Complications

The patient should be watched carefully for hemopericardium, hemothorax, or pneumothorax. Should any of these complications occur they can be treated with direct aspiration or surgery as needed. A vasovagal reaction with bradycardia and hypotension may be encountered. Bleeding complications may result from laceration of the LAD or intercostal arteries. Patients with previous open heart surgery usually have obliterated pericardial space, decreasing the likelihood of cardiac tamponade.

Embolism may occur if an LV clot is displaced from the apex. The detailed methodologic approach to insertion of the direct LV needle can be found in the reference texts. Direct LV puncture is contraindicated in a patient who is receiving anticoagulants.

Indications for Endomyocardial Biopsy

DEFINITIVE

Cardiac transplantation follow-up
Monitoring of athracycline cardiotoxicity

POSSIBLE

Viral myocarditis
Secondary cardiomyopathies (sarcoidosis, hemochromatosis,
    amyloidosis, etc.)
Differentiation of restrictive versus constrictive cardiac disease
Endocardial fibrosis
Hyperesinophilic syndrome
Malignancies involving the heart

ENDOMYOCARDIAL BIOPSY

Endomyocardial biopsy is an increasingly common procedure in the catheterization laboratory. At least 30,000 endomyocardial biopsy procedures were performed in the United States in 1989 for indications other than monitoring of cardiac transplant rejection.

Indications (See the box on page 422)

Monitoring of cardiac transplant rejection and athracycline cardiotoxicity are the only two definitive indications for endomyocardial biopsy. Other indications include diagnosis for secondary causes of cardiomyopathy, myocarditis (when there is a history of congestive heart failure in the past 6 months), and differentiation between restrictive and constrictive cardiomyopathies.

Contraindications

1. Anticoagulation
2. Anatomic abnormality

Biopsy Devices

There are two basic types of bioptomes: (1) stiff shaft devices (Konno, Kawai, and Stanford bioptomes; Fig. 7-4), and

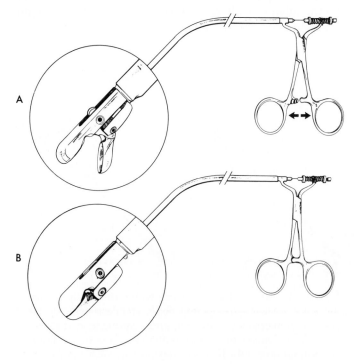

Fig. 7-4.   Scholten bioptome, open **(A)** and closed **(B)**. (From Tilkian AG, Daily EK: *Cardiovascular procedures: diagnostic techniques and therapeutic procedures,* St Louis, 1986, Mosby.)

(2) floppy shaft devices (King and Cordis bioptomes; Fig. 7-5) that are positioned with the aid of a long sheath. The femoral sheath dilator is 94 cm in length and the long sheath is 85 cm in length. Biopsy sheaths come in both 5- and 7-cm curves (for large right atrium or transplanted hearts).

Technique

Endomyocardial biopsy can be performed under fluoroscopic or echocardiographic guidance from the femoral or internal jugular approach.

Femoral approach.   Under local anesthesia the right or left femoral vein is punctured by modified Seldinger technique and a 0.038-inch guidewire is advanced into the femoral vein. A 7 French biopsy sheath with a 7 French dilator is advanced over the guidewire. A large-curve (7-cm) sheath is used when the atrium is dilated, as in cardiac transplantation. The dilator is not completely radiopaque. The sheath with the dilator inside is advanced into the right atrium and then the dilator is withdrawn into the sheath. With the help of the guidewire the sheath is advanced across the tricuspid

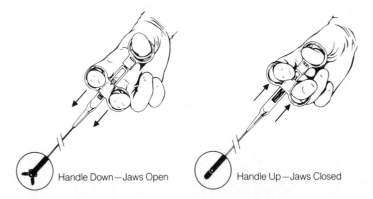

Handle Down—Jaws Open   Handle Up—Jaws Closed

Fig. 7-5.   Disposable biopsy forceps with formable tip, pivoting jaws, a clear wire-braided body, stainless-steel cutting jaws, a stainless-steel wire coil, and a spring-loaded three-ring plastic handle that controls the operation of the jaws. The thumb ring of the handle is flexible and rotates to accommodate any thumb position, thereby reducing manual stress. (Courtesy of Cordis Corporation, Miami, Fla.)

valve and into the right ventricle. The biopsy sheath is equipped with a back-bleed valve and a side arm for flushing. Blood is aspirated and the sheath is flushed and connected to the pressure monitor, identifying an RV pressure tracing. A floppy shaft biopsy forcep is advanced through the sheath and into the right ventricle. The sheath is pointed toward the intraventricular septum, which should be confirmed in the LAO projection to ensure that the bioptome has not entered the CS inadvertently. The RV outflow tract and (usually) the inferior and RV free wall should be avoided.

The bioptome jaws are opened before leaving the sheath to reduce the chance of perforation. The bioptome is advanced carefully with the jaws springing fully open until contact with the ventricular wall is made and there is slight bending of the bioptome shaft. The bioptome jaws are then closed. After 2 to 3 seconds, the "bite" is withdrawn slowly into the sheath as the sheath is advanced. A tugging sensation will often be elicited. After the bioptome is outside the patient, the sheath should be aspirated and flushed to eliminate air bubbles. The same procedure is repeated until an adequate number of specimens (usually four to six) is obtained. RV pressures are measured before and after the biopsy. The biopsy sheath is then removed and hemostasis is secured.

For heterotopic heart transplantation (i.e., piggy back hearts) the donor right atrium will be located in the right hemithorax. Its connection to the recipient atrium may be marked with a radiopaque ring. The biopsy sheath will be advanced over the guidewire and into the donor right ventricle, and biopsy samples will be taken as described above.

Internal jugular approach with echocardiographic guidance (Figs. 7-6 and 7-7). Extensive experience in performing endomyocardial biopsies under echocardiographic guidance as well as fluoroscopy has been reported. An 8 French short sheath is inserted into the right internal jugular vein by standard Seldinger technique. A bioptome (Storz, Inc., Culver City, CA) is inserted through the venous sheath and into the right atrium. Using two-dimensional echocardiography, the tricuspid valve leaflets are readily visible, aiding the passage of the bioptome across the valve with minimal trauma. Usually a counterclockwise (anterior) rotation helps guide the bioptome past the tricuspid valve. Further

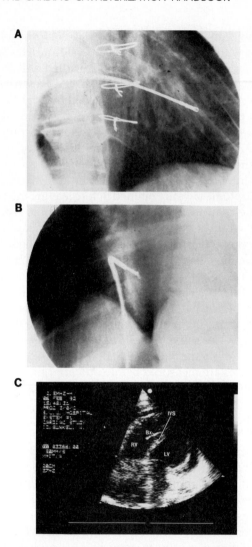

Fig. 7-6. *Left panels:* **A,** Anteroposterior cineangiographic image of femoral endomyocardial bioptome location and **B,** corresponding left anterior oblique view. **C,** Simultaneous two-dimensional echocardiographic image showing position of bioptome (*Bx*) against the right ventricular side of the interventricular septum (*IVS*). *LV,* Left ventricle; *RV,* right ventricle. *Continued on page 427.*

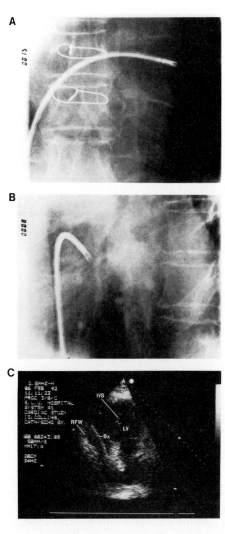

Fig. 7-6. *Continued. Right panels:* Same views in another transplant recipient showing nearly identical angiographic location, but positioning of bioptome and sheath against the right ventricular free wall (*RFW*). (From Bell CA, Kern MJ, Aguirre FV, Donohue T, Bach R, Wolford T, Penick D, Ofili E, Miller L: Superior accuracy of anatomic positioning with echocardiographic-over fluoroscopic-guided endomyocardial biopsy. *Cathet Cardiovasc Diagn* 28:291–294, 1993.)

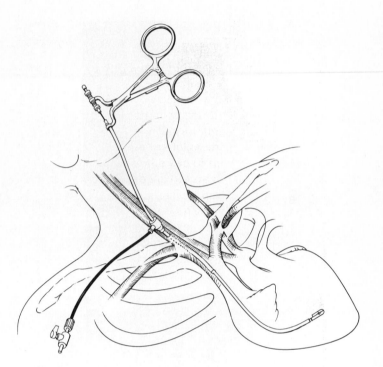

Fig. 7-7. Internal jugular approach. The bioptome tip is in the right ventricular apex, pointing toward the ventricular septum. (From Tilkian AG, Daily EK: *Cardiovascular procedures: diagnostic techniques and therapeutic procedures,* St Louis, 1986, Mosby.)

counterclockwise rotation usually straightens the curve and orients the bioptome toward the central ventricular septum. Under echocardiographic guidance, biopsies can be obtained safely from the intraventricular septum, apex, and free wall. The sheath is then removed and hemostasis secured.

The advantages of echocardiographically guided endomyocardial biopsy are the following:

1. It does not require the use of the angiographic suite.
2. There is no radiation exposure to the patient or operator.
3. Because two-dimensional echocardiography equipment is portable, the procedure can be performed in the intensive care unit or patient room.
4. Biopsies can be obtained from multiple areas, including the intraventricular septum, apex, and free wall, which may increase the diagnostic yield.

5. More accurate positioning of the bioptome is achieved with two-dimensional echocardiography than with fluoroscopy.

At St. Louis University, only two significant complications have occurred in 4700 biopsies performed over a 5-year period under echocardiographic guidance. If present, cardiac tamponade from RV perforation will be apparent 20 to 30 minutes after biopsy. Conduction block and tricuspid leaflet damage have been reported.

Internal jugular approach with fluoroscopic guidance. The same technique and principles as above are used, except that fluoroscopic guidance is substituted for the echocardiogram.

CS CATHETERIZATION (See Chapter 6)

The CS is located in the inferoposterior aspect of the tricuspid valve on the RA side. The CS ostium is approximately 0.5 to 1 cm in diameter and proceeds in a caudal/posterior and then superior direction.

Indications

1. Determination of myocardial oxygen extraction and lactate production
2. Collection of transmyocardial catecholamines and other cardiac metabolites
3. Measurement of CS thermodilution blood flow
4. Electrophysiology studies (particularly for localization of accessory conduction pathways)
5. Retroperfusion in the CS is an investigational technique, using either synchronized counterpulsation or continuous intermittent positive pressure methods

Techniques

The approach to the CS is typically from the right internal jugular vein, left subclavian vein, or the antecubital veins from either arm (as described earlier). Most of the catheters used for CS blood flow measurement and oxygen and metabolite extraction are large-diameter, relatively stiff catheters and do not lend themselves to the curves needed to approach the CS from the femoral direction.

A large-diameter catheter with an occluding balloon for CS retroperfusion (instilling blood or drugs in the heart through pressurized delivery through the CS) involves similar catheter placement technique. Retroperfusion is currently investigational. The same precautionary notes hold when inserting these extra-large-diameter catheters.

PERICARDIOCENTESIS

Indications

Pericardiocentesis may be required for diagnosis and management of acute and chronic pericardial effusions. In cardiac tamponade this is a lifesaving technique. A sufficient degree of skill must be employed in order to prevent further damage to the heart and pericardium.

Procedure

In the cardiac catheterization laboratory, pericardiocentesis often is preceded by echocardiographic confirmation of pericardial fluid. However, in cases in which a large pericardial effusion is suspected, or in which tamponade is acute, echocardiographically assisted positioning is not required, and may be detrimental by delaying needed intervention. Although monitoring of pericardial pressure is not essential, it is important to document evidence of cardiac tamponade and resolution of pericardial pressure restricting cardiac output.

Route to pericardium (Fig. 7-8).   A long 16- or 18-gauge needle connected to a stopcock and tubing to a pressure transducer can be used. The preferred approach is the subxyphoid route, but other sites are acceptable depending on the location and volume of the effusion (Fig. 7-8). The advantage of the subxyphoid approach is a decreased likelihood of coronary and internal thoracic artery laceration.

Setup and positioning.   The patient is set at a 30° to 45° head-up angle to permit pooling of pericardial fluid on the inferior surface of the heart. Local anesthesia is instilled through the pericardial needle as it is advanced initially perpendicularly to the skin and then at a sharp low angle (near parallel with horizontal plane) under the xyphoid toward the left shoulder. If the patient is obese a larger needle and considerable force may be required to tip the syringe under the subxyphoid process toward the heart.

We routinely place a balloon-tipped catheter into the PA via a femoral vein to assess equalization of diastolic right-

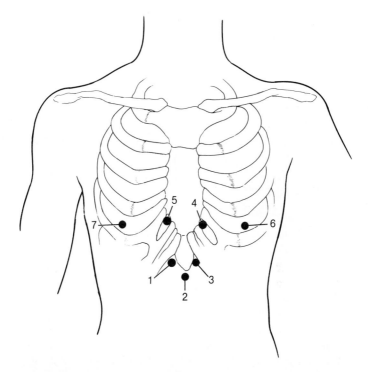

Fig. 7-8. Locations for pericardiocentesis. *1* to *3*, Xiphoid approaches. *4*, Fifth left intercostal space at sternal border. *5*, Fifth right intercostal space at the sternal border. *6*, Apical approach. *7*, Approach for major fluid accumulation on the right side. (Adapted from Spodick DH: *Acute pericarditis*, New York, 1959, Grune & Stratton.)

sided pressures (and to document the change with intervention), then withdraw this catheter into the right atrium for continuous monitoring during pericardial puncture. Often a 5 French sheath placed in a femoral artery is useful for monitoring of arterial pressure.

Puncturing the pericardium (Figs. 7-9 and 7-10).   Aspiration during passage of the needle through the skin may block the needle with subcutaneous tissue. Flush any tissue that may have accumulated in the needle (during aspiration) before passing through the pericardium, a rigid fibrous membrane. The pericardial puncture feels similar to a lumbar

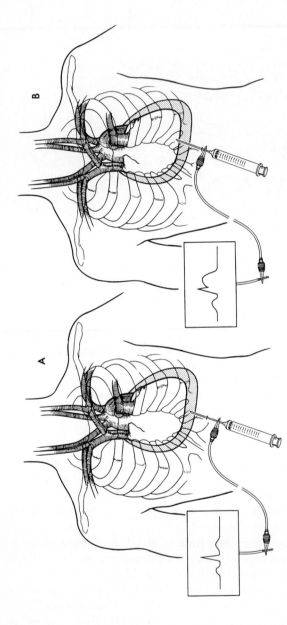

Fig. 7-9. **A,** Electrocardiographic monitoring of pericardial needle tip. Note normal ST segment while tip is not touching the epicardium. **B,** When needle tip touches epicardium, current of injury ("contact" current) with elevated ST segment is seen. (From Tilkian AG, Daily EK: *Cardiovascular procedures: diagnostic techniques and therapeutic procedures,* St Louis, 1986, Mosby.)

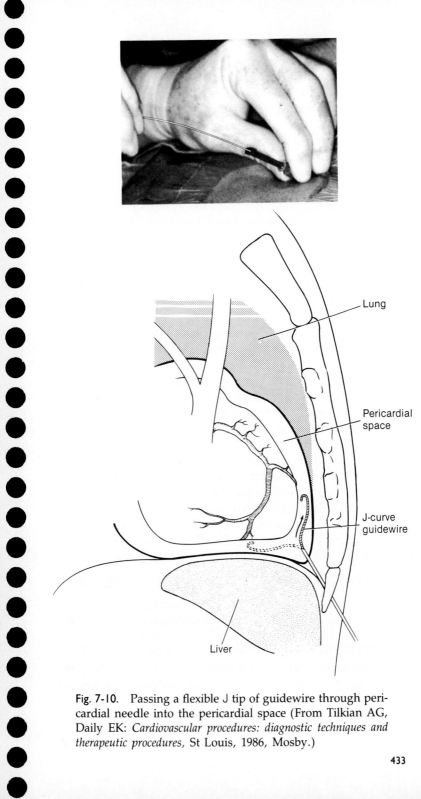

Fig. 7-10. Passing a flexible J tip of guidewire through pericardial needle into the pericardial space (From Tilkian AG, Daily EK: *Cardiovascular procedures: diagnostic techniques and therapeutic procedures,* St Louis, 1986, Mosby.)

Lung

Pericardial space

J-curve guidewire

Liver

puncture. If the pericardial fluid is of a chronic variety, it may have a clear or serosanguineous appearance.

If hemodynamic monitoring is employed, once fluid can be aspirated through the needle, confirmation that the needle tip has entered the pericardial space can be immediately obtained by turning the stopcock and observing the pressure. In this manner, inadvertant RV puncture can be immediately recognized. In cases of tamponade, pericardial pressure will resemble RA pressure. Alternatively, if echocardiographic guidance is utilized, injection of a tiny amount of agitated saline through the needle will appear as microbubbles in the pericardial space to confirm position; if electrocardiographic guidance is used, a current of injury will be seen on contact with the epicardium (Fig. 7-11). Of these methods, we favor hemodynamic monitoring for its ease of application in the catheterization lab.

Once the needle is in the pericardial space it is our practice to pass a small guidewire, under fluoroscopy, high into the pericardial space and exchange the needle for a softer multiple side-hole plastic catheter (or sheath). Pericardial and RA pressures are measured (Figs. 7-12 and 7-13). With moderate to large effusions, fluid usually can be easily extracted from the pericardial space. If there is a question as to the exact position of the needle or catheter, even after measuring the pressure, a small amount of radiographic contrast media may be injected. Contrast media pools in the dependent portion of the pericardial space but will wash out of a vascular space rapidly if a cardiac chamber has been inadvertently entered. Bloody pericardial fluid will be of a lower hematocrit than intravascular blood and will not clot rapidly when placed in a red top tube.

INTRAVASCULAR FOREIGN BODY RETRIEVAL (Fig. 7-14)

Multiple-catheter systems have been designed to retrieve foreign bodies, which are usually fragments of previous catheters or guidewires. Most catheter fragments result from injudicious insertion or removal of catheters inserted from the subclavian, jugular, or rarely inferior vena caval approaches. Most recently, angioplasty guidewire fracture required refined removal techniques for coronary arteries. A catheter-housed wire loop or snare is commonly available.

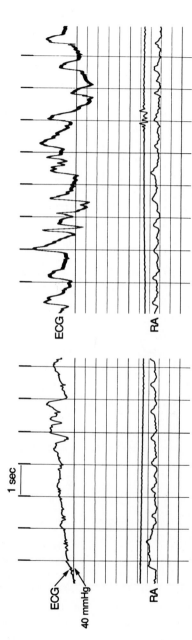

Fig. 7-11. Electrocardiographic method during pericardiocentesis. The electrocardiogram (*ECG*) in the left panel shows normal tracing. The electrocardiographic clip is attached to the pericardial needle. On advancement of the needle through the pericardium, contact is made with the heart, as shown by the electrocardiogram injury current in the right panel. *RA*, right atrial pressure. (From Kern MJ: Hemodynamic rounds: interpretation of cardiac pathophysiology from pressure waveform analysis. New York, 1993, Wiley-Liss.)

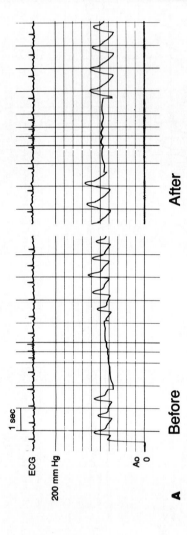

ECG

1 sec

200 mm Hg

Ao
0

A   **Before**   **After**

Fig. 7-12. *Continued on page 437.*

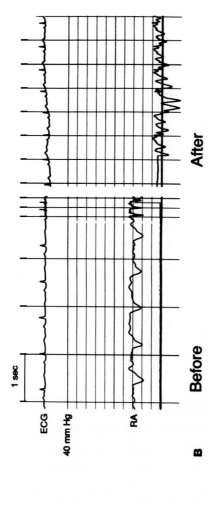

Fig. 7-12. *Continued.* Hemodynamic results of pericardiocentesis. **A,** Aortic (*Ao*) pressure and **B,** right atrial (*RA*) pressure before and after withdrawal of pericardial fluid. Note the elimination of pulsus paradoxus of aortic pressure and return of Y descent of right atrial waveform after pericardiocentesis. (Also, see Chapter 3.)

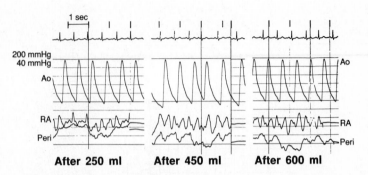

Fig. 7-13. Hemodynamic results of pericardiocentesis after withdrawal of 600 ml of pericardial fluid. This patient did not have tamponade. *Ao*, aortic pressure (0 to 200 mm Hg scale); *RA*, right atrial pressure; *Peri*, pericardial pressure (0 to 40 mm Hg scale).

A loop passing through a very small intracoronary guiding catheter can be applied to retrieve intracoronary guidewire fragments from angioplasty systems. The snare and loop techniques have been successfully used in both venous and arterial applications. Extra care always must be employed with the snare because its rigid tip may damage surrounding structures from which the catheter fragment is to be retrieved. In addition, the type of catheter fragment or guidewire material that is being retrieved also may scratch or tear the cardiac chamber unless it is captured at a distal end with the free, sharp edge of the fragment contained so that it will not produce injury.

SPECIAL CONDITIONS

Cardiac Catheterization in the Heart Transplant Patient

Cardiac transplantation is now a common procedure in most tertiary care centers. Routine yearly follow-up of the post-transplant patient includes cardiac catheterization, coronary angiography and assessment of LV function, PA pressures, and endomyocardial biopsy. Cardiac transplant patients have unique problems that may include altered anatomic relationships, absence of anginal pain, contrast allergic reactions, and high sensitivity to infection, all of which must be considered in the approach to this unusual patient popula-

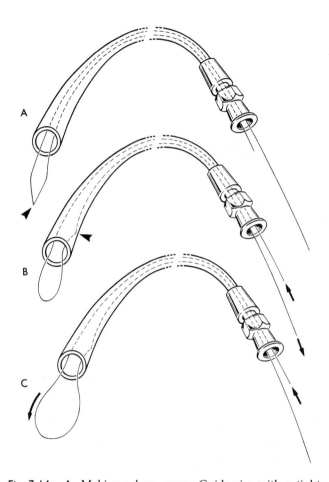

Fig. 7-14. **A,** Making a loop snare. Guidewire with a tight fold (*arrow*) beyond the catheter tip. **B,** Tight fold is withdrawn within the catheter by withdrawing one free end of the guidewire, while advancing the other end, forming a nontraumatic, blunt-tip loop/snare. **C,** The size of loop/snare is enlarged by further advancing of the guidewire end not containing the initial tight fold. *Continued on page 440.*

tion. Routine left and right heart catheterization usually is performed from the femoral approach in the post–heart transplant patient. If femoral scar tissue is excessive on one side, approach from the opposite groin or arm may be necessary. If endomyocardial biopsy is considered the internal

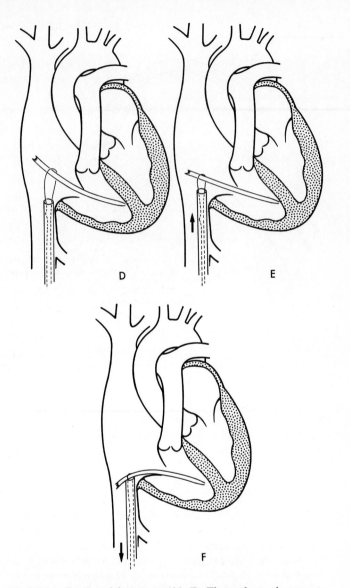

Fig. 7-14. *Continued from page 439.* **D,** The catheter fragment is snared. **E,** The catheter is advanced, while the wire is held so that the catheter rests gently on the fragment, confirming encirclement and securing the fragment. **F,** The loop is closed down tightly and the fragment pulled out with the catheter. (From Tilkian AG, Daily EK: *Cardiovascular procedures: diagnostic techniques and therapeutic procedures,* St Louis, 1986, Mosby.)

jugular or femoral venous approach may be suitable using either fluoroscopy or echocardiographically guided biopsy. (See Endomyocardial Biopsy.)

Angiographic notes for the heart transplant patient.   The transplanted heart is rotated clockwise. Thus the right coronary ostium is anterior and the left coronary ostium is located in a more posterior plane than the normal heart. In addition, a suture ridge in the lower ascending aorta at the site of the aortic anastomosis may be encountered, causing the Judkins catheter to snag or bend as it is advanced. A guidewire may be needed to move the left Judkins catheter across this ridge. To reach the posterior position of the left coronary orifice a Left Judkins 5-cm curved catheter may be useful. In addition, the anterior position of the right coronary ostia may be better engaged using an AP or slightly rightward oblique view. The multipuprose angiographic catheter may be required for unusual positions of the coronary ostia.

Adherence to sterile techniques cannot be overemphasized. An anaphylactoid reaction to contrast media for multiple posttransplant studies must be considered and pretreated.

Adult Complex Congenital Heart Disease

Adults with corrected congenital heart disease will be encountered with increasing frequency by the adult cardiac catheterization physician. Detailed knowledge of previous cardiac surgery and catheterization and echocardiographic findings is necessary for the performance of a complete and efficient catheterization. Residual hemodynamic and electrophysiologic abnormalities must be identified in these patients to maintain long-term survival.

Ventricular septal defects may occur at the muscular septum or the site of an old patch in corrected hearts. Great vessel shunts may occur from collateral supply, especially in those patients with repaired cyanotic heart disease or incompletely occluded shunts. Cyanosis in these individuals may be due to:
1. Persistent left SVC to left atrium shunting with or without CS or septal defect
2. Right pulmonary AV fistula (Glenn anastomosis)
3. Acquired lung disease
4. A combination of the above

To identify shunts in the adult, careful hemodynamic and oximetric measurements are important. Both right and left pulmonary arteries must be sampled for oxygen saturations during the oximetry run. For the most accurate results, the entire oximetry run should be performed in under 10 minutes (see Chapter 3). Patients with cyanosis are placed on 100% oxygen to identify cardiac causes of cyanosis from noncardiac ones.

To obtain optimal ventriculographic results, large-flow (8 French) pigtail catheters with a high-contrast volume load (50 ml at 25/sec) may be required. Large-format image intensifiers (9-inch screen) are needed to display both ventricles simultaneously. Coronary artery abnormalities may occur and contribute to ventricular dysfunction in the adult with congenital heart disease. The late natural history of coronary atherosclerosis in corrected forms of congenital heart disease is unknown. It is recommended that any patient over the age of 35 with evidence of ventricular dysfunction undergo coronary arteriography.

Patients with complex congenital heart disease, such as tetralogy of Fallot with an overriding aorta, ventricular septal defect, and pulmonary stenosis or truncus arteriosus (common arterial trunk with ventricular septal defect), may have abnormally large aortic roots requiring modified coronary catheters. Single coronary arteries or anomalous origins of the left coronary artery from the right coronary artery may be part of the truncus arteriosus (a common pulmonary and aortic outflow tube) and transposition of the great vessels (switching of pulmonary artery and aorta).

Catheter therapy.   Balloon dilation or occluder catheter therapy may be performed in both children and adults with congenital heart disease to dilate narrowed heart valves or to close atrial or ventricular septal defects. Special devices are available to close patent ductus arteriosus (fetal communication between aorta and PA that normally closes at birth). These lesions should be 10 mm in diameter or smaller for catheter therapy.

For aortic and mitral stenosis, balloon-catheter valvulotomy may be performed. Pulmonic valvuloplasty is common in children and also may be practical in adults (see Chapter 9).

SUGGESTED READINGS

Bell CA, Kern MJ, Aguirre FV, Donohue T, Bach R, Wolford T, Penick D, Ofili E, Miller C: Superior accuracy of anatomic positioning with echocardiographic-over fluoroscopic-guided endomyocardial biopsy. *Cathet Cardiovasc Diagn* 28:291–294, 1993.

Berland J, Cribier A, Savin T, Lefebvre E, Koning R, Letac B: Percutaneous balloon valvulopasty in patients with severe aortic stenosis and low ejection fraction: immediate results and 1-year follow up, *Circulation* 79:1189–1196, 1989.

Croft CH, Lipscomb K: Modified technique of transseptal left heart catheterization, *J Am Coll Cardiol* 5:904–910, 1985.

Lock JE, Keane JF, Fellows KE: The use of catheter intervention procedures for congenital heart disease, *J Am Coll Cardiol* 7:1420–1423, 1986.

Mason JW, O'Connell JB: Clinical method of endomyocardial biopsy, *Circulation* 79:971–979, 1989.

McKay RG, Safian RD, Lock JE, Mandell VS, Thurer RL, Schmitt SJ, Grossman W: Balloon dilatation of calcific aortic stenosis in elderly patients: postmortem, intraoperative, and percutaneous valvuloplasty studies, *Circulation* 74:119–125, 1986.

Miller LW, Labovitz AJ, McBride LA, Pennington DG, Kanter K: Echocardiography-guided endomyocardial biopsy: a 5 year experience, *Circulation* 78(suppl 3):99–102, 1988.

Rediker DE, Block PC, Abascal VM, Palacios IF: Mitral balloon valvuloplasty for mitral restenosis after surgical commisurotomy, *J Am Coll Cardiol* 11:252–256, 1988.

8

HIGH-RISK CARDIAC CATHETERIZATION

Eugene A. Caracciolo, Thomas J. Donohue, Morton J. Kern, Richard G. Bach, Carl Tommaso, and Ubeydullah Deligonul

THE HIGH-RISK PATIENT
Definition

Patients classified as high risk are more likely to die or suffer MI or ventricular fibrillation during cardiac catheterization than are other patients. Numerous studies have summarized the clinical and anatomic characteristics of patients at high risk: those with known significant three-vessel or LMCA disease, severe LV dysfunction, diabetes, or poorly controlled hypertension (see the box on p. 445). Markedly abnormal exercise treadmill test results suggesting severe coronary artery disease are also an indication of potential high-risk status. Congestive heart failure, recent acute MI, unstable angina, and severe valvular heart disease (especially critical aortic stenosis) have a high incidence of morbidity/mortality during and following cardiac catheterization. With increasingly complex interventional procedures, the occurrence of major complications in the cardiac catheterization laboratory has increased markedly.

Management of Complications During Cardiac Catheterization (Table 8-1)

Complications of coronary arteriography must be managed immediately. MI during the course of coronary angiography may be the result of an embolism, (air or thrombus), or arterial damage such as a dissection caused by catheter placement.

Patient Characteristics Associated with Increased Mortality from Cardiac Catheterization

---

AGE

Infants (<1 year old) and the elderly (>65 years old). Elderly women appear to be at higher risk than elderly men.

FUNCTIONAL CLASS

Mortality in Class IV patients is more than 10 times greater than in Class I and II patients.

SEVERITY OF CORONARY OBSTRUCTION

Mortality for patients with left main disease is more than 10 times greater than for patients with one- or two-vessel disease.

VALVULAR HEART DISEASE

Especially when combined with coronary disease, this condition is associated with a higher risk of death at cardiac catheterization than coronary artery disease alone.

LEFT VENTRICULAR DYSFUNCTION

Mortality for patients with LV ejection <30% is more than 10 times greater than in patients with ejection fraction ≥50%.

SEVERE NONCARDIAC DISEASE

Patients with
  Renal insufficiency
  Insulin-requiring diabetes
  Advanced cerebrovascular and/or peripheral vascular disease
  Severe pulmonary insufficiency

Modified from Grossman W: Complications of cardiac catheterization: incidence, causes and prevention. In Grossman W, editor: *Cardiac catheterization and angiography,* ed 3, Philadelphia, 1986, Lea & Febiger.

TABLE 8-1. Management of complications during cardiac catheterization

Complications/precautions	Treatment
Myocardial infarction (0.2%)	Intracoronary nitroglycerin (rule out spasm)
	Consider intracoronary thrombolysis or possible coronary angioplasty, or emergency aortocoronary bypass
Cerebrovascular accident (0.1%)	
Systemic heparinization	
Cleaning of guidewires before use	
Limit guidewire-blood exposure (<2 min)	
Use guidewire to cross aortic arch (especially in atherosclerotic aortas) especially for Amplatz, bypass graft catheter	
Aspirate/flush catheters frequently	
Remove air bubbles in any of the tubing, solutions or injection syringe	
All tubing and catheter connections tight	
Dissection (0.1%)	No further coronary injections
Never advance guidewire or catheter against resistance; catheter tip location confirmed by gentle contrast injection	If ischemia produced, emergency aortocoronary bypass
Do not manipulate catheter in coronary ostium, monitoring pressure of catheter tip	If dissection associated with thrombus but no ischemia, use heparin (controversial)
Do not inject with damped pressure	(Consider coronary stenting if available)

Acute pulmonary edema

Treat preexisting CHF optimally

Limit contrast medium in high risk; avoid LV angiography in severe aortic stenosis, marked CHF or pulmonary hypertension

Use nonionic or low osmolar contrast media agents

Avoid hypotension

Limit flush solution volume

Monitoring LV filling pressure (PCW)

Elevate patient's trunk 30 to 45 degrees

Oxygen, morphine (2 to 5 mg IV), nitrates (100 to 200 μg IV), furosemide (20 to 100 mg IV)

Nitroprusside for afterload reduction with dopamine or dobutamine

Intraaortic balloon pumping

Cardiogenic shock

Careful patient selection: (1) left main coronary artery stenosis, (2) aortic stenosis at high risk, and (3) acute infarction

Prophylactic IABP for high-risk left main coronary artery angiography; minimize number of injections; treat hypotension

Stop procedure if hypotension persists

Atropine, adequate volume expansion, intraaortic injection of 0.125 to 0.250 mg Aramine (metaraminol), intraaortic balloon pumping

Rule out pericardial tamponade with RA and RV pressures; consider urgent echocardiogram

Monitor filling pressures

If shock caused by coronary occlusion, treat with emergency PTCA or CABG

Vasopressor support

Intraaortic balloon pump

Intubation/mechanical ventilation

Pacemaker as needed

Continued on pages 448–449.

TABLE 8-1. *Continued from pages 446–447.* Management of complications during cardiac catheterization

Complications/precautions	Treatment
Ventricular tachycardia, asystole, or fibrillation (0.6%)	
Use nonionic contrast agents in high-risk patients	Cough for temporary increase in BP
Do not wedge coronary artery catheter; contrast material washout should be brisk; ECG and blood pressure should be normal before next injection	Remove catheter from RV, LV, or coronary ostium
	CPR followed by prompt defibrillation
	Defibrillation (200 J)
Do not inject when catheter tip pressure is damped	Lidocaine (50 mg bolus, 2 to 4 mg/min IV)
Use atropine, volume expansion, or Aramine (metaraminol) for hypotension	Refractory VF usually as a result of extensive CAD; emergency percutaneous cardiopulmonary bypass should be considered
Limit contrast medium injected into coronary arteries; avoid prolonged injections	
Air embolism	
For prevention and treatment see p. 446	Same as cerebrovascular accident
Hematoma in femoral artery (0.1% major, 1% to 2% minor)	
Puncture below inguinal ligament	Evacuation rarely required
Attention to compression	Surgical consult for enlarging hematoma, compartment syndrome, or cool extremity
Prolonged compression if patient coughing, aortic insufficiency, hypertension, or heparin not reversed	

Retroperitoneal bleeding

Avoid high (above inguinal ligament) femoral artery puncture
Watch for hypotension, low abdominal or flank pain, within 2 to 12 hours of procedure
Low hematocrit, tachycardia (if not receiving beta blockers)

Reverse anticoagulants
Volume replacement
Transfusion if HCT <25

Cardiac tamponade

Avoid stiff catheters in RA or RV; pacing catheters handled gently
Avoid posterior LA wall during transseptal catheterization

Prompt pericardiocentesis with catheter drainage
Cardiovascular surgery consultation
Surgical exploration and closure for persistent bleeding

Contrast agent nephrotoxicity

See p. 17
Hydration, mannitol, furosemide, and nonionic contrast agents

Generally self-limited; dialysis rarely needed

Contrast agent reaction

See p. 13

Vasovagal reaction

See p. 459

Modified from Tilkian AG, Daily EK: *Cardiovascular procedures: diagnostic techniques and therapeutic procedures*, St. Louis, 1986, Mosby.
CHF, congestive heart failure; LV, left ventricular; PCW, pulmonary capillary wedge; RA, right atrial; RV, right ventricular; IV, intravenous; PTCA, percutaneous transluminal coronary balloon angioplasty; CABG, coronary bypass graft surgery; ECG, electrocardiogram; VF, ventricular fibrillation; CPR, cardiopulmonary resuscitation; CAD, coronary artery disease; Hct, hematocrit; BP, blood pressure; LA, left atrial.

Toxic effects of contrast media may contribute to myocardial ischemia. In patients in whom myocardial ischemia develops, rapid assessment of the location and cause (thrombus, dissection, spasm) by coronary arteriography should be made, and reperfusion attempted with intracoronary nitroglycerin (spasm), thrombolytic agents (if a thrombus is identified), or emergency revascularization with angioplasty or bypass surgery.

Peripheral arterial complications such as loss of pulse as a result of thrombi can be treated with thrombolytic agents or Fogarty balloon extraction. If a large dissection has occurred, a vascular surgeon should be consulted immediately. Enlarging hematomas should be drained if they compromise circulation to the extremities.

Arterial thromboembolism to other areas, such as the brain, may not be immediately treatable but may require observation and/or administration of heparin depending on neurologic findings. Occipital blindness, a rare event that is due to hyperosmolarity of the contrast agent, is usually transient and requires no definitive treatment except for hydration and maintenance of blood pressure. Movement of an air embolus to the CNS may demonstrate features of acute stroke with agitation and confusion or aphasia. A small air embolus does not often result in permanent damage. Although hyperbaric oxygen chambers have been used successfully for treatment, these are not widely available.

Hypotension

Hypotension may occur before, during, and after cardiac catheterization from a variety of conditions. Hypotension before cardiac catheterization may be caused by hypovolemia induced by the fasting state (water intake should be allowed) or preprocedural medications. Hypotension during the cardiac catheterization procedure may be secondary to vasovagal reaction or caused by injection of the contrast agent. Vasovagal reactions are also common, leading to irreversible shock if untreated. Vasovagal reactions frequently are elicited by pain at the site of vascular access. In some elderly patients a vagal reaction may occur without bradycardia, appearing as unexplained hypotension. Generally, hypotension following coronary arteriography or left ventriculography is transient and self-limited. However, aggressive treatment is occasionally required. Hypotension after the cardiac catheterization procedure is often caused by hypovolemia secondary to excessive contrast-induced diuresis or myocardial depression.

Cardiac tamponade and hemorrhage from the arterial entry site also should be considered in the postcatheterization hypotensive patient.

Acute myocardial ischemia may result in hypotension at any time before, during, or after the procedure. If hypotension ensues secondary to myocardial ischemia, intraaortic balloon pump (IABP) and/or coronary autoperfusion catheters may be inserted, as appropriate, for myocardial preservation.

Treatment of hypotension depends on the symptomatology of the patient as well as the underlying etiology.

Fluids. Hypotension secondary to hypovolemia is treated with IV saline infusion. Patients often will respond acutely to elevation ($>30°$) of the lower extremities (increased venous inflow, "internal transfusion"). Generally, several hundred milliliters of saline is required to restore adequate blood pressure in patients who are hypotensive secondary to hypovolemia. Hypovolemia in catheterization patients can be avoided by infusing IV saline at a rate of 100 ml/hr before the start of the procedure (particularly in patients who will be fasting for more than 12 hours) as well as for 8 to 12 hours after the procedure. In patients who are hypovolemic from hemorrhage, administration of blood products often will be necessary. Obviously, immediate measures should be taken to obtain adequate hemostasis in such patients. In patients with a history of congestive heart failure, care should be taken to prevent overhydration. Generally, careful monitoring of fluid intake and urine output will be adequate to follow such patients. However, in critically ill patients, the use of a Swan-Ganz catheter for pulmonary artery and pulmonary capillary wedge pressure measurement may be necessary for an accurate determination of their fluid status.

Vasopressors. In patients who develop hypotension without coexisting hypovolemia, pharmacologic therapy may be necessary to restore an adequate blood pressure. Intraarterial (not coronary) aramine bolus (1 mg) will temporarily increase blood pressure to normal range while assessment is continuing and other vasopressors are being prepared. The vasopressor of choice in acute situations is IV dopamine. The initial dose in symptomatic hypotension is 5 μg/kg/min. The dose can be titrated upward until an adequate blood pressure is obtained. In critically ill patients, norepinephrine (Levophed) or epinephrine drips may be required to obtain an acceptable blood pressure.

Other measures. In the case of drug-induced hypotension, treatment is directed toward discontinuation or reversal of the offending medication. In some patients this means stopping or decreasing IV vasodilators, such as nitroglycerin. In hypotensive patients who have received IV narcotics, IV Narcan is the treatment of choice. Patients in whom hypotension is associated with severe bradycardia often will respond to atropine. Finally, hypotension secondary to cardiac tamponade is an emergency condition, which should be treated immediately by pericardiocentesis. Methods to determine accurate doses of drugs are listed on Tables 8-2 to 8-4.

MANAGEMENT OF ARRHYTHMIAS IN THE CATHETERIZATION LABORATORY

Serious arrhythmias (including ventricular fibrillation, ventricular tachycardia, supraventricular tachycardia, asystole, and heart block) occur in approximately 1% of either right or left heart catheterizations. In almost all instances the arrhythmia can be managed successfully by prompt recognition and appropriate treatment. Arrhythmias may result from intracardiac catheter manipulation, coronary artery contrast injections or the use of balloon-tipped catheters for right heart catheterization.

The most important determinant of short- and long-term (neurologically intact) survival is the interval from the onset of hemodynamic collapse to the restoration of effective, spontaneous circulatory and respiratory function. The following section provides guidelines for the optimal treatment of the majority of patients. These guidelines do not preclude other measures that may be indicated on the basis of the specific characteristics of each patient.

TABLE 8-2. Infusion methods of potent drugs

Drug dosages given in different units

mg/min	μg/kg/min	μ/min	units/hour
Lidocaine	Dopamine	Nitroprusside	Heparin
Pronestyl	Dobutamine	Nitroglycerin	
Bretylium	Amrinone		
Amiophylline	Levophed		
Hydralazine			
Amiodarone			

Common concentrations

Nitroprusside (50 mg/250 ml) = 200 μg/ml
Nitroglycerin (50 mg/250 ml) = 200 μg/ml
Levophed (8 mg/250 ml) = 32 μ/ml
Dobutamine (1 g/250 ml) = 4000 μ/ml
Dopamine (800 mg/250 ml) = 3200 μg/ml
Hydralazine (100 mg/100 ml) = 1 mg/ml
Lidocaine (2 g/250 ml) = 8 mg/ml
Heparin (2500 units/250 cc) = 100 units/ml

Converting desired dose (in μg/kg/min) to infusion rate (in ml/hr):

1. Weight (in kg) × desired dose/kg/min = μg/min

2. $\dfrac{\mu g/ml}{60}$ = μg/ml/min

3. $\dfrac{\mu g/min}{\mu g/ml/min}$ = ml/hr infusion rate

Example: Dopamine (assume 70 kg at 3μg/kg/min)
1. Compute dose for weight

$$70 \times 3 = 210 \ \mu g/min$$

2. Compute drug concentration per minute (from common concentrations)

$$\frac{320 \ \mu g/ml}{60^*} = 53.3 \ \mu g/ml/min$$

3. When using IVAC delivery in ml/hr, compute dose of IVAC

$$\frac{210 \ \mu g/min}{53.3 \ \mu g/ml/min} = 3.9^* \ ml/hr$$

*Round off to nearest whole number when setting infusion pump.

Converting infusion rates (ml/hr) to dose (μg/min)

$$\frac{Rate \ (ml/hr) = \mu g/ml}{60} = \mu g/min$$

Converting infusion rate (ml/hr) to dose for weight (μg/kg/min)

$$\frac{rate \ (ml/hr) \ \times \ \mu g/ml}{60} = \mu g/min$$

$$\frac{\mu g/min}{kg \ weight} = \mu g/kg/min$$

Automatic Infusion Pump, IVAC Corporation.

TABLE 8-3. The quick Millerau method

1 μg/kg/min = 1 ml/hr
Drug dose (mg = 3 $\times$ body weight kg in 50-ml solution)

Example 1: Dobutamine for 50-kg patient
3 $\times$ 50 kg = 150 mg in 50 ml
$\qquad$ = 1 ml/hr
$\qquad$ = 1 μg/kg/min
(If 0.1 μg/kg/min is needed, use 0.3 $\times$ body weight.)

Example 2: Norepinephrine for a 80-kg patient
Need range of 0.1 to 3μg/kg/hr, use 0.3 $\times$ body weight
0.3 $\times$ 80 = 24 mg in 50 ml
$\qquad$ = 0.1 μg/kg/min
$\qquad$ = 1 ml/hr
If infusion rate = 2.5 ml/hr, dose infused = 0.25 μg/kg/min

From Millereau M: Dilution of potent drugs, *Am J Cardiol* 68:418, 1991.

TABLE 8-4. Converting infusion rates

Converting DESIRED DOSE (μg/min) to infusion rate (ml/min or ml/hr)

$$\frac{\text{Desired dose } (\mu g/min)}{\text{Drip concentration } (\mu g/ml)} = ml/min$$

If using a volume infusion pump that uses a ml/hr format such as an IVAC Model 560, convert μg/min to μg/hr.

$$\frac{\text{Desired dose } (\mu g/min)}{\text{Drip concentration } (\mu g/ml)} \times 60 = ml/hr$$

Converting desired dose (mg/min) to infusion rate (ml/min or ml/hr)

$$\frac{\text{Desired dose } (\mu g/min)}{\text{Drip concentration } (\mu g/ml)} = ml/min$$

If using a volume infusion pump that uses a ml/hr format such as an IVAC Model 560, convert μg/min to μg/hr.

$$\frac{\text{Desired dose } (mg/min)}{\text{Drip concentration } (mg/ml)} \times 60 = ml/hr$$

Automatic Infusion Pump, IVAC Corporation.

Primary Prevention of Arrhythmias

Electrocardiographic monitoring. Continuous electro-cardiographic monitoring is essential in performing a safe cardiac catheterization. Should a problem develop with the electrocardiographic leads or equipment during the procedure, it must be remedied before continuing the procedure.

IV access. All patients should have a functioning 18-gauge peripheral IV line established with normal saline as the infusing solution before starting the procedure. If peripheral venous access is a problem, a femoral venous sheath large enough to accommodate a pacing wire and allow the rapid flow of saline should be placed. A 6 French or larger femoral venous sheath should be placed routinely in potentially unstable or acutely ill patients.

Standby transvenous pacing. The need for prophylactic pacemaker insertion is determined by the patient's risk of developing a bradyarrhythmia and the patient's ability to tolerate the arrhythmia should it occur. Risk factors for the developing of bradyarrhythmia include the following:

1. Preexisting right bundle branch block during left heart catheterization
2. Preexisting left bundle branch block during right heart catheterization, particularly with stiff catheters (e.g., Cournand)
3. Heart block greater than first degree
4. Marked sinus bradycardia
5. Coronary artery angioplasty involving the (dominant) artery supplying the AV node

Flexible balloon-tipped, flow-directed pacemaker wires have the lowest risk for cardiac perforation.

Limiting cardiac catheter manipulations. Catheter passage through the heart always should be performed with cautious and smooth motion. Particular note should be made of ventricular ectopy during catheter manipulation.

Limiting coronary artery contrast. Injections should be sufficient to opacify the arterial tree without excessive volume or rates of injection. Ionic contrast media predisposes a patient to bradycardia and ventricular fibrillation, especially during injection of the RCA.

Giving atropine.   Before coronary contrast injections with ionic contrast in patients with heart rates less than 60 bpm, 0.6 mg atropine may be administered.

Components of Arrhythmia Management

Immediate modalities

Catheter removal. Removal of stimulating catheters most often terminates the arrhythmia.

Cough. When sustained hypotension is recognized before loss of consciousness (and cardiac arrest), forceful coughing can generate sufficient blood flow to the brain to maintain consciousness until definitive treatment can be initiated.

Precordial thump. A solitary precordial thump can be accomplished quickly and may terminate ventricular tachycardia, ventricular fibrillation, asystole, marked bradycardia with hemodynamic instability, or convert complete AV block to a more stable rhythm. It should not delay defibrillation in a patient without a blood pressure.

Defibrillation and cardioversion. Definitive electrical treatment has the highest priority of any modality. A defibrillator should be strategically placed in each cardiac catheterization laboratory suite. During procedures the power should be turned on and conductive jelly should be applied to the defibrillator paddles to minimize any delays in the event that defibrillation is required. The time from the onset of the arrest to successful defibrillation is the major determinant of survival in cardiac arrests caused by ventricular fibrillation. If pulseless ventricular tachycardia or ventricular fibrillation is present, defibrillation should be performed immediately. An algorithm for treatment of ventricular fibrillation with CPR is provided in Fig. 8-1.

Proper technique, including paddle placement (Fig. 8-2) and the use of proper conducting material, is essential to the success of defibrillation. One paddle should be placed along the upper right sternal border, below the clavicle, and the other lateral to the nipple with the center of the electrode in the midaxillary line. The paddles should be applied with firm pressure (about 25 lb). The individuals using the paddles must make sure that no one is touching the bed or the patient during defibrillation.

Continuing modalities

Securing adequate routes for drug administration. A central venous (internal jugular or subclavian) line should be used for drug administration. If an antecubital vein is being used, rapid entry of drugs into the central circulation can be facilitated by the following:

1. Large volume of flush solutions (50 ml)
2. A long line into the central circulation

The distal wrist, hand, and saphenous veins provide poor access to the central circulation and thus are not appropriate for resuscitative efforts. The femoral venous route will provide prompt access to the central circulation with a long catheter that reaches above the diaphragm. *Intracardiac injections are not indicated.*

Cardiopulmonary resuscitation. Chest compressions (1.5- to 2-inch depression; 5:1 compression/breath ratio) should be performed if no blood pressure is present (Fig. 8-3). Remember to adjust the catheterization laboratory table to accommodate chest compression (Fig. 8-4).

IV fluids. Volume expansion is not recommended in the routine cardiac arrest patient unless there is an indication of preexisting volume depletion. Volume expansion may diminish blood flow to the cerebral and coronary circulations.

The use of sodium bicarbonate early in a code sequence should be predicated on a clearly defined metabolic derangement (e.g., hyperkalemia or preexisting acidosis), which is not generally the case with the routine patient with cardiac arrest in the catheterization laboratory. Adequate ventilation may correct acidosis better than sodium bicarbonate. Sodium bicarbonate only should be administered after rhythm- and contractility-stabilizing interventions have been employed. The dosage is 1 mEq/kg initially, followed by 0.5 mEq/kg every 10 minutes. Sodium bicarbonate should not be given in the same IV line as catecholamines (inactivation) or calcium (formation of precipitates). Postresuscitation sodium bicarbonate administration should be guided by knowledge of arterial blood gases.

Administration of calcium does not improve the chances of survival of cardiac arrest. High serum calcium levels induced by calcium administration may be detrimental, espe-

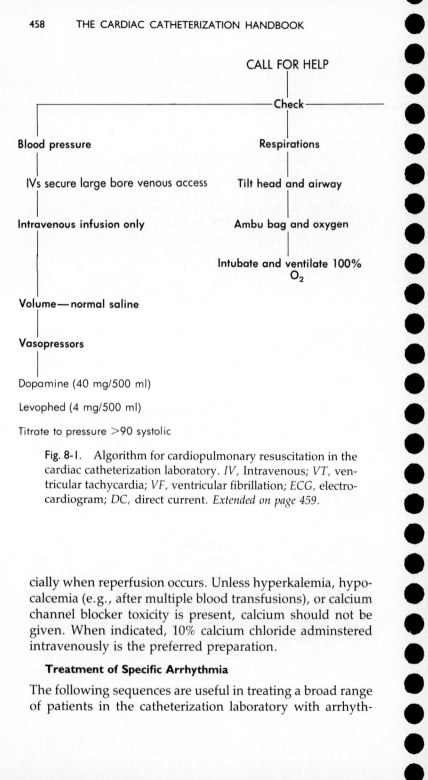

CALL FOR HELP

Check

Blood pressure

IVs secure large bore venous access

Intravenous infusion only

Volume—normal saline

Vasopressors

Dopamine (40 mg/500 ml)

Levophed (4 mg/500 ml)

Titrate to pressure >90 systolic

Respirations

Tilt head and airway

Ambu bag and oxygen

Intubate and ventilate 100%
O_2

Fig. 8-1. Algorithm for cardiopulmonary resuscitation in the cardiac catheterization laboratory. *IV,* Intravenous; *VT,* ventricular tachycardia; *VF,* ventricular fibrillation; *ECG,* electrocardiogram; *DC,* direct current. *Extended on page 459.*

cially when reperfusion occurs. Unless hyperkalemia, hypocalcemia (e.g., after multiple blood transfusions), or calcium channel blocker toxicity is present, calcium should not be given. When indicated, 10% calcium chloride adminstered intravenously is the preferred preparation.

Treatment of Specific Arrhythmia

The following sequences are useful in treating a broad range of patients in the catheterization laboratory with arrhyth-

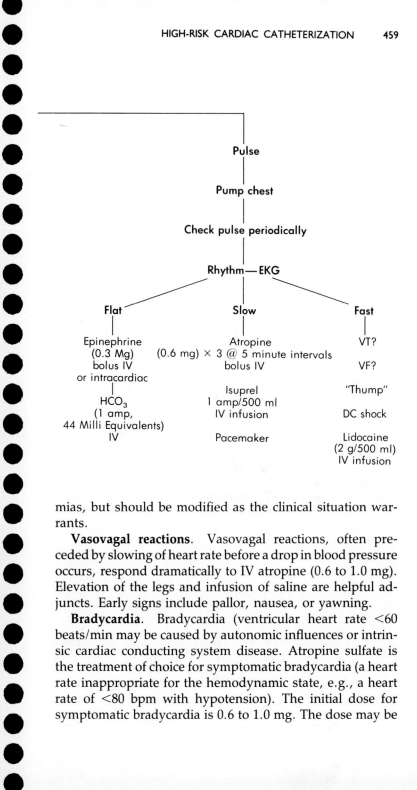

Pulse

Pump chest

Check pulse periodically

Rhythm—EKG

Flat	Slow	Fast
Epinephrine (0.3 Mg) bolus IV or intracardiac	Atropine (0.6 mg) × 3 @ 5 minute intervals bolus IV	VT?
		VF?
HCO₃ (1 amp, 44 Milli Equivalents) IV	Isuprel 1 amp/500 ml IV infusion	"Thump"
		DC shock
	Pacemaker	Lidocaine (2 g/500 ml) IV infusion

mias, but should be modified as the clinical situation warrants.

Vasovagal reactions. Vasovagal reactions, often preceded by slowing of heart rate before a drop in blood pressure occurs, respond dramatically to IV atropine (0.6 to 1.0 mg). Elevation of the legs and infusion of saline are helpful adjuncts. Early signs include pallor, nausea, or yawning.

Bradycardia. Bradycardia (ventricular heart rate <60 beats/min may be caused by autonomic influences or intrinsic cardiac conducting system disease. Atropine sulfate is the treatment of choice for symptomatic bradycardia (a heart rate inappropriate for the hemodynamic state, e.g., a heart rate of <80 bpm with hypotension). The initial dose for symptomatic bradycardia is 0.6 to 1.0 mg. The dose may be

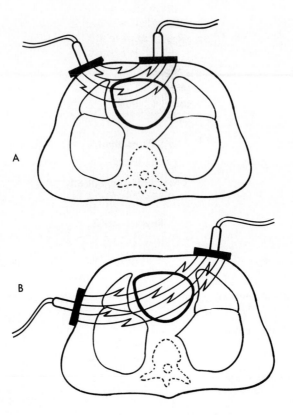

Fig. 8-2. Cardioversion paddle positions. **A,** Avoid too close positioning of electrode paddles (a substantial amount of current shunts between them and an insufficient amount reaches the heart). **B,** Space paddles widely, allowing a sufficient amount of current to reach the left ventricle. (**A** and **B,** Adapted from Ewy GA: Defibrillating cardiac arrest victims, *J Cardiovasc Med 7:44, 1982.*) *Continued on page 461.*

repeated every 5 minutes as needed to a maximal dose of 2 mg. Doses of less than 0.5 mg may induce vagotonic effects. Rarely will a pacemaker be needed for bradycardia. Isoproterenol is a pure beta-adrenergic agonist with positive chronotropic (heart rate) and inotropic (contractility) properties. Beta-adrenergic vasodilation leads to a reduction in arterial pressure and thus is contraindicated during cardiac arrest. The only indication for isoproterenol is for the immediate,

C

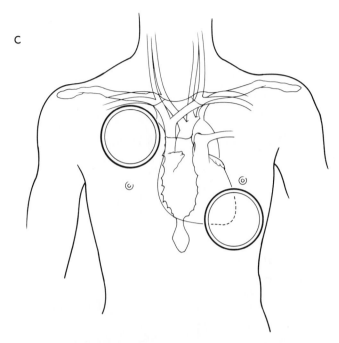

Fig. 8-2. *Continued from page 460.* **C,** Anteroapical position for cardioversion or defibrillation. See text for details. (**C,** From Tilkian AG, Daily EK: *Cardiovascular procedures: diagnostic techniques and therapeutic procedures,* St. Louis, 1986, Mosby.)

temporary control of hemodynamically significant bradycardia that is refractory to atropine, and only until a pacemaker can be inserted. The dose is 2 to 10 μg/min.

Sinus or junctional rhythm and second degree AV block (type I) often does not require specific treatment. However, in symptomatic patients these rhythms usually respond to atropine. Atropine should be given as needed, up to 2 mg in divided doses (0.5 mg). If symptomatic bradycardia persists after the second dose of atropine (i.e., a third dose is needed) a transvenous pacemaker should be placed. An external pacemaker or isoproterenol can be used in the symptomatic patient if atropine fails to maintain the patient until a transvenous pacemaker can be placed.

Second degree AV block (type II) and *third degree AV block* is treated with a temporary transvenous pacemaker even in

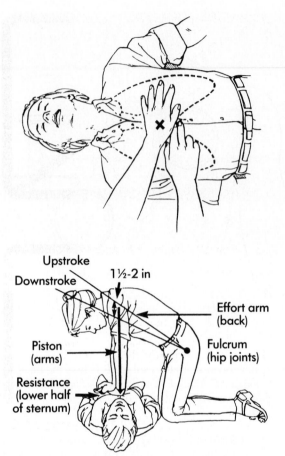

Fig. 8-3. Techniques for external chest compression. *Top,* Locating the correct hand position on the lower half of the sternum. *Bottom,* Proper position with shoulders directly over the sternum and elbows locked. (From Standards and guidelines for cardiopulmonary resuscitation [CPR] and emergency cardiac care [ECC], *JAMA* 255:2905, 1986. Copyright 1986, American Medical Association.)

the absence of symptoms. If bradycardia is associated with adverse hemodynamics or symptoms (e.g., hypotension, congestive heart failure, ischemia, infarction), atropine can be used to temporize the situation in divided doses of up to 2 mg until the pacemaker can be inserted. If atropine fails

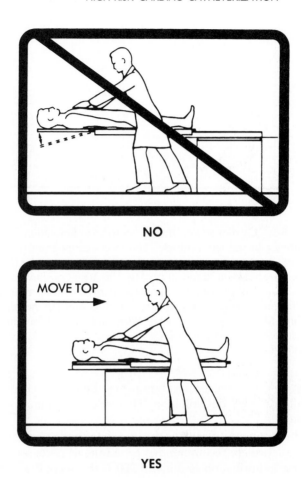

NO

MOVE TOP

YES

Fig. 8-4. Emergency cardiopulmonary resuscitation procedures on the cardiac catheterization table. CPR may not be effective with the table top extended. Position the top caudally to the end of travel to provide additional support and minimize the possibility of table damage or failure. The patient load capacity of this carbon fiber top is 350 lb (159 kg). (Courtesy of Phillips Radiographic, Inc., Shelton, Conn.)

an external pacemaker or isoproterenol can be used to maintain the patient until a transvenous pacemaker can be placed.

Ventricular fibrillation (Fig. 8-5). Intracardiac and intracoronary catheters should be removed quickly and definitive treatment with defibrillation should be carried out immedi-

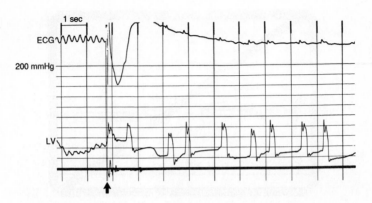

Fig. 8-5. Cardioversion during ventricular fibrillation with catheter in the left ventricle. The electrocardiogram (*ECG*) shows coarse ventricular fibrillation with left ventricular (*LV*) pressure between 30 and 40 mm Hg. The *Arrow*, cardioversion with 200 J is performed. The normal rhythm then returns with generation of LV pressure (70 to 80 mm Hg systolic). (Kern MJ: *Hemodynamic rounds: Interpretation of cardiac pathophysiology from pressure waveform analysis*, New York, 1993, Wiley-Liss.)

ately. A single precordial thump may be employed only if it will not delay defibrillation. Thereafter, guidelines are as follows:

1. Three consecutive unsynchronized defibrillations in rapid sequence are recommended for adults as necessary. The first defibrillation is done at 200 J, the second at 200 to 300 J, and the third at 360 J. For children, 2.5 to 50 J (2 J/ kg) is used.
2. If these defibrillations are unsuccessful, begin CPR, give 1 mg epinephrine, intubate if possible, and ventilate the patient manually. If intubation is not possible, a mouthpiece should be inserted and the patient ventilated by face mask. Epinephrine administration should be repeated at least every 5 minutes until a pulse is established. The success of treatment at this point depends in large part on adequacy of CPR. CPR should not be stopped for more than 5 seconds except to defibrillate or intubate. Treatment of underlying abnormalities (e.g., hypokalemia, hypomagnesemia, ischemia, infarction, airway ob-

struction, or hypoxia) that may be causing the arrhythmia is critical.

3. Defibrillate again with 360 J.
4. If unsuccessful, administer lidocaine (1 mg/kg bolus), and defibrillate again with 360 J.
5. If unsuccessful, administer bretylium (5 mg/kg bolus) and defibrillate with 360 J. Additional doses of lidocaine may be preferred.
6. At this time, the use of bicarbonate should be considered, particularly if there has been a delay in ventilating the patient.
7. Finish loading with either lidocaine or bretylium. Defibrillate with 360 J after each dose of antiarrhythmic agent.
8. If ventricular fibrillation is refractory to the above measures, one may consider Pronestyl, propranolol, or emergency cardiopulmonary bypass.
9. If ventricular fibrillation recurs during the arrest sequence, defibrillation should be reinitiated at the energy level that had previously resulted in successful defibrillation.

Nonsustained ventricular tachycardia. Nonsustained ventricular tachycardia usually can be eliminated by repositioning or withdrawing intracardiac or coronary catheters. Frequent nonsustained ventricular tachycardia secondary to acute myocardial ischemia, rather than catheter irritation, should be treated with lidocaine.

Sustained ventricular tachycardia. If sustained ventricular tachycardia persists after removing intracardiac catheters, management proceeds according to the stability of the patient. A single precordial thump may be employed by the operator before cardioversion.

In the absence of a blood pressure, sustained ventricular tachycardia is treated the same as ventricular fibrillation. In patients who are hemodynamically unstable (e.g., conditions of hypotension [systolic blood pressure <90 mm Hg], pulmonary edema, or unconsciousness), synchronized cardioversion with 50 J is the treatment of choice.

Synchronized cardioversion uses the largest R wave. If the QRS cannot be distinguished, use the unsynchronized mode:

1. Lubricate paddles with conduction gel.

2. Avoid excessive gel that may conduct energy to the operator or bystanders.
3. Clear all personnel before discharing paddles.
4. Position paddles properly (see Fig. 8-2).

Sedation may not be given in critically ill patients. If cardioversion is unsuccessful, successive synchronized attempts with 100, 200, and then 360 J are appropriate. If electrical cardioversion alone is unsuccessful, lidocaine should be administered, followed by bretylium. If these two drugs fail an infusion of Pronestyl should be tried. Repeat synchronized cardioversion with 360 J after each dose of antiarrhythmic agent.

In stable patients the first approach used is antiarrhythmic therapy. Lidocaine followed by Pronestyl are the drugs of first choice. If these two drugs fail a slow infusion of bretylium should be tried. If still unsuccessful, synchronized cardioversion, beginning with 50 J as described above, is indicated. The patient should be sedated.

Antiarrhythmic agents for ventricular tachycardia. *Lidocaine* is the drug of choice for the management of ventricular ectopy, including ventricular tachycardia and ventricular fibrillation. Lidocaine initially should be given as a bolus of 1 mg/kg. Additional boluses of 0.5 mg/kg can be given subsequently (every 8 to 10 minutes) to a total dose of 3 mg/kg in the arrest setting. In the nonarrest setting the initial bolus should be reduced by half if any of the following conditions are present: congestive heart failure, shock, hepatic dysfunction, or age greater than 70 years. After a successful resuscitation a constant infusion of lidocaine at a rate of 2 to 4 mg/min should be initiated if lidocaine has been successful during the resuscitation.

Bretylium tosylate, 5 mg/kg, is given as an IV bolus for refractory ventricular fibrillation or refractory pulseless (or hemodynamically unstable) ventricular tachycardia. For hemodynamically stable patients, 5 to 10 mg/kg of bretylium tosylate should be diluted to 50 ml with 5% dextrose in water and administered by slow IV infusion over 8 to 10 minutes to reduce the acute hypotensive effects of the agent. Subsequently a constant infusion can be initiated at a dose of 1 to 4 mg/min if bretylium has been successful during the resuscitation.

Procainamide requires a relatively long time to achieve therapeutic levels. In the urgent situation, 1 g of procainamide hydrochloride can be administered over 30 minutes. A constant infusion rate (1 to 4 mg/min) is then administered and later titrated to serum drug levels. In situations that are not urgent, 1 g should be given over at least 1 hour. The rate of drug administration should be reduced or discontinued if hypotension is induced or if there is a greater than 50% prolongation of the QRS complex or QT interval.

NOTE: Wide complex tachycardia of uncertain etology (i.e., ventricular tachycardia versus paroxysmal supraventricular tachycardia [PSVT] with aberrancy) should be treated as ventricular tachycardia until proven otherwise. *Verapamil is contraindicated.*

Asystole is usually the result of extensive myocardial ischemia. Right ventricular pacing should be instituted as quickly as possible. *Atropine* (1 mg) should be given and can be repeated in 5 minutes if necessary. Asystole should be confirmed in two leads because it can be difficult to distinguish fine ventricular fibrillation from asystole. If the diagnosis is unclear, one should assume that fine ventricular fibrillation is present and treat accordingly. External pacing can be employed if right ventricular pacing cannot be established immediately. Metabolic abnormalities, including hyperkalemia or severe preexisting acidosis, may contribute to the genesis of the arrhythmia and may respond to the use of buffers. A solitary precordial thump may be employed. *Epinephrine* is the catecholamine of choice for cardiac arrest. Its cardiac and vasoconstrictor alpha-adrenergic properties make it superior to other alpha-adrenergic agents (methoxamine and phenylephrine), which have comparable effects on the heart but fail to increase central nervous system blood flow as much as epinephrine. The dose of epinephrine is 0.5 to 1 mg given at least every 5 minutes. During cardiac arrest, higher rather than lower doses may be more efficacious. If asystole is refractory to the above measures, emergency cardiopulmonary bypass should be considered.

Electromechanical dissociation (EMD) is a rhythm disturbance that is almost uniformly fatal unless the underlying cause can be identified and immediately treated. General treatment includes the use of epinephrine (1 mg) every 5 minutes. Bicarbonate may be considered. If EMD is refractory, emergency cardiopulmonary bypass may be considered. Emergency cardiopulmonary bypass (see Chapter 9) may be lifesaving in certain cases of circulatory arrest, such as massive pulmonary embolism or acute coronary occlusion when the coronary anatomy is known and an operating room is immediately available.

Underlying causes of EMD include the following:

1. Hypovolemia, especially that resulting from bleeding. Once the diagnosis is made, aggressive volume repletion is indicated.

2. Pericardial tamponade, especially in patients with either acute infarction, recent cardiac biopsy, recent endocardial pacer insertion, or uremia. If tamponade is suspected, blind pericardiocentesis is warranted (see Chapter 7).

3. Enhanced vagal tone may occur in patients with ischemic heart disease and should be suspected whenever the heart rate is inappropriate for the degree of hypotension. Atropine is required.

4. Massive pulmonary embolism may precipitate EMD. On rare occasions, the embolus may break up during prolonged resuscitative efforts.

5. Tension pneumothorax in patients with central venous access above the diaphragm. Fluoroscopy may be helpful if immediately available. If there is any suspicion of tension pneumothorax, the operator carefully should insert a needle attached to a glass syringe into the pleural space. If a tension pneumothorax is present, air under pressure will push the plunger out of the syringe.

Supraventricular arrhythmias.   In cases of *paroxysmal supraventricular tachycardia* and *atrial fibrillation,* therapy depends on the hemodynamic stability of the patient.

1. In patients who are unstable (e.g., as a result of hypotension, chest pain, congestive heart failure, acute ischemia, or infarction), the therapy of choice is immediate synchronized cardioversion. Sedation with a rapidly acting IV agent (e.g., diazepam) is recommended for conscious, nonhypotensive patients as long as it does not delay the procedure. The recommended energy for the initial discharge is 75 to 100 J. If conversion occurs but PSVT or atrial fibrillation immediately recurs, repeated electrical

cardioversion is not indicated. If conversion does not oc-cur, then increasing energy levels (e.g., 200 J, 360 J) should be employed. If these maneuvers fail, treatment with IV Pronestyl followed by repeated attempts at cardioversion are recommended. Relative contraindications to cardio-version include overt digitalis toxicity because severe bradycardia or asystole may occur after cardioversion. In stable patients with atrial fibrillation the ventricular response can be controlled with digitalis, verapamil, or beta blockers. The rhythm can be converted with pro-cainamide or elective cardioversion.

2. Stable patients with PSVT initially should be treated with vagal maneuvers. The Valsalva maneuver is usually the most successful. In the absence of known carotid disease or carotid bruit, carotid sinus massage can be employed. If vagal maneuvers are unsuccessful, a stable patient should receive pharmacologic therapy. Verapamil and recently adenosine (5- to 12-mg IV bolus) are the drugs of choice. Patients who fail to respond to verapamil or adenosine can be treated with any of the following: overdrive pac-ing, Pronestyl, elective cardioversion, digitalis, or beta blockers.

Verapamil (for reentrant supraventricular tachycardia) is a calcium channel blocker with electrophysioloigic effects on the AV node and, to a lesser extent, the SA node. It also has negative inotropic properties. It is a common agent used for the conversion of narrow QRS complex paroxysmal su-praventricular tachycardia in stable patients if maneuvers that increase vagal tone are unsuccessful. Verapamil is also useful for rate control in patients with atrial fibrillation and a rapid ventricular response. Initially, a 5-mg dose should be given IV over 1 minute and, additional doses of 2.5 to 5 mg given in 5- to 10-minute intervals up to a maximal dose of 20 mg if PSVT persists without an adverse response to the initial dose. Contraindications to verapamil include his-tory or presence of bradycardia, hypotension, decompen-sated congestive heart failure, or concomitant use of an IV beta blocker. The following adverse reactions to verapamil can occur: severe bradycardia, hypotension, congestive heart failure, and facilitated accessory conduction in patients with Wolff-Parkinson-White syndrome. Hypotension frequently can be reversed by the IV administration of 0.5 to 1.0 g of calcium chloride.

Adenosine is a naturally occurring agent increasing AV nodal blockade as well as coronary blood flow. It is 90% to 100% effective in terminating reentrant supraventricular or AV nodal tachycardia in 5- to 12-mg IV bolus doses. It has a 30-second onset of action and a 60-second offset of action. Transient flushing is the only major side effect.

Digitalis is useful for controlling a rapid ventricular response in patients with atrial fibrillation, atrial flutter, or PSVT. The toxic/therapeutic ratio is narrow and the onset of action is slower than verapamil (i.e., digitalis is not useful for acute situations).

Beta blockers (including *propranolol*) can be used to control recurring episodes of PSVT. Beta blockers may be particularly hazardous when cardiac dysfunction is present. The dosage for propranolol is 1 mg every 5 minutes intravenously up to a total of 0.1 mg/kg. Short-acting beta blockers (esmolol) are administered in 1- to 5-mg boluses and have 5 to 10 minute half-lives.

CARDIAC SUPPORT DEVICES
IABP (See the box on p. 472)

Intraaortic balloon counterpulsation is an important adjunct to diagnostic cardiac catheterization and interventional cardiology. Before a diagnostic cardiac catheterization or interventional procedure, the patient should be medically treated to optimize hemodynamics and reduce myocardial ischemia. IABP counterpulsation increases myocardial oxygen supply and decreases myocardial oxygen demand. Inflation at the onset of diastole (at the dicrotic notch on the central arterial pressure tracing) results in diastolic pressure augmentation, which increases coronary artery and systemic perfusion. Deflation of the balloon just prior to systole (end diastole on the arterial pressure tracing) results in decreased ventricular afterload, which decreases myocardial oxygen consumption and increases the cardiac output (CO) (Fig. 8-6).

In unstable patients, an IABP may be required before proceeding with the catheterization. During diagnostic cardiac catheterization or interventional procedures, hypotension (not responding to volume loading or IV vasopressors)

A. Diastole: Balloon Inflation
Augmentation of
Diastolic Pressure
• Coronary perfusion↑

B. Systole: Balloon Inflation
Decreased Afterload
• Cardiac work↓
• Myocardial oxygen
  consumption↓
• Cardiac Output↑

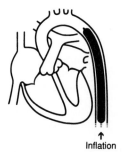

↑
Inflation

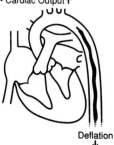

Deflation
↓

Fig. 8-6.   A schematic representation of balloon inflation **(A)** during diastole and deflation **(B)** just before the onset of systole. Diastolic augmentation increases coronary artery perfusion while deflation of the balloon just before the onset of systole decreases afterload, which results in decreased myocardial oxygen demand, decreased cardiac workload, and increased cardiac output.

and medically refractory angina are important indications for IABP placement.

Technique.   Before the percutaneous insertion of an intraaortic balloon, careful assessment of physical contraindications to insertion of large-diameter (9.5 to 10 French) over-the-wire catheters is required. If clinically indicated a low abdominal aortogram will help identify the course and disease of iliac and femoral vessels before the insertion of an intraaortic balloon.

Procedural complications of intraaortic balloon placement most commonly result from low site of puncture, perforation of the superficial femoral artery, or forceful advancement of the guidewire and damage to the arterial entry site. The puncture site should be 2 cm below the inguinal ligament, similar to or slightly more proximal to a standard femoral puncture for cardiac catheterization. Puncture lower than the prescribed site may introduce the balloon in a superficial

Indications and Contraindications for Intraaortic
Balloon Counterpulsation

INDICATIONS

Refractory unstable angina
Cardiogenic shock
Postoperative hemodynamic compromise
Acute myocardial infarction with mechanical impairment as a
    result of mitral regurgitation or ventricular septal defect
Intractable ventricular tachycardia as a result of myocardial
    ischemia
Patients with left main (LM) coronary stenosis or severe three-
    vessel disease undergoing anesthesia for cardiac surgery
High risk PTCA
Maintenance of vessel patency after PTCA of a total occlusion

CONTRAINDICATIONS

Anatomic abnormality of femoral-iliac artery
Iliac or aortic atherosclerotic disease impairing blood flow run off
Moderate or severe aortic regurgitation
Aortic dissection or aneurysm
Patent ductus (counterpulsation may augment the abnormal
    pathway of aortic to pulmonary artery shunting)
Bypass grafting to femoral arteries or aorta
Bleeding diathesis
Sepsis

artery too small to accept this large catheter, which can lead
to ischemia of the extremity.

The balloon is inserted into either groin using standard
Seldinger technique; the needle puncture provides access to
the artery, and the guidewire advances smoothly up the
femoral and iliac arteries to the central aortic area. The needle
is withdrawn, and a small 7 or 8 French dilator is inserted
into the artery. The dilator is removed and the balloon sheath
with the large 9.5 to 10 French dilator is inserted. (Some
manufacturers are making "sheathless" balloon catheters.)
The operator should carefully maintain tension and extension on the guidewire for easy passage of this assembly.
Once the assembly has been positioned, the guidewire and
introducer are removed if the sheath has no valve. Pinching

the sheath beneath the hub will seal blood within the sheath while the IABP catheter, preloaded with a second guidewire, is inserted. Occluding the hub with a finger prevents a copious amount of blood from escaping during insertion of the balloon. Most intraaortic balloons now no longer need manual wrapping or unwrapping and are inserted easily over a preloaded guidewire to the central aortic position. However, it is important to obtain a negative vacuum in the balloon using a large syringe and the one-way valve provided in the IABP insertion kit. The marker at the tip of the balloon should be left 1 to 2 cm below the top of the aortic arch. The guidewire is then removed and the central lumen is aspirated carefully, flushed, and connected to a pressure transducer. Fluoroscopic observation of the balloon inflated above the renal arteries confirm optimal placement.

Once the balloon has been positioned at the aortic arch, it is connected to the console and automatically filled. Counterpulsation is then initiated. In smaller people, pumping may not begin if the distal end of the balloon remains in the sheath. In this case, *partial* withdrawal of the sheath should remedy this problem. The sheath seal is then placed over the sheath hub to ensure complete hemostasis. The balloon is secured with umbilical tape and the femoral artery sheath is sutured to the leg. The position of the balloon is checked frequently to make sure that it remains stable. X-ray confirmation is recommended after the patient has returned to the intensive care unit.

The timing cycle of the balloon should initially begin at 1:2 pumping (one inflation for every two beats), while adjusting the timing of the balloon inflation so that augmented and nonaugmented pressure waveforms can be compared (Fig. 8-7). The central aortic pressure is used to assess hemodynamic effects (Fig. 8-8). A peripheral radial line may be used if the central balloon pressure tracing is inadequate, but the delay in timing (50 ms) should be considered.

Inflation of the balloon should occur at the aortic dicrotic notch (T wave on ECG), and deflation should occur immediately before systole (at or before the R wave) to provide maximal augmentation of diastolic flow and maximal reduction of "presystolic" diastolic pressure (Fig. 8-9). The electrocardiogram is used to trigger the balloon console. However,

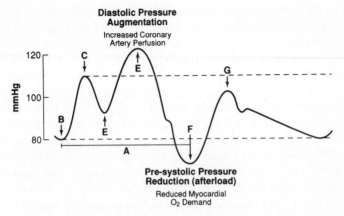

Fig. 8-7.   Arterial waveforms during 2:1 intraaortic balloon pump counterpulsation. **A,** One complete cardiac cycle; **B,** unassisted aortic end-diastolic pressure; **C,** unassisted aortic systolic pressure; **D,** dicrotic notch (balloon inflation); **E,** diastolic augmentation; **F,** assisted aortic end-diastolic pressure; **G,** assisted systole. Diastolic augmentation occurs during balloon inflation, which results in increased coronary artery perfusion. Reduction in the presystolic pressure (afterload) occurs with balloon deflation and reduces myocardial oxygen demand. The assisted systolic pressure (**G**) should be lower than the unassisted aortic systolic pressure (**C**) due to a reduction in the aortic end-diastolic pressure (**F**).

optimal management of balloon timing and volume is guided by direct pressure reading. If no pressure wave is available, the ECG may be used for timing the balloon; however, this practice is discouraged. After proper adjustment of balloon inflation/deflation, the timing cycle is set at 1:1 pumping. Factors that affect diastolic augmentation are listed in Table 8-5.

The effects of intraaortic balloon pumping on coronary blood flow depend on the degree of coronary arterial obstruction. In patients undergoing coronary angioplasty, flow distal to severe stenoses showed no effect of intraaortic balloon pumping. After coronary angioplasty, flow was markedly increased and further augmented with intraaortic balloon pumping (Fig. 8-10).

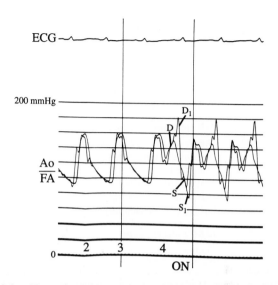

Fig. 8-8. Hemodynamic tracings of femoral artery (*FA*) and central aortic (*Ao*) pressure during intraaortic balloon pumping, demonstrating the augmentation in diastole in the central position (*D*) and femoral artery position D_1) and reduction in systolic load in the central position (*S*) and the femoral artery position (S_1). Moving the timing of inflation toward the dicrotic notch and the timing of deflation away from systolic upstroke will augment the diastolic pressure and optimally reduce systolic load. *ON*, the point at which the balloon pump is turned on.

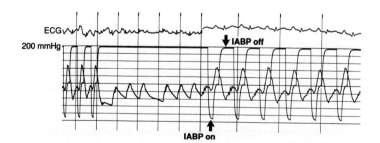

Fig. 8-9. Arterial pressure wave and influence of intraaortic balloon pumping (*IABP*). A timing signal from the balloon pump demonstrates effective diastolic pressure augmentation and systolic pressure reduction.

TABLE 8-5.   Factors affecting diastolic augmentation

Patient hemodynamics
Heart rate
Stroke volume
Mean arterial pressure
Systemic vascular resistance

IAB mechanical factors
IAB in sheath
IAB not unfolded
IAB position
Kink in IAB catheter
IAB Leak
Low helium concentration

IABP console factors
Timing
Position of IAB augmentation dial

IAB, Intraaortic balloon; IABP, intraaortic balloon pump.

Assessment of the patient during counterpulsation includes evaluation for infection, thrombocytopenia, hemorrhage, hemolysis, and vascular obstruction with limb ischemia. Thrombus or dissection may be present at the puncture site or proximally. Heparin administration (5000-Unit bolus with 1000 Units/hr) is standard practice in most institutions. Aortic dissection may occur if the balloon has not been positioned carefully over a guidewire. *We do not recommend insertion of a counterpulsation balloon without a leading guidewire*

Fig. 8-10.   Effects of intraaortic balloon pumping (IABP) on distal coronary flow (velocity) before and after angioplasty. *Top panels, Pre,* Before angioplasty, severe narrowing in the circumflex coronary artery (*open arrow*) is associated with minimal flow velocity (by Doppler guidewire) and no effect of intraaortic balloon pumping. *Bottom panels, Post,* After angioplasty (*open arrow*) distal coronary flow velocity is markedly increased and further augmented by intraaortic balloon pumping; these findings are nearly identical to flow patterns in a normal adjacent reference artery. CFX, circumflex artery. (From Kern MJ, Aguirre F, Bach R, Donohue T, Segal J: Augmentation of coronary blood flow by intra-aortic balloon pumping in patients after coronary angioplasty, *Circulation* 87:500–511, 1993.)

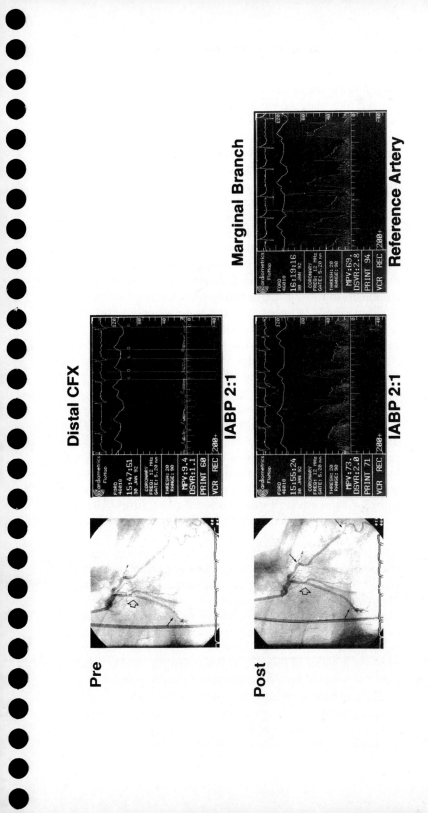

under any circumstances. The patient must remain comfortable and relatively supine while the balloon is inplaced, although some degree of hip flexion may be permitted (30°). Where performing angiography from the contralateral femoral artery, a J-wire is used. The balloon is placed on standby while the wire and catheter pass the balloon, so that damage is minimized.

Intraaortic balloon removal. When clinically indicated the balloon can be removed by aspirating negative pressure on the balloon lumen and jointly withdrawing the sheath and balloon assembly while compressing the puncture site. The femoral artery should be compressed below the puncture site as the catheter and sheath are removed to avoid embolism to the leg. Once the balloon has been inflated, its deflated profile is larger than the sheath lumen, and therefore it cannot be completely withdrawn into the sheath prior to removal. Pressure over the groin must be maintained for 30 to 60 minutes with frequent assessment of distal pulses. Anticoagulation should be discontinued four hours prior to removal of the balloon catheter. A PTT or activated clotting time should be checked before the balloon is removed.

Percutaneous cardiopulmonary support (CPS). CPS is used in the catheterization laboratory as an adjunct to high-risk angioplasy for maintenance of adequate perfusion in hemodynamic catastrophes instead of, or in conjunction with an IABP, and for rescue of an unexpected catastrophe during diagnostic and interventional procedures. The CPS system utilizes a conical rotating centrifugal pump that provides negative pressure for venous outflow as well as positive pressure for arterial inflow. A flow probe, heat exchanger, and membrane oxygenator are all in series in the circuit. There are two cannulae, venous and arterial, that are inserted either percutaneously or by cutdown. The venous cannula is 16 to 20 French, 75 cm in length, and inserted over a tapered dilator. It is positioned with the distal end in the right atrium for venous blood withdrawal. The arterial cannula is 16 to 20 French, 32 cm in length, and is inserted into the femoral artery for retrograde aortic perfusion.

The cannula are relatively easily inserted using the percutaneous technique by an experienced invasive cardiologist. If a cutdown is employed, either a surgeon or cardiologist proficient with this technique is required.

A separate arterial access is necessary to monitor blood pressure. During an operator's early experience, the procedure should be performed with a perfusionist and cardiac anesthesiologist in attendance.

TECHNIQUE FOR ELECTIVE PERCUTANEOUS CARDIOPULMONARY SUPPORT

For elective insertion, iliac/femoral angiography is performed via the femoral artery where the cannulae will be inserted to ascertain patency of the vessel, to identify the femoral rather than the profunda artery, and to assess vessel tortuosity which may interfere with insertion of the cannula and the flow rate. A single wall puncture is made in each vessel. After the vein is punctured, it is sequentially enlarged with 8, 12, and 14 French dilators; the cannula and dilator assembly is inserted and positioned so the distal end lies in the upper portion of the right atrium. An extra stiff 0.038-inch guidewire, held in position by an assistant, will facilitate passage through a tortuous femoral system. An alternative to the sequential dilator method is the use of a 5- or 6-mm balloon, which may be considerably faster.

As the inner dilator is removed from the sheath, the patient should be asked to perform a Valsalva maneuver, or pressure should be applied to the abdomen to create positive pressure, filling the sheath with blood and avoiding an air embolism. The sheath is then locked using the attached thumb clamp. The sheath and connector tubing are filled by an assistant with a large syringe filled with saline while the operator mates the tubing and sheath taking care to eliminate any air in the circuit.

The arterial cannula is inserted in a similar manner. The artery is dilated subsequently with 8, 12, and 14 French dilators (or a 5- or 6-mm balloon); the cannula and dilator assembly is inserted. The arterial sheath and connector are mated in a similar fashion as the venous system. A side port and stopcock allow the arterial system to be purged of air.

After the cannulae are inserted, 300 units/kg heparin is administered for full anticoagulation. Activated clotting times are frequently measured (approximately every 20 minutes) with additional heparin administered to keep the activated clotting time >400 seconds.

Once the interventional procedure has been concluded, the patient is weaned from CPS by the method used in the cardiac operating room. CPS flow is reduced gradually while observing the patient's hemodynamic status. When flow reaches 0.5 L/min, the venous line is closed with the thumb clamp. At this time, if volume repletion is needed, fluids are infused via the arterial line. Once volume repletion is complete, the clamp on the arterial line is clamped off. The recirculation line is then opened to prevent stasis in the circuit. If it is necessary to return to CPS, the recirculation line is closed with reinstitution of CPS. Destruction of blood elements and activation of clotting factors by the oxygenator precludes (using traditional oxygenators) having patients on CPS for greater than 6 hours.

The large amount of fluid required for the priming circuit and connecting lines will result in a significant drop in the patient's hematocrit during the procedure. Therefore, following the procedure, blood remaining in the circuit is retrieved using a cell saver and returned to the patient.

If the system was inserted percutaneously, the patient is transferred to a stretcher with a full metal base and positioned near the edge of the stretcher. The cannulae are withdrawn with hemostasis achieved manually. A C-clamp compressor system is used to compress the vessels to the point where no bleeding is noted but where pulses are still present either by palpation or by Doppler. The patient can then be transported to the intensive care unit for further monitoring. The C-clamp is left in place for 6 hours or until the PTT has reached 70 seconds. At this time, the C-clamp can be gradually released, and if no further bleeding is noted, the patient is usually maintained at bed rest on the same stretcher for another 12 to 24 hours. Some operators keep the cannulae in for 4 to 6 hours after the procedure to allow for metabolism of heparin and then remove the cannulae and maintain hemostasis by manual compression (1 to 1.5 hours).

Emergency Percutaneous CPS

Percutaneous femoral-femoral CPS can be lifesaving in refractory cardiac arrest when initiated within 30 minutes in a patient with surgically or angioplasty-remediable disease or in a candidate for cardiac transplantation. In a patient who does not fulfill these criteria, CPS should *not* be considered. Safe and effective application of CPS in the catheterization laboratory requires teamwork between the cardiologist, the cardiac surgeon, and the perfusionist. Once initial attempts to resuscitate the patient fail, the patient's eligibility for CPS and further treatment should be determined, and CPS initiated without delay if appropriate.

Cautionary Notes

CPS cannulae are large-bore catheters. When CPS is utilized, the likelihood of vascular problems is high, especially in the elderly or in those with peripheral vascular disease. In an emergency situation, a quick evaluation of the extremity circulation is performed and the artery and vein are approached as described above. While the cannulae are inserted, the external circuit is prepared, primed, and purged of all air. When adequate flow is established, the resuscitation can be stopped. Arrhythmias are treated by standard methods. Ventricular fibrillation is defibrillated by DC shock. Further treatment (e.g., bypass surgery of PTCA) is planned immediately.

Elective Use of CPS: High-Risk Coronary Angioplasty

The elective use of CPS in high-risk PTCA patients may provide stable hemodynamics during the procedure. The indications for elective use of CPS are yet to be determined. In most high-risk PTCA patients (e.g., those with poor LV function, dilatation of only remaining vessel, dilatation of a territory supplying ≥50% of the myocardium), standby CPS seems a reasonable approach. In this method, 5 French sheaths are placed into the contralateral femoral artery and vein. These small sheaths allow easy placement of the cannula, saving valuable time. Angiography is performed to document the patency of the iliac/femoral artery. In patients with obstructive disease in the iliofemoral system, elective percutaneous CPS should not be attempted. The external circuit is primed and purged of air and is kept ready for immediate use should a hemodynamic catastrophe occur during angioplasty. It is important to remember that because CPS will not increase regional myocardial blood flow or alleviate myocardial ischemia, acute coronary dissection or occlusion should be treated immediately with perfusion catheters, distal perfusion, stenting, or emergency coronary artery bypass graft surgery.

The complications of percutaneous CPS are primarily vascular in nature: bleeding, thromboembolism, and pseudoaneurysm formation. Complications specific to CPS (e.g., thrombocytopenia, disseminated intravascular coagulation) are seen especially in patients where long-term support (>6 hours) was necessary.

SUGGESTED READINGS

Caldwell G, Millar G, Quinn E, Vincent R, Chamberlain DA: Simple mechanical methods for cardioversion: defence of the precordial thump and cough version, *Br Med J* 291:627–629, 1985.

Eisenberg MS, Hallstrom AP, Copass MK, Bergner L, Short F, Pierce J: Treatment of ventricular fibrillation: emergency medical technician defibrillation and paramedic services, *JAMA* 251:1723–1726, 1984.

Kahn JK, Rutherford BD, McConahay DR, et al.: Supported "high risk" coronary angioplasty using intraaortic balloon pump counterpulsation, *J Am Coll Cardiol* 15:1151–1155, 1990.

Kern MJ, Aguirre F, Bach R, Donohue T, Segal J: Augmentation of coronary blood flow by intra-aortic balloon pumping in patients after coronary angioplasty. *Circulation* 87:500–511, 1993.

Millereau M: Dilution of potent drugs, *Am J Cardiol* 68:418, 1991.

Ohman EM, Califf RM, George DS, et al.: The use of intraaortic balloon pumping as an adjunct to reperfusion therapy in acute myocardial infarction. The thrombolyses and angioplasty in myocardial infarction (TAMI) study group, *Am Heart J* 1218:895–901, 1991.

Pennington DG, Merjavy JP, Codd JE, et al.: Extra-corporeal membrane oxygenation for patients with cardiogenic shock, *Circulation* 70:I-130–I-137, 1984.

Reichman RT, Joyo CI, Dombitsky WP, et al.: Improved patient survival after cardiac arrest using a cardiopulmonary support system, *Ann Thorac Surg* 498:101–105, 1990.

Shawl FA, Domanski MJ, Wish MH, Davis M: Percutaneous cardiopulmonary bypass support in the catheterization laboratory: technique and complications, *Am Heart J* 120:195–203, 1990.

Standards and guidelines for cardiopulmonary resuscitation (CPR) and emergency cardiac care (ECC), *JAMA* 255:2905–2914, 1986.

Stueven HA, Tonsfeldt DJ, Thompson BM, Whitcomb J, Kastenson E, Aprahamian C: Atropine in asystole: human studies, *Ann Emerg Med* 13:815–187, 1984.

Tommaso CL, Johnson RA, Stafford JL, Zoda AR, Vogel RA: Supported coronary angioplasty and standby coronary angioplasty for high-risk coronary artery disease. *Am J Cardiol* 66:1255–1257, 1990.

Vignola PA, Swaye PS, Gosselin AJ: Guidelines for effective and safe percutaneous intra-aortic balloon pump insertion and safe percutaneous intra-aortic balloon pump insertion and removal, *Am J Cardiol* 48:660–664, 1981.

Vogel RA: Femoral-femoral cardiopulmonary bypass assisted coronary angioplasty, *Cardiac Surg* 78:213–220, 1993.

Vogel RA, Shawl F, Tommaso C, O'Neill W, Overlie P, O'Toole J, Vandormael M, Topol E, Tabari KK, Vogel J, Smith S Jr, Freedmann R Jr, White C, George B, Teirstein P: Initial report of the National Registry of Elective Cardiopulmonary Bypass Supported Coronary Angioplasty, *J Am Coll Cardiol* 15:23–29, 1990.

Voudris V, Marco J, Morice M-C, Fajadet J, Royer T: "High-risk" percutaneous transluminal coronary angioplasty with preventive intra-aortic balloon counterpulsation, *Cathet Cardiovasc Diagn* 19:160–164, 1990.

9

INTERVENTIONAL TECHNIQUES

Ubeydullah Deligonul, Morton J. Kern, Richard G. Bach, Thomas J. Donohue, Eugene A. Caracciolo, Frank V. Aguirre, and J. David Talley

PTCA

Until 1977, coronary artery bypass surgery was the only alternative to medicine for the treatment of coronary artery disease. Coronary artery bypass surgery attaches a segment of leg vein (or chest wall artery) to the heart in order to detour blood around the narrowed portion (i.e., stenosis) of the coronary artery. PTCA provides an alternative procedure in which the narrowed portion of the artery can be enlarged selectively without surgery.

The acronym PTCA stands for

P, percutaneous—refers to the insertion of a catheter into a body through a small puncture site in the skin

T, transluminal—refers to the procedure being performed from the inside of the artery lumen

C, coronary—identifies the specific artery to be dilated

A, angioplasty—a technique for remodelling a blood vessel through the introduction of an expandable balloon catheter

A thin, steerable guidewire is introduced into the coronary artery and positioned across the stenosis into the distal aspect of the artery. An angioplasty balloon catheter, which is considerably smaller than the guiding catheter, is inserted through the guiding catheter and is positioned (in the artery) across the stenotic area by tracking over the guidewire. Once the balloon is correctly placed within the area to be dilated, it is inflated several times for periods ranging from 45 seconds to several minutes. The inflation and deflation of the balloon in the blocked artery alleviates the arterial stenosis and restores blood flow to an area of the heart previously deprived by the stenosed artery. If no complications occur, only 1 to 2 days of hospitalization are required, and the patient commonly returns to work shortly (<7 days) thereafter.

How Angioplasty Works

Several theories regarding the mechanisms of angioplasty have been proposed.

Disruption of plaque and the arterial wall.   The inflated balloon exerts pressure against the plaque and the arterial wall, causing fracturing and splitting. The concentric lesion fractures and splits at its thinnest and weakest point. Eccentric lesions will split at the junction of the plaque and the arterial wall. Dissection or separation of the plaque from the medial wall releases the splinting effect that is caused by the lesion and results in a larger lumen. This is the major effective mechanism of balloon angioplasty.

Loss of elastic recoil.   Balloon dilatation causes stretching and thinning of the medial wall. Stretching causes the medial wall to lose its elastic properties. The degree of elastic recoil loss will be affected by the balloon size/artery size ratio. Over time (1 to 6 weeks) there may be some return of elastic recoil.

Redistribution and compression of plaque components.   During angioplasty, shear pressures cause denudation or stripping of endothelial cells and the extrusion or pushing out of plaque components. There may be some molding of the softer lipid material, but this effect accounts for a very small part of the overall effect of angioplasty.

Indications

1. Angina pectoris causing sufficient disability to warrant coronary artery bypass graft surgery in spite of optimal medical therapy

2. Mild angina pectoris with objective evidence of ischemia (abnormal stress test or abnormal stress thallium) and high-grade lesion of a vessel supplying a large area of myocardium
3. Unstable angina
4. Acute MI in patients who have contraindications to thrombolytic therapy or have evidence of persistent or recurrent ischemia despite thrombolytic therapy (in some institutions, direct PTCA without thrombolytic therapy is used as the primary therapy)
5. Angina pectoris after coronary artery bypass graft surgery
6. Restenosis after successful PTCA

Contraindications

1. Unsuitable coronary anatomy
2. Extremely high-risk coronary anatomy in which closure of vessel would result in patient death
3. Contraindication to coronary bypass graft surgery (some patients will have PTCA as their only alternative to revascularization)
4. Bleeding diathesis
5. Patient noncompliance with procedure and post-PTCA instructions
6. Multiple PTCA restenoses

Complications

1. Death (<1%)
2. MI (<3% to 5%)
3. Emergency coronary artery bypass grafting (<5%) and abrupt vessel closure (3% to 8%)
4. All the complications that can occur during cardiac catheterization can also occur during PTCA; access site bleeding is not uncommon
5. Restenosis—intimal hyperplasia at the site of PTCA occurs in approximately 30% to 40% of patients after successful PTCA leading to recurrence of anginal symptoms; typically, restenosis occurs within the initial 6 months after PTCA

PTCA Equipment

PTCA equipment consists of three basic elements: the guiding catheter, the balloon catheter, and the coronary guidewire (see Appendix VIII) (Fig. 9-1).

Guiding catheter.   A special large-lumen catheter is used to guide the coronary balloon catheter to the vessel of the lesion to be dilated.

As compared to the diagnostic catheters, the guiding catheters have thinner walls and larger lumens, allowing contrast injections while the balloon catheter is in place. The guiding catheters are stiffer to provide support for advancing the balloon catheter into the coronary artery and, therefore, respond differently to manipulation than diagnostic catheters. The guiding catheter tip is not tapered, occasionally causing pressure dampening upon engaging the coronary ostium. Size 8 or 10 French guiding catheters are available for PTCA. Size 7 and even 6 French guiding catheters are also available but will not generally accept stents (see below). Some catheters have relatively shorter and more flexible tips to decrease catheter-induced trauma.

Functions of the guiding catheter (Figs 9-2 and 9-3). There are four major functions that a guiding catheter serves during PTCA:

1. *Balloon catheter delivery and guidance.* The guiding catheter provides a method for delivery of the balloon catheter to the coronary ostium. If the guiding catheter is not seated properly in a coaxial manner, it may not be possible to transmit the force needed to advance the balloon across the stenotic area.
2. *Power transmission.* After seating (cannulation) and delivery of the balloon catheter to the coronary ostium, the guiding catheter provides the necessary backup support or "platform" to push the balloon catheter across the stenosis.
3. *Contrast injection.* The guiding catheter also permits contrast administration with or without the balloon catheter in place. New large-lumen guide catheters no longer require the balloon catheter to be removed from the guiding catheter to allow adequate opacification of the vessel during angiography.
4. *Pressure monitoring.* The guiding catheter lumen measures aortic pressure proximal to the stenotic area for determination of the transstenotic pressure gradient.

Guiding catheter terminology. Several terms that commonly are used when referring to guiding catheters are important.

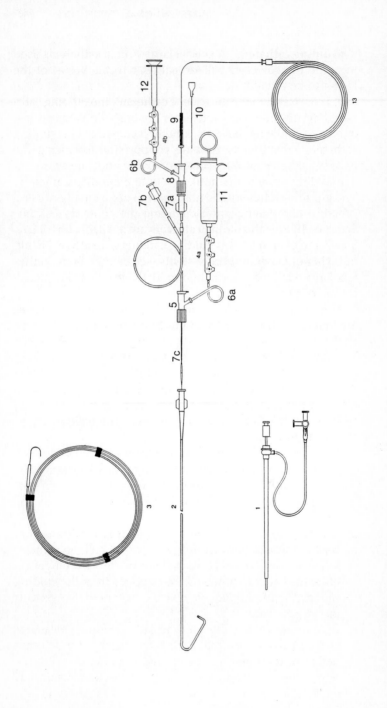

Backing out. The guiding catheter is being ejected from the coronary ostium into the aortic root when pressure is applied to the balloon in an attempt to cross the lesion. This is caused by insufficient backup and/or a very tight stenosis.

Backup. A stable position of the guiding catheter at the orifice of the coronary ostium provides the necessary platform to advance the balloon across the lesion.

"Deep throat." This refers to the process of manipulating the guide over the balloon catheter shaft past the ostium, further into the vessel, to obtain increased backup support for crossing difficult lesions. This maneuver typically is used as a *last resort* because there is an increased chance of guide-induced dissection of the proximal vessel.

Balloon catheters

Development of coronary angioplasty balloon catheters. Technological refinements of balloon catheter equipment as well as increased operator experience have dramatically improved the primary success rate of coronary angioplasty. In the initial National Heart, Lung and Blood Institute series in which the experience of 105 centers from 1977 to 1981 was compiled, less than two thirds of angioplasty procedures were successful. In 1985 and 1986, an additional National Heart, Lung and Blood Institute survey was performed and showed that the clinical success rate of angioplasty had improved to 78%. Since then, the use of ultra-low-profile devices, flexible, steerable guidewires, improved radiological imaging equipment, and more specific selection criteria by experienced operators has led to success rates of greater than 90%.

Fig. 9-1. The equipment for a percutaneous transluminal coronary angioplasty (PTCA) system. *1,* Catheter sheath introducer; *2,* guiding catheter; *3,* diagnostic guidewire; *4,* manifold (three-port); *5,* adjustable hemostasis valve (Tuohy-Borst or Y adaptor); *6a,b,* extension tubing (short); *7a,* guidewire port of PTCA balloon catheter; *7b,* contrast port of balloon catheter; *7c,* inflation port of PTCA balloon catheter; *8,* adjustable hemostasis valve (Tuohy-Borst or Y adaptor); *9,* steering device; *10,* insertion tool; *11,* control syringe (three-ring); *12,* inflation device.

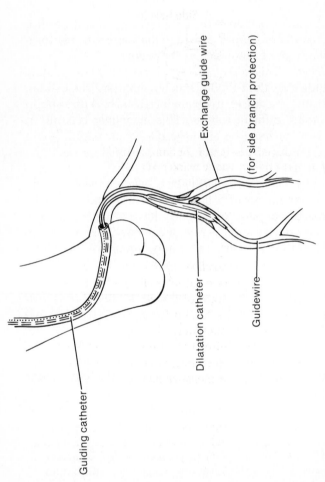

Fig. 9-2. Angioplasty procedure with technique to protect side branches. An exchange guidewire is positioned across the bifurcation in the vessel to be protected. The dilatation catheter, with its own guidewire, is used for the principal lesion. (From Oesterle SN and others: Angioplasty at coronary bifurcations: singleguide, two-wire technique, *Cathet Cardiovasc Diagn* 12:57, 1986.)

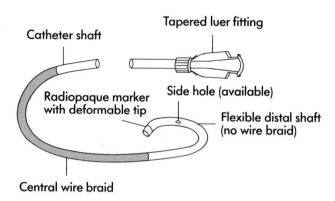

Fig. 9-3. Illustration of a guiding catheter showing variable position of central wire braid, optional distal sidehole, deformable tip, and radiopaque marker. (From Avedissian MG and others: Percutaneous transluminal coronary angioplasty: a review of current balloon dilatation systems, *Cathet Cardiovasc Diagn*, 18:263, 1989.)

Over-the-wire angioplasty balloon catheters. A standard over-the-wire angioplasty balloon catheter (Fig. 9-4) has a central lumen throughout the length of the catheter for the guidewire and another separate lumen for the balloon inflation. These balloons are approximately 145 to 155 cm long and can be used with guidewires of various dimensions (0.010 to 0.018 inch). The balloon catheter may have a wire lumen large enough for pressure measurement and distal contrast injection.

The advantages and limitations of over-the-wire angioplasty balloon catheters are listed in Table 9-1. These catheters accept multiple guidewires, which allow for the exchanging of additional devices that may require stronger, stiffer guidewires. Although on some catheters the guidewire lumen is available for pressure measurement or contrast injection, current ultra-low-profile over-the-wire angioplasty balloon catheters do not have this feature. In addition, the inability to inject through the distal end interferes with the evaluation of the patency of distal arteries by analysis of contrast runoff. Maintenance of distal wire position is of paramount importance in coronary angioplasty. For over-

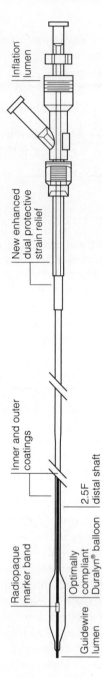

Fig. 9-4. Schematic design of a typical over-the-wire angioplasty balloon catheter. Note that the guidewire extends the entire length of the catheter. (From Talley JD, Joseph A, Kupersmith J: Preliminary results utilizing a new percutaneous transluminal coronary angioplasty balloon catheter, *Cathet Cardiovasc Diagn* 20:108–113, 1990, with permission.)

TABLE 9-1. Advantages and limitations of angioplasty balloon types

Advantages	Limitations
Over the wire	
Distal wire position	Two experienced personnel required
Distal port available for pressure measurement or contrast media injection	Larger profile
Acceptable multiple guidewires	
Rapid exchange	
Distal wire position	Excellent guiding catheter support
Enhanced visualization	Exchanging balloons at hemostatic valve can be technically demanding
Low-profile balloons	Poor balloon tracking if wire lumen not flushed with heparinized saline
Single-operator system	
Fixed wire	
Enhanced visualization	Lack of through lumen
Single-operator system	Inability to recross lesion without removing system
Flexibility	
Access to distal lesions	
Use with small guiding catheters	
Low-profile balloons	

the-wire balloon catheters, the guidewire can be extended to help maintain distal position while the balloon catheter is completely withdrawn over the guidewire to permit another balloon catheter to be exchanged and introduced over the same guidewire for additional dilatations.

Over-the-wire angioplasty balloon catheters have few limitations. These catheters are, in general, slightly larger than the rapid-exchange and fixed-wire catheter types and their use with smaller size (6 French) guiding catheters may be difficult. Also a primary operator and experienced personnel are required to facilitate guidewire, balloon placement, and catheter exchanges.

Rapid-exchange (monorail) angioplasty balloon catheters. To improve on ease of exchanging over-the-wire angioplasty balloon catheters by single operators, "rapid-exchange" balloon catheters were developed. This catheter differs in that only a variable length of the shaft has two lumens (Fig. 9-5A). One lumen is for balloon inflation and the other, which extends only a portion of the catheter shaft, houses the guidewire. Because only a limited portion of the balloon requires dual lumens, the catheters can be made smaller to optimize artery visualization.

Rapid-exchange balloon catheters address certain inherent limitations of over-the-wire systems. First, over-the-wire balloon exchanges requiring extension of the distal wire are unnecessary because the rapid-exchange portion of the catheter is short. Second, a single operator can use rapid-exchange balloon catheters without the aid of other assistants to maintain distal guidewire position or facilitate balloon navigation.

However, monorail catheters also have limitations. These include the need for excellent guiding catheter support, difficulty with simultaneous manipulation of the guidewire, balloon catheter, and guiding catheter, and blood loss during removal of the balloon catheter at the rotating hemostatic valve because of an open Y connector during the balloon backout. Additionally, the balloon may be difficult to track across the wire if the distal lumen is not properly flushed with heparinized saline solution. Finally, care must also be exercised when the balloon and guidewire are advanced through the guiding catheter to the coronary ostia. If the balloon is advanced in front of the wire, the wire may come out of its lumen, necessitating repeated assembly of the balloon and guidewire.

Fixed-wire angioplasty balloon catheters. The "fixed-wire" catheter has the balloon mounted on the wire with a distal flexible steering tip (Fig. 9-5B). The proximal end of the catheter consists of a single nonremovable port connected to a hollow metal tube (hypotube). A core wire extends from the hypotube to the end of the distal steerable tip. This assembly is coated with a thin plastic shaft that enhances flexibility. Fixed-wire balloons have only one enclosed lumen for balloon inflation.

The advantages and limitations of fixed-wire angioplasty balloon catheters are listed in Table 9-1. The small shaft

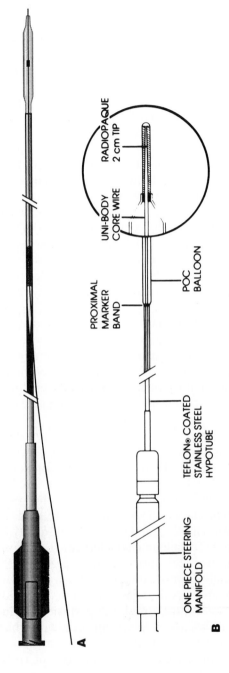

Fig. 9-5. **A,** Schematic design of a typical rapid-exchange angioplasty balloon catheter. Note that the guidewire extends on "through" the distal part of the catheter allowing for single-operator use. (Courtesy of SciMed Life Systems, Maple Grove, Minn.) **B,** Schematic design of a standard fixed-wire angioplasty balloon catheter. This design has only one "through" lumen for balloon inflation, and the device itself serves as a "steerable guidewire." *POC,* polyolefin copolymer. (From Talley JD, Joseph A, Killeavy ES, Garratt KN, Hodes ZI, Linnemeier TJ, Yussman ZA, Brier ME, Kupersmith J: Multicenter evaluation of a new fixed-wire coronary angioplasty catheter system: clinical and angiographic characteristics and results, *Cathet Cardiovasc Diagn* 22:310–316, 1991, with permission.)

size of the single-lumen design provides excellent coronary visualization. Because the balloon is mounted on the distal guidewire, the device can easily be used by a single operator. Fixed-wire balloon catheters are particularly useful for distal lesions, subtotal stenoses, and lesions located in tortuous vasculature. In addition, they may be particularly beneficial when small guiding catheters are used.

However, fixed-wire catheters have significant limitations. These catheters lack the inherent safety advantage of over-the-wire and rapid-exchange systems because the balloon is mounted on a guidewire. To exchange this catheter for a different balloon size, the catheter is removed completely and recrossing with a new size catheter is performed. A narrowed or dissected lesion may not permit balloon advancement or may even close the vessel. The lack of a distal lumen prevents measuring of distal pressure or injection of contrast media to evaluate distal vessel runoff.

Summary. A variety of coronary angioplasty balloon catheters are currently available. All existing models have intrinsic advantages and limitations based on their design. Selection of an appropriate balloon catheter for angioplasty should consider these design characteristics as well as the anatomic problems to ensure a technically and clinically successful procedure.

The balloon is inflated and deflated using a hand-held syringe device with a pressure gauge. The balloon catheters come in different sizes (1.5 to 4 mm for coronary dilatations), which refer to the inflated diameter of the balloon. The balloon diameter is selected according to the size of the vessel to be dilated. The coronary balloon catheters are made of different plastic materials that determine the flexibility of the catheter shaft and the balloon characteristics (e.g., burst pressure and actual diameter under different pressure levels). There are special-purpose coronary balloon catheters, such as those with preshaped angles and those with side holes in the shaft, permitting distal autoperfusion during prolonged balloon inflations. A perfusion catheter, which contains multiple side holes in the shaft but no balloon, allows perfusion of the coronary vessel in cases of vessel closure during PTCA. This prevents or minimizes myocardial ischemia until bypass surgery can be performed. Perfusion balloon catheters along with stents are currently used to reduce the need for emergency bypass.

Steerable guidewires (Fig. 9-6).   Coronary guidewires, very small-caliber (0.014- to 0.018-inch) steerable wires, are advanced into the coronary artery or branches beyond the lesion to be dilated. A J tip of varying degree usually is shaped by the operator to allow steerability in negotiating side branches and tortuous artery curves. The balloon catheter is advanced over the wire and, after artery dilatation, removed safely with the wire remaining in place beyond the dilated lesion. Extra long guidewires (300 cm) are utilized to exchange balloon catheters. The tip flexibility and torque control characteristics of these coronary guidewires vary. Generally the softer wires are safer and easier to advance into the tortuous branches, whereas the stiffer wires give better torque control and may be useful for crossing difficult or total occlusions.

Other equipment.   *Y connector (adjustable hemostasis device).* The Y connector is an accessory device that minimizes back-bleeding while the balloon catheter is inserted into the guiding catheter. This setup allows the injection of contrast and pressure monitoring through the guiding catheter, regardless of balloon catheter position.

Inflation device. A syringe device inflates the balloon on the balloon catheter with precise measurement of the inflation pressure in atmospheres. These devices are disposable. Generally, balloons are inflated at pressures of 4 to 12 atm. Typically the balloon is inflated with sufficient pressure to compress the plaque and fully expand the "dumbbell," which is an indentation in the partially inflated balloon due to the undilated stenosis. Occasionally, very hard lesions (caused by calcium or fibrosis) may require very high pressure atmosphere levels (>14 atm) to remove the dumbbell. Needless overinflation of the balloon increases the risk of dissection and balloon rupture.

Torque (tool) device. A small cylindrical pin vise clamp slides over the proximal end of the steerable guidewire, permitting the operator to perform fine manipulations of the guidewire.

Long sheath. The longer-length (23 cm) femoral arterial sheath allows one to negotiate a tortuous artery more easily than with the standard 10-cm sheath used for diagnostic

Standard Tip Flexibility

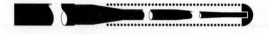

Dia. Inches	Length cm	Tip Shape
.014	175	Straight
.018	175	Straight
.014	175	J

Soft Tip Flexibility

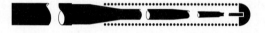

Dia. Inches	Length cm	Tip Shape	Remarks
.014	175	Straight	
.018	175	Straight	
.014	175	J	
.014	300	Straight	Exchange

SuperSoft Tip Flexibility

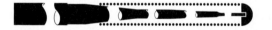

Dia. Inches	Length cm	Tip Shape	Remarks
.012/.014	175	Straight	
.012/.014	175	J	
.012/.014	300	Straight	Exchange
.014	175	Straight	
.014	175	J	
.014	300	Straight	Exchange
.018	175	Straight	
.018	300	Straight	Exchange

Fig. 9-6. Characteristics and specifications of angioplasty guidewires.

catheterization, and it improves the torque of the guiding catheter.

Exchange and extension guidewires. An exhange guidewire is similar to those mentioned above except that its length is 280 to 300 cm. This long wire replaces the initial wire when the exchange of the balloon catheter is necessary (e.g., upsizing balloon or insertion of perfusion catheter). Alternatively, and more conveniently, a 120- to 145-cm extension wire can be connected to the initial guidewire to allow balloon catheter exchanges.

The "Trapper" guidewire exchange system uses a special short balloon on a wire that is not long enough to leave the guide. When inflated, it traps the guidewire inside the guide catheter permitting the balloon catheter to be pulled off without moving the guidewire. A different-size balloon catheter can then be advanced over the wire, the trapper deflated, and the balloon catheter readvanced into the artery.

PTCA Clinical Procedure

I. Pre-PTCA workup
   A. Noninvasive testing for ischemia
      1. ECG (evidence of resting ischemia/recent infarction)
      2. Exercise treadmill with/without thallium as indicated; pharmacologic stress study (e.g., Dipyridamole)
      3. Two-dimensional echocardiogram (as indicated for LV function or valvular heart disease)
   B. Coronary angiography evaluation
   NOTE: Order of tests depends on clinical presentation; demonstration of ischemia is important.
II. Pre-PTCA preparation
   A. Patient preparation
      1. Cardiothoracic surgeon consultation, particularly for multivessel disease or decreased LV function
      2. Patient teaching
      3. Appropriate laboratory work (type and cross match, complete blood cell and platelet counts, PT, PTT, electrolytes, BUN, creatinine)
   B. Patient preparation in catheterization suite
      1. ECG (inferior and anterior wall leads): 12-lead (radiolucent) ECG

2. Skin prep; both inguinal areas
3. Venous access for temporary pacing for RCA or dominant circumflex artery
4. Premedications
   a. Aspirin (325 mg PO): failure to administer aspirin before PTCA is associated with a two to three times higher acute complication rate
   b. Persantine (75 to 100 mg PO; optional)
   c. Calcium antagonist (30 mg PO diltiazem or 10 mg PO nifedipine); avoid doses producing hypotension
   d. Diazepam (5 mg IV or PO)
   e. Benadryl (25 mg IV or PO)
   f. Heparin (10,000 units or 100 units/kg IV bolus; 1000 units IV/hr)
   NOTE: Check activated clotting time, >300 seconds.
   g. Demerol (25 to 50 mg IV) before balloon inflation

C. Guiding coronary arteriograms (perform after giving 100 to 200 µg nitroglycerin intracoronary)
   1. Definition of coronary anatomy and collateral supply (if any)
   2. Guiding shots to use as reference maps for guidewire and balloon positioning
   3. Size of the artery relative to known guide catheter diameter used to select the balloon catheter.
   NOTE: 8 French = 2.87 mm = 3.0 balloon. If the artery is smaller, use 2.5, 2.0-mm balloon. If the artery is larger, use 3.5, 4.0-mm balloon catheter.

III. PTCA procedure
   A. Seating guiding catheter
      1. Guiding catheter selected for angle of vessel take-off and optimum backup
      2. Cannulation of target vessel
   B. Insertion of balloon catheter
      1. Size of PTCA dilatation catheter to fit vessel (based on normal reference; balloon/artery ratio <1:1.2)
      2. Steerable guidewire with appropriate tip softness

      3. Balloon and guidewire inserted through hemostasis valve and pin vise connected to guidewire

      4. Flush systems for pressure monitoring (when applicable)

  C. Crossing the lesion with the wire and balloon

      1. Maintain seating of guiding catheter

      2. Pass guidewire beyond lesion as far distal as possible

      3. Advance dilatation balloon into center of lesion

      4. Measure transstenotic gradient (when feasible)

  D. Dilating the lesion

      1. Maintain centering of the balloon (use radio-opaque markers on balloon)

      2. Use adequate inflation pressure (to remove dumb-bell) and time (60 to 120 seconds as tolerated)

  E. Assessing the dilatation result

      1. Reduced transstenotic gradient (<15 mm Hg)

      2. Enlarged artery lumen ($>20\%$ change in diameter with $\leq40\%$ residual lesion), no thrombus

      3. Good angiographic flow

      4. Observe for lesion stability

      5. No residual ischemia

      6. Acceptably stable dissection (if any)

  F. Post-PTCA arteriograms

      1. Removal of dilatation catheter and wire

      2. Obtain target vessel arteriograms (after additional intracoronary nitroglycerin)

      3. Collateral supply arteriograms (optional)

IV. Discharge from catheterization suite after PTCA

      1. Suturing of arterial and venous sheaths in place

      2. Sterile bandages

        Check PTT and adjust heparin infusion (heparin often maintained 1000 unit/hr until next morning)

      3. Teaching on hospital course and bleeding problems

      4. Notification of departments

        a. Intensive care (or other appropriate patient care area)

        b. Operating room and surgical team

        c. Lab and ECG

V. Post-PTCA: day 1
  A. Sheaths out after heparin stopped for 2 to 4 hours
  B. Post-PTCA medications
    1. Calcium antagonists (30 mg PO tid diltiazem; 10 mg PO tid nifedipine) for 4 weeks
    2. Aspirin (325 mg PO daily)
VI. Discharge post-PTCA: day 2 (home)
  A. Follow-up schedule
    1. Exercise treadmill test (usually performed 2 to 6 months after PTCA)
    2. If symptoms or signs of recurrent ischemia, repeat coronary angiography
  B. Discharge teaching
    1. Adherence to medications and testing
    2. Return to activities of daily living
    3. Early symptoms of restenosis and contributing factors (e.g., smoking, diet)

Equipment needed for measuring translesional pressures. The following equipment is required in order to measure pressures during PTCA:
1. Two pressure manifolds and transducers
2. Pressure tubing with Y connectors
3. Hemodynamic monitor and recorder

On occasion proximal and distal pressures are to be measured before and after angioplasty. The guiding catheter is used for proximal pressure that represents aortic pressure. The balloon dilatation catheter is used for distal pressure, measured at the distal tip of the balloon catheter beyond the lesion.

Different properties of wall flexibility and stiffness of guiding catheters and balloon dilatation catheters cause them to transmit pressures differently.

Technique for pressure monitoring during PTCA (see Chapter 3). Once the angioplasty catheters are connected to the pressure monitoring systems, the balloon catheter is advanced until both the guiding catheter and balloon catheter are at the ostium of the vessel. The pressure transmitted through each catheter is measured and recorded. The pressure at this location should be the same. Any small difference between the two pressures before crossing the lesion is called the *intrinsic gradient*.

In Fig. 9-7 the angioplasty system is in place in the patient's left anterior descending artery. The proximal aortic pressure is obtained through the guiding catheter. In the example the proximal pressure is 150/80 mm Hg. The distal pressure is measured through the balloon catheter at 95/58 mm Hg.

[Mean proximal (aortic)
$-$ mean distal (coronary)] pressure $=$ initial gradient

105 mm Hg $-$ 65 mm Hg $=$ 40 mm Hg

As the procedure continues, repeated inflations will be performed and the gradient between the proximal and distal pressures will decrease. Ultimately a gradient of less than 15 mm Hg is considered a successful result (Fig. 9-7).

The risk of abrupt closure and restenosis increases with higher residual gradients. A persistent pressure gradient, especially if the angiographic result is suboptimal, is an indication for further inflations (either prolonged inflations or upsizing of the balloon). Pressure measurements and the evaluation of gradients are valuable if a reliable pressure tracing can be obtained. The reliability of pressure gradients is questioned when one is dealing with small vessels, acute bends in vessels, or multiple lesions in a vessel. Although gradients are not routinely used, this information, as well as distal coronary flow velocity data (see Chapter 6), has value when questionable angiographic results are obtained.

Clinical examples of PTCA are given in Figs. 9-8 to 9-11.

Peripheral Arterial Balloon Angioplasty (PTA) (Fig. 9-12)

Peripheral arterial disease is a common manifestation of atherosclerosis. Generally, peripheral arterial disease can be managed conservatively, although some patients will require revascularization therapy (either surgery or PTA). Certain anatomic considerations often make a given patient a better candidate for one procedure than the other. As for coronary artery disease, discrete localized lesions usually are best treated by balloon angioplasty, while diffuse disease and long total occlusions often do better with bypass surgery. A team approach involving input from both the vascular interventionalist and vascular surgeon will result in optimal treatment for a given patient.

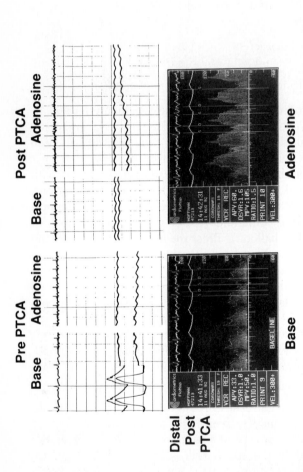

Pre PTCA
Base   Adenosine

Post PTCA
Base   Adenosine

Distal
Post
PTCA

Base

Adenosine

Fig. 9-7. *Top,* Pressure gradient (aortic and distal coronary pressures distal artery flow on a 0 to 200 mm Hg scale) before and after percutaneous transluminal coronary angioplasty (*PTCA*). *Bottom,* velocity signal is shown after PTCA. Adenosine increases the flow after PTCA. Note the change in post-PTCA adenosine pressure during high flow. (From Kern MJ, Flynn MS, Carraciolo EA, Bach RG, Donohue TJ, Aguirre FV: Use of translesional coronary flow velocity for interventional decisions in a patient with multiple intermediately severe coronary stenoses, *Cathet Cardiovasc Diagn* 29:148–153, 1993.)

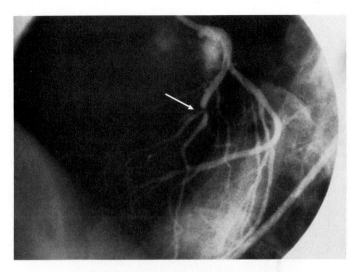

Fig. 9-8. Angiogram of bifurcation lesion in the left anterior descending artery and diagonal arteries requiring simultaneous double balloon technique. (See Fig. 9-9.)

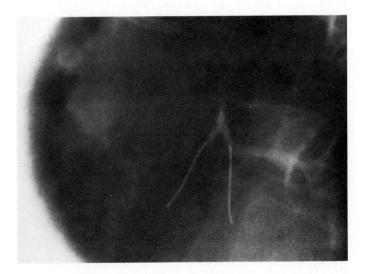

Fig. 9-9. Simultaneous double (fixed-wire) balloons (probes) dilating the bifurcation stenosis.

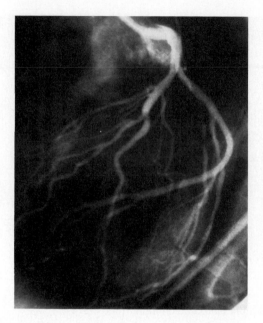

Fig. 9-10. The postangioplasty procedure demonstrating good result with the bifurcation lesion without complications.

Indications

1. Intermittent (life-style–limiting) claudication for more than 6 months
2. Severe limb ischemia
3. Pain while resting
4. Nonhealing ulcer

Contraindications

1. Nonsignificant arterial disease based on Doppler studies and ankle/brachial flow index
2. Medically unstable
3. Long (>15 cm) arterial occlusion
4. Lesion jeopardizes supply of critically dependent collaterals

Technique

1. Angiography of vessel in question
2. Insert arterial sheath (antegrade or retrograde approach,

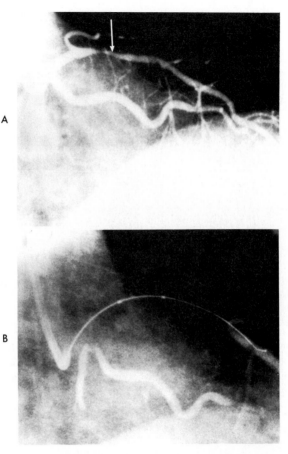

Fig. 9-11. **A,** An angiogram showing proximal left anterior descending stenosis. **B,** A guidewire across the stenosis with balloon markers in place. Note persistent stain of contrast in the circumflex consistent with left main coronary dissection. This complication required emergency bypass surgery.

depending on lesion); heparin (10,000 units IV, 1000 units/hr infusion)
3. Pass guidewire (e.g., Wholey or Terumo guidewires are very useful for PTA)
4. If small coronary-size balloon catheter used, a guiding catheter is used
5. Advance balloon catheter over wire through lesion and

A   B

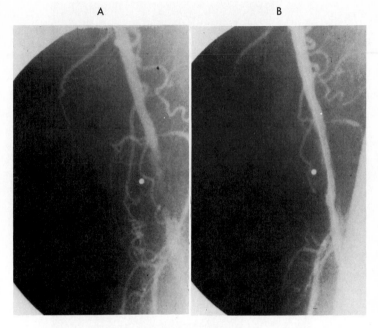

Fig. 9-12. **A,** A superficial femoral artery showing midvessel total occlusion. **B,** A femoral arteriogram after dilatation with guidewire in place showing good result and patent vessel.

dilate (usually two or more inflations); inflated balloon diameter size based on adjacent nondiseased vessel segment

6. Remove balloon catheter and then check patency; redilate as necessary
7. Final angiogram with guidewire removed
8. Postprocedural care as with PTCA, with Doppler and ankle/brachial indices of peripheral pulses for lower extremity procedures

Complications

1. Vasospasm—use 100 to 200 μg intraarterial nitroglycerin (also may use 2 to 10 mg papaverine intraarterially or 50 mg lidocaine)
2. Thrombus—increase heparin; consider thrombolytics (see later in this chapter)
3. Arterial dissection

4. Vessel perforation (1%)
5. Death (<0.5%)

Renal Balloon Angioplasty

Nonsurgical opening of narrowed renal artery may alleviate renovascular hypertension and/or improve renal function.

Indications

1. Renovascular hypertension caused by atherosclerotic or fibromuscular narrowing of renal artery (approximately 1 in 50 hypertensive patients) after
   a. Failed medical therapy
   b. Increased renal vein renin on side of arterial disease
2. Renal transplant artery stenosis
3. Renal artery/vein bypass graft stenosis
4. Renal insufficiency with >50% artery stenosis

Contraindications

1. Unstable medical condition
2. Borderline lesion (<50% or no pressure gradient without elevated lateralized renin)
3. Long segment (>2 cm) of total occlusion
4. Aortic plaque extending into renal artery

Technique

1. Lower aortic approach
   a. Femoral arterial access; sheath and guiding catheter (renal artery guide) inserted; initial angiograms
   b. Heparin 5000 to 10,000 units IV and 100 to 200 μg intraarterial nitroglycerin
   c. Advance guidewire across lesion; watch for small-vessel spasm
   d. Advance 2- to 5-mm balloon dilation catheter across lesion
   e. Dilate at 4 to 10 atm
   f. Deflate and withdraw balloon; check patency
   g. Final angiogram
2. Brachial or axillary arterial approach for down-pointing renal arteries
   a. Entry of brachial or axillary artery by cutdown or percutaneous technique
   b. Apply steps b through g above

Postprocedural Care

1. Monitor blood pressure for 48 hours; may be high or low
2. Post-PTCA care regimen

Complications

1. Death (1%)
2. Thrombus (1%)
3. Nonocclusive dissection (2% to 4%)
4. Worsening renal failure (1.5% to 6.0%)
5. Embolus to peripheral artery (1.5% to 2.0%)
6. Embolus to distal renal artery (2%)
7. Rupture of artery (1%)

VALVULOPLASTY
Percutaneous Balloon Valvuloplasty

Percutaneous techniques as alternatives to surgery for the treatment of valvular and congenital heart disease were introduced in the early 1980s and have now undergone sufficient investigation to define their roles in interventional cardiology. In the pediatric population, balloon valvuloplasty is frequently used to relieve selected congenital valvular disorders, including pulmonic and aortic stenosis. In the adult population, balloon aortic valvuloplasty has been relegated to a palliative role in the management of aotric stenosis in patients who are not surgical candidates, while balloon mitral valvuloplasty for mitral stenosis has emerged as an excellent alternative to surgical commissurotomy or valve replacement and, in selected patients, is now considered by many as the treatment of choice.

Percutaneous balloon aortic valvuloplasty (PBAV) (Fig. 9-13). PBAV has been employed successfully in the pediatric management of congenital aortic stenosis. PBAV for the treatment of adult calcific aortic stenosis was first introduced in 1985. It initially held promise in the treatment of adult calcific aortic stenosis, with encouraging acute hemodynamic results. With a disappointingly high restenosis rate (which may approach 50%), however, PBAV now must be considered a short-term palliative procedure to be applied to a highly selected group of patients.

Indication in adults. The indications for the procedure have evolved since its introduction.

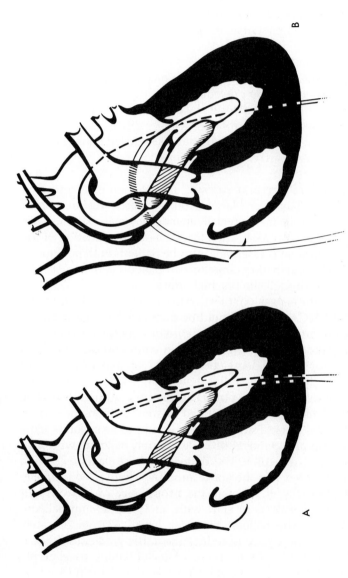

Fig. 9-13. A diagram of two techniques of aortic balloon valvuloplasty. **A,** The retrograde approach. **B,** The antegrade, transseptal approach.

1. PBAV use should be limited to symptomatic patients who are not candidates for valve surgery. The age of the patient per se is not a contraindication for surgery.
2. In selected patients with poor LV function, PBAV can be used as a bridge to surgery.
3. PBAV has a palliative use in symptomatic aortic stenosis patients scheduled to undergo major noncardiac surgery or other invasive procedures.

NOTE: Prior to PBAV, an evaluation for severe coronary artery disease and peripheral vascular disease is warranted. Significant aortic regurgitation and severe left main coronary artery disease are contraindications to PBAV.

Procedure

EVALUATE ARTERIAL ACCESS. The balloon catheters used for PBAV have very large profiles, increasing the risk of vascular problems, especially in elderly female patients with fragile small arteries. Therefore, a careful evaluation of the arterial system is essential. In some patients with poor lower extremity circulation, smaller-size balloon catheters can be inserted through the brachial artery.

EXCLUDE SEVERE CORONARY ARTERY DISEASE. The possibility of LMCA disease should be excluded by angiograms.

EXCLUDE SIGNIFICANT AORTIC INSUFFICIENCY. An aortic regurgitation of more than 2+ is a contraindication for the procedure, as the degree of regurgitation may increase after PBAV.

USE OF SINGLE OR DOUBLE BALLOONS. Although double balloon use has been advocated by some authors the current practice is to use a single balloon. Low-profile balloons allow insertion and removal of 23- to 25-mm balloons with relatively less difficulty. The diameter of the balloons should not be larger than the aortic annulus. There is no generally accepted way of selecting the proper size of balloon. Our practice usually is to start with an 18- to 20-mm balloon, increasing the balloon diameter up to 23 mm or rarely 25 mm as necessary to reduce the aortic gradient >50%.

POSITIONING THE BALLOON. After obtaining baseline hemodynamics the aortic valve is crossed and a stiff (Amplatz 300-cm) guidewire with a large pigtail-type curve is positioned in the left ventricle. The patient is anticoagulated with 5000 units of heparin. The skin puncture site is enlarged.

The balloon catheter (prepared by flushing diluted contrast solution, then applying negative pressure) is advanced into the left ventricle over the wire and positioned across the aortic valve. Longer balloons (4 to 5 cm) give better stability during inflation.

VALVE DILATION. The balloon catheter is inflated and deflated by hand with continuous monitoring of arterial pressure and cardiac rhythm. The patient should be observed carefully for syncope and seizures during brief hypotension. Several inflations are performed until disappearance of the balloon "waist." Before each inflation the arterial pressure and pulmonary artery oxygen saturation (monitored with an oximetric pulmonary catheter) should return to baseline.

FINAL RESULT. Following documentation of satisfactory reduction in gradient ($\leq$30 mm Hg) and increase in valve area ($\geq$25% of baseline), the procedure is terminated (Fig. 9-14). The balloon catheter and sheaths are removed after reversal of heparin with protamine sulfate.

AFTER THE PROCEDURE. After sufficient dilatations, the balloon catheter is exchanged for a LV pigtail catheter and hemodynamic measurements repeated. A satisfactory result usually yields a mean gradient of <30 mm Hg and >25% increase in valve area. Ascending aortography is indicated to determine the presence of postdilatation aortic regurgitation. Following reversal of anticoagulation with protamine sulfate,

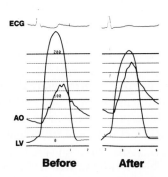

Fig. 9-14. Simultaneous aortic (*AO*) and left ventricular (*LV*) pressures before and after aortic valvuloplasty in an 86-year-old woman, showing marked reduction in aortic valve gradient and increase in aortic valve area from 0.4 to 0.9 cm^2.

the balloon catheter and sheaths are removed and the site managed with manual compression. The patient should be carefully monitored for bleeding, hematoma, pseudoaneurysm and AV fistula. Patients can be ambulated and discharged the day after the procedure if no complications arise. REMEMBER: Significant aortic stenosis, albeit of a lesser severity, is still present after PBAV.

Complications. The most frequent complications of PBAV are vascular, usually involving the percutaneous entry site. Significant vascular trauma or bleeding problems can occur in approximately 5% to 20% of cases. Embolic phenomena are infrequent (1 to 2%). Procedural and total in-hospital mortality is low at 4% to 7%. LV perforation, cardiac tamponade, and precipitation of severe aortic regurgitation are rare (<2%) but serious complications.

Follow-up. Although the average increase in valve area after PBAV is only approximately 0.5 cm^2, most patients report reduction in dyspnea and angina. In approximately 50% of patients with poor LV function the ejection fraction improves during follow-up. The reduction in syncope is more difficult to document. The 1-year mortality is up to 25%, especially in the very elderly and in those patients with New York Heart Association class IV symptoms. Although this mortality figure seems more favorable than the natural history of untreated symptomatic calcific aortic stenosis (1-year mortality of 40% to 50%), a survival benefit with PBAV has yet to be proven. The recurrence of symptoms and/or renarrowing of the valve is a frequent occurrence in the first 6 to 12 months (up to 50% of patients) after PBAV. The follow-up data emphasize the palliative nature of the procedure.

Percutaneous balloon mitral valvuloplasty (PBMV). PBMV for the treatment of mitral stenosis has been studied extensively over the past ten years, and when successful has been found to yield both marked immediate hemodynamic improvement and sustained clinical benefit. Prospective comparisons of PBMV with surgical commissurotomy in selected patients have shown similar hemodynamic and clinical results in follow-up. Not all patients, however, are optimal candidates for PBMV, and echocardiography remains essential to evaluate mitral valve structure which may predict a successful outcome.

Indications

SYMPTOMATIC MITRAL STENOSIS. (Isolated or combined with mixed valvular disease with less than moderate mitral regurgitation). Patients with suitable valvular characteristics who are surgical (or nonsurgical) candidates can be offered balloon valvuloplasty because of the comparable risk and the relative ease of the procedure.

Immobile, severely thickened and fused valve leaflets may not respond well to balloon valvuloplasty. Severe calcification of the leaflets is another negative predictor for success. However, symptomatic patients with these unfavorable characteristics who are not candidates for surgery may still benefit from the procedure. PBMV is contraindicated in the presence of atrial thrombus, best detected with high sensitivity by using transesophageal echocardiography.

Procedure. Although retrograde mitral valvuloplasty methods have been described, two techniques utilizing antegrade transseptal access to the mitral valve have been developed and more widely applied. The first involves use of a single, specially designed balloon catheter (Inoue balloon), while the second employs a double-balloon technique. The hemodynamic results are usually comparable, although in some studies the double-balloon procedure shows a tendency to greater valve area increase. Clinical success is high with either technique and complication rates are low and similar. Due to its single-balloon design and relative ease in crossing of the mitral valve, use of the Inoue balloon in general requires less fluoroscopic and procedural time. It is not yet widely available in the United States.

LEFT ATRIAL ACCESS. Following baseline hemodynamic measurements, transseptal catheterization is performed (see Chapter 7, p. 414). Care should be exercised not to perform the puncture too high on the septum. This location will present great difficulty in crossing the mitral valve and positioning the balloons. Sometimes it may be necessary to float a balloon catheter through the mitral valve to enter the left ventricle.

A long Mullins sheath is then advanced into the left ventricle and two stiff (Amplatz) guidewires with pigtail-type curves (made by the operator) are advanced into the left ventricular apex.

DILATING THE INTERATRIAL SEPTUM. Following placement of the guidewires the atrial septum is dilated with a 6- to 8-mm balloon to allow easy passage of the larger dilatation catheters. These small atrial septal defects are not generally clinically important.

INOUE SINGLE BALLOON TECHNIQUE. The Inoue balloon catheter has a unique design allowing inflation of the tip of the balloon to facilitate crossing the mitral valve and a 4-mm-diameter size range allowing stepwise incremental valve dilatation. Simplified selection of balloon size is based on patient height. Once LA access is obtained, the interatrial septum is dilated and the Inoue balloon tracked over the guidewire into the left atrium. The tip of the balloon is then inflated, and with steering by the stylet the balloon is floated across the mitral valve. Care should be taken that the balloon catheter is free within the ventricular cavity and not entangled in chordae tendineae. The partially inflated balloon is then withdrawn to engage the mitral valve leaflets and fully inflated to achieve commissural splitting. The transmitral pressure gradient and an echocardiographic assessment of commissural separation and valvular regurgitation have been recommended after each dilating step to monitor the need for continued larger dilatation in an effort to safely obtain the maximum mitral orifice possible without severe mitral regurgitation.

DOUBLE BALLOON TECHNIQUE. Selection of conventional double-balloon size has often been based on body size or surface area, with a balloon dilating area to BSA ratio of $3.1:4.0$ cm^2/m^2, or on estimates of mitral annular size by echocardiography. In an average adult, two 20-mm balloons are usually required, although thin or small individuals may need one or both to be 18-mm balloons. Following transseptal puncture, a long Mullins sheath or an Arrow double-lumen balloon catheter is used to enter the left ventricle and two stiff (Amplatz) guidewires with pigtail-type distal curves are advanced into the LV apex. If desired, by use of a double lumen balloon-tipped catheter, the guidewires may be advanced into the descending aorta. Two balloon catheters are then advanced over the wires and positioned across the mitral valve side by side. Care must be taken that the balloons are not across the interatrial septum or too far forward into the left ventricle. With fluoroscopic guidance and close monitoring of arterial pressure and cardiac rhythm, the balloons are then rapidly simultaneously inflated and deflated. Inflations are repeated until the valve indentation or "waist" in the balloons disappears (Fig. 9-15). For monitoring during the procedure, PCW and LV pressure can be continuously observed. A 5 French pigtail can be placed via a 6 French femoral arterial sheath (See Figs. 9-16 to 9-19).

FINAL RESULT. In addition to final LA − LV pressure measurements, a right-sided oxygen saturation run and/or dye dilution are performed to detect left-to-right shunting at the atrial septal level. It is important to take any left-to-right

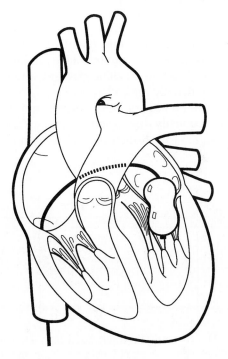

Fig. 9-15. Diagram of Inoue balloon catheter in position across the mitral valve during mitral valvuloplasty.

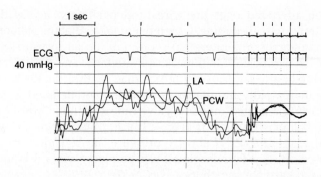

Fig. 9-16. When monitoring percutaneous balloon mitral valvuloplasty a pulmonary capillary wedge (*PCW*) pressure is often used. Differences between pulmonary capillary wedge and left atrial (*LA*) may introduce error into final gradient measurements. (From Kern MJ: *Hemodynamic rounds: Interpretation of cardiac pathophysiology from pressure waveform analysis,* New York, 1993, Wiley-Liss.)

shunt into consideration while calculating the final valve area. The average decrease in mitral valve gradient is approximately 50% to 75% of the baseline gradient, and the increase in valve area is usually around 100%.

Complications. Procedural and hospital mortality is rare (0% to 2%) and usually due to ventricular perforation. Complications of transseptal puncture, such as hemopericardium

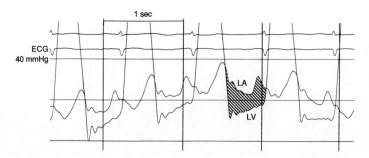

Fig. 9-17. Directly measured left atrial (*LA*)-left ventricular (*LV*) gradient before a percutaneous balloon mitral valvuloplasty shows gradient of 18 mm Hg. (From Kern MJ: *Hemodynamic rounds: Interpretation of cardiac pathophysiology from pressure waveform analysis,* New York, 1993, Wiley-Liss.)

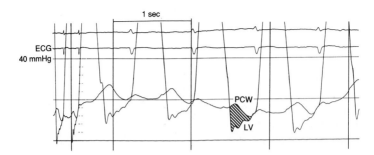

Fig. 9-18. After a percutaneous balloon mitral valvuloplasty pulmonary capillary wedge (*PCW*)-left ventricular (*LV*) gradient remains >8 to 10 mm Hg. The pulmonary capillary wedge waveform is damped. (From Kern MJ: *Hemodynamic rounds: Interpretation of cardiac pathophysiology from pressure waveform analysis,* New York, 1993, Wiley-Liss.)

or tamponade, are also rare (<2%), and systemic emboli may occur in 1% to 2%. Mitral regurgitation increases in between 20% and 50% of patients but is significantly increased (more than angiographic grades) in only 8% to 10%. Significant mitral regurgitation may appear late following PBMV. Mitral regurgitation severe enough to require valve replacement occurs in 0.9% to 3% of patients following PBMV and is usually due to noncommissural tearing of the mitral leaflets and/or chordal rupture. An atrial septal defect with left-to-

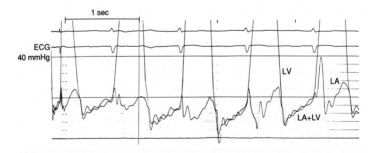

Fig. 9-19. In the same patient as Figure 9-18, left atrial (*LA*)-left ventricular (*LV*) pressure after a percutaneous balloon mitral valvuloplasty now has no gradient, a highly successful result. (From Kern MJ: *Hemodynamic rounds: Interpretation of cardiac pathophysiology from pressure waveform analysis,* New York, 1993, Wiley-Liss.)

right shunting is detectable in 8% to 87% (depending on the sensitivity of the method used for detection), the majority of which are less than 1.4 to 1, clinically unimportant, and decrease or disappear in follow-up.

Follow-up. In general, the symptomatic status of most patients starts improving immediately and improves further during follow-up. Short-term symptomatic improvement is present in the vast majority. Long-term follow-up ($\geq$5 years) in a large series of PBMV patients has recently been published. The long-term outcome remains very good in selected patients, especially those with less evidence of valve deformity (mobility, thickening, calcification, subvavlular disease) reflected in low preprocedural echocardiographic scores (see above) and with low LV end-diastolic pressure. In such patients event-free 5-year survival is >80%. Patients with more deformed valves and higher echocardiographic scores have a higher rate of restenosis. However, the incidence of restenosis and long-term outcome following PMBV appears comparable to closed mitral commissurotomy.

Pulmonary Valvuloplasty

Pulmonary stenosis can now be easily treated by percutaneous balloon valvuloplasty. The technique is similar to mitral valvuloplasty. Femoral venous access is obtained. Guidewire placement across the pulmonic valve is followed by balloon dilation. Success is determined by the reduction of pulmonary gradient and reduced RV pressure (Fig. 9-20).

Combined interventional procedures. In selected patients, combined interventional methods have been successfully utilized in the treatment of coexistant coronary and valvular disease or multivalvular disease. The sequence of the procedures should be determined so as to increase the patient's safety. In combined aortic stenosis and coronary artery disease it may be reasonable to perform PTCA several days after PBAV has been successfully performed. On the other hand, in a patient with very critical coronary stenosis, PTCA may be done first to avoid significant myocardial ischemia in case of profound hypotension, which may occur during PBAV. In combined aortic stenosis and mitral stenosis the aortic stenosis is relieved first to avoid the possibility of increasing diastolic loading with worsened aortic gradient as a result of increased SV.

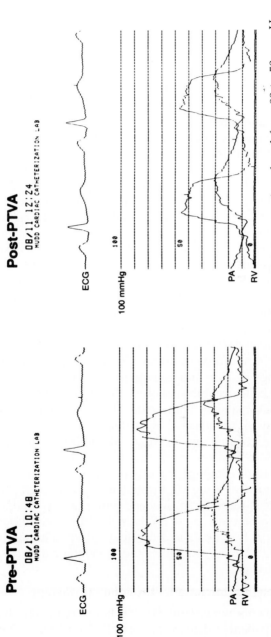

Fig. 9-20. In a patient with pulmonic stenosis, right ventricular (*RV*) pressure is reduced from 80 to 50 mm Hg after a single-balloon technique of pulmonic valvuloplasty. *PA*, Pulmonary artery pressure.

Thrombolytic Therapy

Thrombolytic therapy involves pharmacologic lysis of thrombus formed at the site of an intravascular obstruction. In most hospitals, IV thrombolytic therapy for patients with acute MI presenting within 6 to 12 hours of the onset of symptoms has become the standard of care in patients without contraindications to thrombolytic therapy. Intracoronary administration of thrombolytic agents for acute MI also has been performed in the past. Intracoronary thrombolytic therapy offers the advantage of angiographic confirmation of an occlusion (Figs. 9-21 and 9-22), an approximately 10% to 20% higher reopening rate, lower dose of thrombolytic agent required, and the ability to monitor the result of thrombolysis angiographically. These advantages, although attractive, are outweighed by the substantial delay in time required to initiate intracoronary versus IV therapy (generally 60 to 90 minutes), the higher rate of significant bleeding secondary to vascular access in the intracoronary group, and the fact that most patients with acute MI initially present in hospitals without cardiac catheterization facilities. For these reasons, IV thrombolytic therapy for acute MI has almost completely replaced intracoronary administration. In hospitals with cardiac catheterization and angioplasty facilities, direct PTCA (without concurrent thrombolytic therapy) can be offered to appropriate patients with acute MI. In addition, patients with acute MI complicated by cardiogenic shock also should be referred for emergency cardiac catheterization, and possible PTCA, regardless of whether thrombolytic therapy was administered. Although the urgency to achieve reperfusion is not as great as acute MI, thrombi may also form in peripheral vessels, resulting in ischemic complications. Peripheral arterial thrombosis generally is treated first with selective intraarterial thrombolytic drugs (e.g., streptokinase, urokinase 250,000 to 500,000 units) and, if symptomatic, surgical embolectomy.

Indications for intraarterial thrombolytic therapy

1. In patients with acute MI (<6 hours optimally, but in some patients as late as 24 hours), IV thrombolytic therapy is more timely but may be less effective.
2. In certain patients with subacute thrombosis (<30 days)

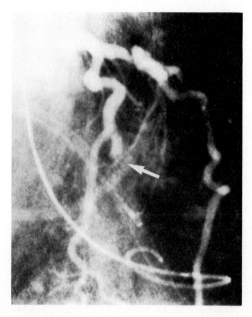

Fig. 9-21. Angiogram of acute occlusion of the circumflex coronary artery consistent with acute myocardial infarction (*arrow*).

intraarterial (or intragraft) selective thrombolytic therapy may be indicated.
3. Intraarterial thrombosis occurring as a complication of coronary or peripheral angioplasty usually responds to intraarterial thrombolysis

Contraindications

1. Active internal bleeding
2. Recent surgery or major trauma (within 2 months)
3. Recent stroke (<6 months)
4. CNS malignancy
5. Bleeding diathesis (check PT, PTT, platelets, hematocrit)
6. Severe uncontrolled hypertension (diastolic blood pressure > 120 mm Hg, systolic blood pressure > 200 mm Hg)
7. Pregnancy

Thrombolytic agents.   At this time there are three thrombolytic agents available that can be used for selective intraart-

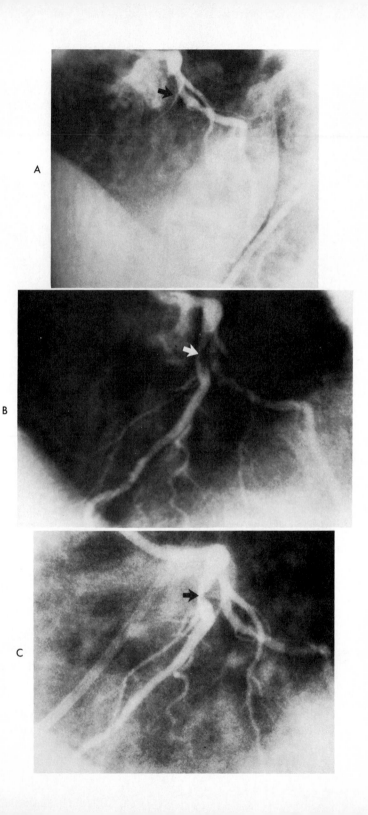

erial thrombolysis: streptokinase, urokinase, and tissue plasminogen activator (t-PA).

Streptokinase is a nonenzymatic protein derived from beta-hemolytic streptococci that indirectly converts plasminogen to the active form plasmin. Streptokinase is a non-fibrin specific agent in that it degrades not only fibrin, but also fibrinogen and other systemic coagulation factors. This results in a systemic fibrinolytic state. In addition, because of the fact that streptokinase is a bacterial protein, patients may develop neutralizing antibodies after the initial administration.

Urokinase is also a direct activator of plasminogen (i.e., does not require binding to fibrin for activation). Thus it also may cause significant systemic fibrinogenolysis; however, unlike streptokinase, urokinase is not antigenic. This agent is commonly used for intracoronary or intragraft infusions (250,000 to 500,000 units over 15 to 30 minutes).

t-PA is produced by recombinant DNA technology. Because t-PA requires binding to fibrin to activate plasminogen, it was initially hoped that it would lead to less bleeding. However, clinical studies have not demonstrated an advantage in terms of bleeding side effects with t-PA use relative to streptokinase. t-PA is not antigenic. IV t-PA does appear to be more efficacious in opening occluded coronary arteries than IV streptokinase for acute MI. However, whether or not this translates into a decrease in mortality remains unproven.

For selective intraarterial thrombolysis there is a general consensus that urokinase is more effective than streptokinase and t-PA. There is less data available for selective intraarterial thrombolysis with t-PA. In our laboratory urokinase is used for selective intraarterial thrombolysis.

Procedure

1. Perform arteriogram to document thrombus and branch vessel anatomy and patency.

Fig. 9-22. **A,** Acute occlusion of the left anterior descending artery before thrombolysis (*arrow*). **B,** Left anterior descending artery now patent after coronary lysis with intracoronary thrombus in place (*arrow*). **C,** After intracoronary administration of thrombolytic agent the shaggy nature of the clot has resolved (*arrow*).

2. Position catheter selectively in vessel to receive thrombolytic agent.
3. For saphenous vein bypass grafts and peripheral vascular vessels, a 2.0 to 4.0 French infusion catheter (with side holes or slits) can be positioned adjacent to the thrombus through which the thrombolytic therapy is infused.
4. Heparin therapy should be administered concurrently with thrombolytic therapy (5000- to 10,000-unit bolus and 1000 units/hr infusion). The PTT should be monitored (aim for PTT 2 to $2\frac{1}{2}$ times control).
5. Thrombolytic administration via catheter:
   a. *Urokinase:* 10,000 to 25,000-unit bolus, infuse at 1000 to 4000 units/min; total dose, 500,00 units.
   b. *Streptokinase:* 25,000 to 50,000-unit bolus, infuse at 500 to 3000 units/minute; total dose, 500,000 to 1,500,000 units.
   c. *t-PA:* 5- to 10-mg bolus, infuse at 0.05 to 0.10 mg/kg/hr; total dose, 30 to 50 mg.
6. The duration of thrombolytic infusion is variable and dependent on a particular patient's presentation. Generally, acute thrombi, such as those that occur as a complication of angioplasty, will require a shorter infusion duration (<1 hour) than subacute thrombi, which often require prolonged infusions (8 to 12 hours). In peripheral arteries and bypass grafts, the catheter may be left in a stable position and the patient transferred to the intensive care unit for several hours while the infusion is continued. Assessment of results requires repeat angiography.
7. After thrombolytic infusion is complete, consider angioplasty or surgery as appropriate if significant ischemia or a stenosis persists.

Complications

1. *Emboli.* A downstream occlusion results from a dislodged thrombus. This complication usually can be managed by continued thrombolysis or laceration by guidewire and/or balloon inflation.
2. *Bleeding.* Serious or life-threatening hemorrhage mandates termination of thrombolytic and heparin infusions. Protamine can be given to reverse heparin. Blood products, including fresh-frozen plasma also may be necessary.

NEW INTERVENTIONAL TECHNIQUES
(See the box on p. 527)

Improved balloon catheter technology has greatly facilitated the application of PTCA to lesions located in tortuous and/or distal vessels. However, the efficacy of PTCA continues to be limited by restenosis, abrupt closure, and poor success in chronic total occlusions. In order to overcome these limitations, investigators worldwide are studying the utility of various new angioplasty technologies. Although several of these devices appear promising, particularly for treatment of acute complications, it appears that balloon angioplasty will remain with us for a number of years.

Cardiac Interventional and Imaging Technologies under Evaluation
in 1994

INTERVENTIONAL TECHNOLOGIES

Laser

Laser balloon angioplasty
Direct laser ablation (excimer most promising)
Fluorescence-guided laser angioplasty
Directional laser atherectomy
Laser-assisted thrombolysis

Electrical/radiofrequency

Spark erosion
Radiofrequency and microwave-heated balloon angioplasty

Atherectomy

Directional (Simpson AtheroCath)
Rotational (Rotoblator, catheter)
Extraction (transluminal extraction catheter)

Stents

Metallic (self-expanding mesh, balloon expandable)
Biodegradable
Polymeric endoluminal paving and sealing

High-energy ultrasound

IMAGING TECHNOLOGIES (See Tables 9-2 and 9-3)

Angioscopy
Intravascular ultrasound (two-dimensional and Doppler)
Atherosclerotic plaque fluorescence

TABLE 9-2.   Imaging technologies as adjuncts to endovascular intervention

Advantages	Disadvantages
Angioscopy	
1. Best method to identify thrombus	1. Requires blood displacement by constant flushing
2. Excellent detail of surface characteristics	2. Limited image acquisition time (≤60 seconds)
3. Forward viewing	3. Potential for vascular damage
4. Potential combination with angioplasty	4. Does not provide quantitative data
Doppler floWire	
1. On-line assessment of coronary flow before, during, and after intervention	1. Nonimaging modality
2. Easily combined with angioplasty device	2. Complexity in interpretation
3. Assesses significance of stenoses	
4. Assesses coronary flow reserve	
5. Small-diameter guidewire	
Intravascular ultrasound imaging	
1. Quantifies wall thickness	1. Need miniaturization
2. Qualitative tissue characterization	2. Not forward viewing
3. Provides a 360° tomographic view	3. Potential for vascular damage
4. Potential combination with angioplasty	

Modified with permission from Siegel RJ, Forrester, JS: *ACC Curr J Rev*, p. 77, March/April 1993.

The limitations of angiography for assessment of true atherosclerotic narrowing, intraluminal thrombus, and intimal tears is well known. With the advent of PTCA and development of new angioplasty technologies, it has become apparent that improved catheter-based systems for evaluation of vessel morphology and physiology are needed. There are several technologies being evaluated for the assessment of coronary arterial disease (see the box on p. 527). The most promising new techniques involve intracoronary two-dimensional ultrasound for imaging and Doppler ultrasound measurement of coronary flow velocity. The latter has been described previously (Chapter 6, pp. 385–399, and Table 9-3).

TABLE 9-3. Specifications of current intravascular diagnostic devices

Type of sytem (company)	Catheter size	Frequency (MHz)
Angioscopy		
Coronary angioscope (Baxter)	4.5 French	Resolution 50 µm at 2 mm
Doppler		
FloWire (Cardiometrics)	0.018-inch guidewire	12
Ultrasound		
Mechanical (Cardiovascular Imaging Systems)	Peripheral 5 French	20
	Coronary 4.3 French	30
	10 French intracardiac	10 to 15
	2.9 French coronary prototype	30
	3.9 French sheath*	20
Phased array (Endosonics)	3.5 French	20
Mechanical (Hewlett-Packard, Boston Scientific)	6.2 French intracardiac or peripheral	12.5 or 20
	4.8 French	20 or 30
	Coronary 3.5 French	20 or 30

Reproduced with permission from Siegel RJ, Forrester JS: Advantages and limitations of intravascular imaging devices in clinical applications, *ACC Curr J Rev*, p. 80, March/April 1993.

Coronary Atherectomy

Because atherosclerotic plaque remains in the artery after balloon dilatation, physical removal of the plaque from inside the coronary artery is thought to improve the results of angioplasty. Three devices developed for this purpose are approved for coronary intervention: the directional atherectomy catheter, high-speed rotablator, and transluminal extraction catheter (TEC).

Directional Coronary Atherectomy (DCA)

DCA is performed using a specially designed catheter with a metal cutting chamber that contains a cylindrical cutter. The cutting chamber is pushed against the lesion by a posteriorly located supporting balloon. The cutter is rotated by a hand-held motor at 2000 rpm and is advanced within the cutting chamber to shave the plaque and deposit it to the nose cone of the catheter (Fig. 9-23).

The DCA works via three interactive mechanisms: Dotter (pushing) effect created by the bulk of the catheter (5 to 7 French), balloon dilatation effect caused by inflation of supporting balloon, and actual cutting and removal of the plaque. The latter is usually the dominant mechanism.

Equipment for DCA. Because of the large size of the DCA catheter and rigid cutter housing, large lumen guide catheters with specially designed curves are needed. The right coronary catheters are 9.5 French and the left coronary catheters are 10 or 11 French. An appropriately sized long sheath and a large-bore rotating hemostatic adapter are required.

Selection of the device. Selection of device size depends on the diameter of the vessel lumen: 5 French for 2.5- to 2.9-mm diameter vessels, 6 French for 3.0- to 3.4-mm, 7 French for 3.5- to 3.9-mm, and 7 French "graft" for 4-mm or larger vessels.

Preparation of the device. The supporting balloon is a direct negative pressure preparation similar to most standard PTCA balloon catheters. Then heparinized saline is injected into the flush port. Subsequently, the guidewire is loaded in either forward (cutter forward) or backward (cutter in the middle). Finally, the motor drive unit is attached. It is

Lesion Characteristics	PTCA	DCA	ELCA	Rotoblator	TEC	Stenting
Type A	■	■				
Complex, eccentric	■	■				■
Ostial		■	■	■		
Diffuse			■	■		
Total Occlusion	■		■			
Calcified				■		
Diff. vein graft			■		■	
Dis. vein graft, focal		■				■
Bifurcation	■					
Thrombus	■	■			■	
Acute closure						■
Excess. recoil		■				■

Fig. 9-23. Scheme for niche application of coronary interventional procedures. *PTCA,* Percutaneous transluminal coronary angioplasty; *DCA,* directional coronary atherectomy; *ECLA,* excimer laser coronary angioplasty; *TEC,* transluminal extraction catheter. Dark box denotes best niche uses.

important to keep the wire at the nose cone level and advance several centimeters when the device is in the guide catheter.

Placement of the guide catheter.   The guide catheter is straightened with a 7 or 8 French long introducer catheter to avoid large-vessel trauma. This system is advanced into the aortic root with the guidewire several centimeters in front of the introducer catheter tip, then the guidewire and inner introducer are removed. The catheter is connected to a manifold similar to the balloon angioplasty setup. Because of the size and stiffness of the guide catheter, extreme care should be taken in manipulation, avoiding deep engagement of the coronary vessel.

Atherectomy (cutting the plaque).   The coronary narrowing is crossed in the usual manner with coronary guidewire (0.014-inch diameter). The DCA device is advanced over the guidewire slowly by keeping constant forward tension and rotating slightly. Do not "jackhammer" the device. The guide catheter may be backing up in the aorta at this time. Do not try to bring the guide catheter deeply in the vessel. Slight removal of the coronary guidewire while advancing the DCA device is helpful. Rarely, it may be necessary to predilate a tight lesion to allow easy passage of the device. While advancing over the artery curves, keep the cutting chamber opening toward the outer curvature and keep the cutter in forward locked position at all times.

Once the device is in place, the balloon is inflated at 10 psi (not atm) pressure and the cutter retracted by using the thumb lever on the motor. The balloon pressure is increased now to 20 to 30 psi. The motor is turned on. The cutter is advanced in a slow and steady manner until it is at the end of the cutting chamber and locked in and the motor is then stopped. The balloon is deflated, the catheter is rotated about a quarter turn, and the sequence is repeated. During cutting, it is important to keep the wire a few centimeters distal to the catheter tip, avoiding entrapment in a small vessel.

Several cuts in different directions can be made during a single passage of the device. An assistant should be watching the pressure and ECG for the signs of ischemia. If ischemia is severe, the device should be removed promptly to allow distal perfusion. If the cutter stops before the end of the cutting chamber or if the guidewire becomes difficult to move in the catheter, then the nose cone might be packed full of shaved material. At this time, the device is removed to empty the contents of the atherectomy catheter cone. A guidewire may be left across the lesion to allow easy introduction of the device if further cuts are necessary. When there is residual narrowing (more than 20%), the same device can be reintroduced to make cuts by applying higher balloon pressures, or a larger-size device can be introduced. However, attempts by overinflating the balloon or oversizing the device increase the risk of perforation.

Anticoagulation and sheath removal.   During the procedure, the patient should be well heparinized with an activated clotting time (ACT) of 300–350 seconds. Although some users advocate early sheath removal (a few hours after the procedure), the occurrence of some late subacute occlusions has convinced many practitioners to keep the sheath in place with systemic heparinization overnight.

Because of the large size of the sheaths, distal leg pulses should be checked frequently. In case of leg ischemia, the sheath should be removed. Longer arterial puncture site compression and longer bed rest are necessary after atherectomy sheath removal. The large size of the sheaths are a significant source of morbidity and mortality, especially in elderly patients.

Routine follow-up is similar to that for regular balloon angioplasty. Restenosis occurs at a similar rate and timing after both angioplasty and DCA procedures. A recent randomized study suggested a small restenosis benefit with DCA as compared to balloon angioplasty in patients with proximal LAD artery lesions. Restenosis after DCA is less in patients with <20% residual narrowing or in those with a normal vessel lumen diameter of 3 mm or larger.

Since some studies indicated increased complications with DCA, the risk/benefit ratio should be carefully evaluated in each patient. Patients with large vessels (>3.0 mm) and ostial or eccentric lesions, which decrease the success with balloon dilatation, seem suitable candidates for DCA. Calcified, angulated, long (<20 mm) narrowings, spiral dissections, and friable graft lesions are not suitable for DCA. Significant iliofemoral occlusive disease precludes insertion of large catheters and, therefore, is a relative contraindication for coronary DCA. It should be emphasized that operator experience is an important factor in patient selection.

Rotational Atherectomy (Rotablator)

The Rotablator is made of a steel burr (1.25 to 2.5 mm in diameter) that is embedded with microscopic diamond particles in the front half and is rotated with a torque wire at up to 200,000 rpm by an external air turbine. The device is inserted through 9 to 10 French guide catheters over a special 0.009-inch guidewire. A continuous pressurized heparin saline infusion is given through the device to aid lubrication and heat dissipation (Fig. 9-24). After the burr is placed just proximal to the lesion, the system is activated and the burr is advanced through the lesion in a slow and steady manner. The abrasive surface of the burr will selectively ablate (pulverize) the hard plaque while sparing the softer normal wall. Several burr passes are performed before removal of the burr

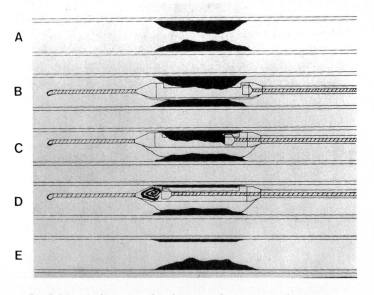

Fig. 9-24. A diagram of a directional coronary atherectomy catheter. The sequence *A* to *E* shows mechanism of cutting a plaque. *A,* Plaque; *B,* the cutting window of the nose cone is positioned; *C,* the support balloon is inflated and cutter is advanced; *D,* cutting is complete with material stored in nose cone; *E,* final result.

and decision for larger-size burr or complementary balloon inflation is made. Most cases require additional angioplasty balloon inflations to decrease the residual stenosis. The maximum burr diameter should be no larger than 70% to 80% of the normal arterial luminal diameter.

The Rotablator is suitable for rigid calcified and long lesions in which the balloon angioplasty success is expected to be low. The complication and restenosis rates are similar to balloon angioplasty, however, there is no randomized comparisons published. A specific complication of Rotablator is temporary no-reflow phenomenon with creatine kinase enzyme rise in some patients. This problem necessitates insertion of a prophylactic pacemaker wire, especially for right coronary lesions.

TEC Atherectomy

TEC is a hollow tube with a conical cutter at the tip. Rotation (750 rpm) and aspiration are applied to the device by means of a complex hand-held drive unit while advancing through the lesion over the special ball-tipped 0.014-inch guidewire. The large size of the device (from 5.5 to 7.5 French) necessitates specially designed 10 French guide catheters. Although the lesion selection is not well defined for TEC, long saphenous vein bypass graft lesions and lesions with thrombus appear to be suitable for treatment with this device. Avoiding complications such as dissection and perforation requires careful patient selection and device handling. The maximum cutter size should be 0.5 mm less than the arterial lumen diameter (Fig. 9-25).

STENTS

Scaffolding the artery wall from inside the lumen to achieve wide and stable patency is an old concept. Several types of stents (coil, mesh, or cage type and metallic or polymer) have been invented and are used in experimental and clinical procedures.

Early application of a stent after the occurrence of occlusion and/or dissection decreases the need for emergency bypass surgery and the risk for MI. Most stents currently available for coronary artery disease are balloon expandable. Some of them require a protective sheath to avoid dis-

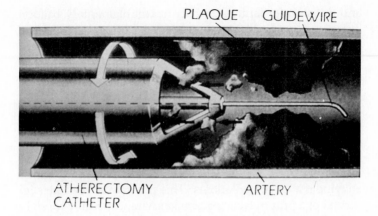

Fig. 9-25. A diagram of a transluminal extraction catheter. Triangular cutting windows rotate while cut material is drawn into catheter by suction. This device is most commonly used for old, thrombosed saphenous vein grafts.

lodgement of the stent from the balloon. Because of their large profile, stent-balloon combinations require larger (large lumen 8 or 9 French) catheters and accordingly larger adapters and sheaths. To facilitate passage of the balloon through tortuous proximal vessels, stiffer angioplasty guidewires are used.

The Cook Flexstent is approved for the treatment of acute or threatened closure complicating balloon angioplasty (Fig. 9-26).

Anticoagulation

The most important part of the stent implantation is the management of anticoagulation. Inadequate or overzealous use of anticoagulants is responsible for most morbidity and mortality associated with stent implantation. The patients should be premedicated with aspirin, dipyridamole, and IV dextran before stent implantation.

Implantation

The implantation is similar to the balloon angioplasty technique. It is important to place the stent to cover the whole length of the dissection or lesion without leaving any inflow and outflow obstructions behind. An appropriately sized balloon will ensure complete expansion of the stent struc-

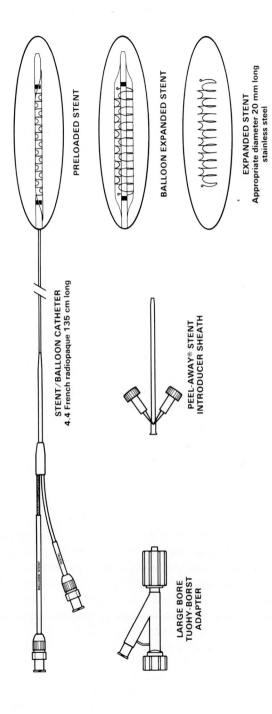

PRELOADED STENT

BALLOON EXPANDED STENT

EXPANDED STENT
Appropriate diameter 20 mm long
stainless steel

STENT/BALLOON CATHETER
4.4 French radiopaque 135 cm long

PEEL-AWAY® STENT
INTRODUCER SHEATH

LARGE BORE
TUOHY-BORST
ADAPTER

Fig. 9-26. The Cook flexstent. (Courtesy of Cook, Inc.)

ture against the wall without leaving empty spaces which may be a source for thrombus formation. Artery side branches usually will not be affected by a stent. In case of multiple stent implantations, the most distal one is placed first to avoid dislocation of the more proximal stent.

If there is inflow or outflow obstruction or residual narrowing, a freshly prepared balloon catheter could be advanced into and through the stented area for further dilatations. If there is residual thrombus, urokinase is infused into the coronary artery.

Postprocedural Care

Sheath removal and resumption of anticoagulation are very important aspects of the poststent care. Sheaths are usually removed on the same day, after allowing the ACT to decrease to 150 seconds. Prolonged manual and assisted femoral artery compression (i.e., 45 to 60 minutes) as well as bed rest (strict bed rest for 24 hours after sheath removal with minimal activity allowed for the next 24 hours) are necessary. Heparin infusion is resumed after puncture site hemostasis is obtained. The PTT is kept between 60 and 80 seconds for several days until an international normalized ratio (INR) of 3 to 4 units is achieved by oral daily doses of coumadin. Heparin should be continued for another 24 hours after the PT is in the desired range for two successive measurements 24 hours apart. Despite all efforts, some patients may develop late bleeding, hematoma, retroperitoneal bleeding, and false aneurysms of the femoral artery.

Subacute thrombotic occlusion may occur in a small but significant proportion of the patients, usually about the third to fifth day of the implantation but may also happen within the week following discharge. Risk factors for the subacute occlusion include small vessels (<3 mm), presence of dissection after stenting, presence of filling defects, and stent placement in infarct-related vessels. Emergency (for treatment of acute closure) rather than elective (primary) implantation itself is a risk factor for subacute occlusion. Patients with these risk factors may require prolonged simultaneous IV and oral anticoagulation. Subacute occlusion is treated with repeat balloon dilatations and urokinase infusion.

Patients are discharged on aspirin, dipyridamole, and cou-

madin. PT is checked every week. Generally, it is not necessary to continue coumadin after 2 months, in which time
complete endothelization will take place.

Restenosis rates after stent implantation are similar to
balloon angioplasty. However, the peak restenosis rate may
be delayed. Restenosis can be managed by repeat angioplasty. Restenosis and reocclusion are affected by the artery
diameter and the degree of residual narrowing. Achieving
a residual narrowing <20% in a 3-mm or larger artery decreases the risk of restenosis after elective implantation.

SUGGESTED READINGS

Avedissian MG, Killeavy ES, Garcia JM, Dear WE: Percutaneous
    transluminal coronary angioplasty: a review of current balloon
    dilatation systems, *Cathet Cardiovasc Diagn* 18:263–275, 1989.

Bonzel T, Wollschläger H, Meinertz T, et al.: The steerable monorail
    catheter system—a new device for PTCA (abastract), *Circulation*
    74:II-459, 1986.

Cowley MJ, Dorros G, Kelsey SF, van Raden M, Detre KM: Acute
    coronary events associated with percutaneous transluminal coro-
    nary angioplasty, *Am J Cardiol* 53:56C–64C, 1984.

Detre K, Hulubkov R, Kelsey S, Cowley M, Kent K, Williams D,
    Myler R, Faxon D, Holmes D Jr, Bourassa M, Block P, Gosselin
    A, Bentivoglio L, Leatherman L, Dorros G, King S III, Galichia J,
    Al-Bassam M, Leon M, Robertson T, Passamani E. Percutaneous
    transluminal coronary angioplasty in 1985–1986 and 1977–1981.
    The National Heart, Lung, and Blood Institute Registry, *N Engl
    J Med* 318:265–270, 1988.

George BS, Voorhees WD, Roubin GS, et al.: Multicenter investiga-
    tion of coronary stenting to treat acute or threatened closure after
    percutaneous transluminal coronary angioplasty: clinical and an-
    giographic outcome, *J Am Coll Cardiol* 22:135–143, 1993.

Gruntzig A, Senning A, Siegenthaler WE: Nonoperative dilatation
    of coronary artery stenosis: percutaneous transluminal coronary
    angioplasty, *N Engl J Med* 301:61–68, 1979.

Kern MJ, Talley JD, Deligonul U, Serota H, Aguirre F, Gudipati C,
    Ring M, Joseph A, Yussman ZA, Kulick D, Salinger M: Prelimi-
    nary experience with 5 and 6 French diagnostic catheters as guid-
    ing catheters for coronary angioplasty, *Cathet Cardiovasc Diagn*
    22:60–63, 1991.

Myler RK, Mooney MR, Stertzer SH, Clark DA, Hidalgo BO, Fish-
    man J: The balloon on a wire device. A new ultra-low-profile
    coronary angioplasty system/concept, *Cathet Cardiovasc Diagn*
    14:135–140, 1988.

Simpson JB, Baim DS, Robert EW, Harrison DC: A new catheter system for coronary angioplasty, *Am J Cardiol* 49:1216–1222, 1982.

Stertzer SH, Rosenblum J, Shaw RE, et al.: Coronary rotational ablation: initial experience in 302 procedures, *J Am Coll Cardiol* 21:287–295, 1993.

Talley JD, Joseph A, Killeavy ES, Garratt KN, Hodes ZI, Linnemeier TJ, Yussman ZA, Brier ME, Kupersmith J: Multicenter evaluation of a new fixed-wire coronary angioplasty catheter system: clinical and angiographic characteristics and results, *Cathet Cardiovasc Diagn* 22:310–316, 1991.

Talley JD, Joseph A, Kupersmith J: Preliminary results utilizing a new percutaneous transluminal coronary angioplasty balloon catheter, *Cathet Cardiovasc Diagn* 20:108–113, 1990.

Topol E, Leya F, Pinkerton C, et al.: A comparison of directional coronary atherectomy with coronary angioplasty in patients with coronary disease, *N Engl J Med* 329:221–227, 1993.

Vogel JHK, King SB III: *Interventional cardiology: future directions;* St. Louis, 1989, Mosby.

10

DOCUMENTATION IN THE CARDIAC CATHETERIZATION LABORATORY

Aileen O'Rourke and Diane Brown

MEDICAL MALPRACTICE

Although the number of medical malpractice claims has remained relatively constant since 1987, it is reported that the amount awarded by juries continues to rise. Medical malpractice actions are frequently initiated due to unresolved anger and frustration on the part of the patient. Time and time again, statements that "no one would answer my questions," "no one took time to explain anything," "no one returned my calls," and so on are made. At a plaintiff's deposition, the defense counsel awaits the disclosure that indicates the underlying motivation that provoked the patient to become a plaintiff. The plaintiff, after the initiation of the lawsuit, sits confident in the solace that "they'll answer my questions now," "they'll explain it all to me now," or "they'll return this call."

It is unfortunate to see the deterioration in the health-care provider–patient relationship. The best advice in this area is to try always to keep lines of communication open between the provider (doctor, nurse, technologist) and the patient. Remember to take the time to let your patient know that he or she is important to you.

THE MEDICAL RECORD: GENERAL POINTS

Despite efforts of health-care providers to deliver the highest-quality patient care and remain available and approachable to patients, litigation will continue to be initiated. Therefore, the importance of an accurate and legible medical record in protecting the interests of patients, physicians, and staff cannot be underestimated. The reasons are twofold. First, and most important, this record may serve as the basis for determining future medical management of the patients. Illegible, imprecise, or unclear entries may result in medical error and injury to the patient. Second, this record may form the basis for either the patient's lawsuit or the medical staff's defense in the event of a medical malpractice action.

In the great majority of medical malpractice cases, the medical record is not only entered into evidence, but also is a determining factor in the outcome of the litigation. Although the parties may introduce many types of evidence to support their respective positions, the medical record is often considered the most reliable, trustworthy, and unbiased piece of evidence because the record was made contemporaneously with the patient's care and prior to the thought of litigation.

The entire medical record, including x-ray films, is generally maintained by the medical records department and is the property of the hospital or privately owned cardiac catheterization laboratory. Although the patient or legal representative/guardian has the legal right to access his or her medical record, each facility has specific policies governing access to medical records.

The information contained within the hospital record, since obtained in the course of providing service to a patient, is confidential except as otherwise provided by law. Medical information from the record or a copy of the record may be released only with the written consent of the patient or legally authorized representative/guardian, court order, or duly executed subpoena.

General Guidelines for Documentation

Proper charting in a medical record for the catheterization laboratory is generally no different than charting in all other areas of the hospital.

1. The most important aspect of documentation in the hospital record relates to handwriting and organization. Write legibly and in an organized fashion when you make entries in the medical record. Include your signature and indicate your professional status (MD, RN, LVN, LPN, NA, etc.). An illegible record can serve as the basis for a lawsuit and result in either a settlement or verdict for the plaintiff even though there may be no merit to the claim. Imagine the impact an illegible and unorganized medical record entry can have when the attorney magnifies the entry, mounts it as a poster, and presents it to the jury. It is easy to believe that a jury will equate sloppy charting with poor care and side with the plaintiff.

2. Use proper spelling, grammar, and punctuation. Errors such as these create an overall negative impression as to the quality of care. Whenever in doubt, look it up. Make sure that the patient's name is on *every* sheet entered into the record.

3. Only use symbols and abbreviations authorized by the facility. The facility maintains and constantly updates its approved abbreviation list, keeping in mind that each symbol or abbreviation should have only *one* meaning. If in doubt regarding the approved abbreviation, write it out. Be careful with the use of symbols; the mistaken use of the letter M instead of F implies that if the staff is not sure about the sex of the particular patient, then they cannot be sure about the quality of the care administered.

4. The frequency of chart entries depends on the individual hospital's department policies, acuity of the patient, changes in the patient's condition, national and state standards, standards of the community, and common sense. Charting should occur as soon as possible to the time of the observation or care provided.

5. Information in the medical record should reflect only accurate facts regarding the particular patient. Avoid generalizations and speculation by charting only what you see, hear, feel, and smell. Do not use words such as *inadvertently, unfortunately, appears, resembles,* and the like. The medical record is a legal document and is not

the proper forum for dispute resolution. It is not the appropriate place to settle grudges with other personnel, nor should the chart contain flippant or humorous remarks. The professionalism of the hospital staff should be reflected in the medical record entries.

6. Chart after the delivery of care, not before. Never make an entry in anticipation of something to be done. Chart only what actually has taken place, including accurate dates and times. It is never appropriate to leave blank spaces on forms designated for chronological, sequential notes.

7. If it is necessary to add an entry at a later time, clearly identify the date and time of the entry as well as the date and time of the occurrence (e.g., 3/10/94 1015 hours charting for 3/8/94 0900 hours). Pertaining to medications, if it becomes necessary to document out of sequence during a normal shift, make certain that the appropriate times are entered into the medical record. Follow hospital policy and procedures as to the method of recording the entry and explanation of why the drug was given late or not given.

8. All entries in the medical record must be made in permanent ink, and no portion of the medical record is to be obliterated, erased, altered, or destroyed.

9. If a charting error is made, do not obliterate the error or remove it from the chart. An appropriate way to correct the error is to draw one line through the entry, and initial, date, and enter the time at which the correction was made. Note the reason for the correction, and then chart the correct information. NOTE: Most facilities have a policy that addresses the issue of charting errors.

10. The chart note should identify precautionary or protective measures that have been taken for the safety of the patient, including the use of side rails and restraints. Hospital policies and procedures should mandate the types of restraints to be used and the need for close observation and documentation. State laws vary on the authorization required for use of restraints in acute facilities, skilled nursing facilities, and mental health facilities.

11. Review your documentation to be certain that the entries in the medical record reflect what is meant.

General Documentation in the Catheterization Laboratory

1. Chart the date, time, method of admission, and transfer or discharge of a patient from the facility.

2. Document on admission and discharge all valuables that are in the patient's possession and their disposition. Include the full name of the person receiving the valuables if they are sent home.

3. Routine documentation should include a concise and accurate record of the care administered, including pertinent observations, psychosocial and physical manifestations, incidents, unusual occurrences, abnormal behavior, treatments, intake and output, vital signs, and the like.

4. Changes in medical orders should be noted in a timely fashion, including date, time, and signature of person noting the order. The orders are to be carried out promptly and recorded as they are completed.

5. Document your participation in treatments rendered by physicians and the reaction of the patient following the treatment.

6. If a change in the patient's condition is identified, the physician should be notified promptly. The date, time, physician involved, way of communicating (e.g., telephone or in person), exactly what was communicated, all instructions received from the physician, all actions taken, and the response of the patient should all be documented.

7. The physician must be informed of all incidents or unusual occurrences related to his or her patient. The medical record should include a factual account of the incident, the reaction of the patient, the name of any physician contacted, and any follow-up. Do not indicate in the medical record that an incident report or quality assurance monitoring form was completed. Do not include a copy of either form in the medical record.

8. At the time of discharge from the laboratory, carefully note the patient's status, the final assessment, including all teaching efforts, and the response from the patient and/or family. Document all take-home instructions and take-home medications, prescriptions, or equipment. Whether handwritten or preprinted take-home instructions are used, have the patient or legal representative/

guardian acknowledge the receipt of the instructions in writing and keep a copy in the record.

9. Do not routinely chart for another person. However, *during emergency situations,* such as a cardiac arrest, designate one person to be in charge of making a detailed account. The recorder should carefully document all treatments, medications, responses of the patient, and personnel involved in the emergency situation. Remember that cosigning someone elses note generally presumes that you agree with the information contained in the note.

Medication and IV Documentation

A physician's orders should be accurately transcribed by the appropriate personnel. Although the registered nurse may not actually transcribe the physician's orders, this nurse has both the legal responsibility to assure the accuracy of the transcription and the professional responsibility to verify the appropriateness of the orders and make an inquiry of the physician when an error is suspected.

1. Include in the medical record the name of the medication, dose, route of administration, and site of injection as well as the date and time of administration. For IV fluids, also include the type and amount of solution, medication added, rate of infusion, type of needle or catheter used, the site of the IV, and assessment of the IV site. A catheterization laboratory flow sheet is often helpful.

2. Document the use of special equipment such as filters, automatic infusion devices, or monitoring equipment used as required by individual hospital policy.

3. Include in the medical record the signatures of both persons checking blood, blood by-products, and any medication designated by hospital policy to be checked by two licensed personnel.

4. Number and accurately record the IVs and blood units that are hung and infused.

5. Document vital signs that are taken before administration of medications and changes in the vital signs as a result of medications.

6. Promptly notify the physician, and document any adverse reactions that the patient experiences as a result

of medications or IVs, including transfusion reactions, infiltrations, rashes, etc. Complete an incident report or quality assurance monitoring form.

7. Follow hospital policies regarding the changing of IV sites, dressing, and tubings, and document those changes. Also document site care rendered.

8. Reasons for and effects of administering PRN medications should be indicated clearly.

9. Carefully note in the medical record if you have clarified or questioned a physician's order and the response of the physician or other person that you have contacted through the chain of command. Keeping an accurate record of the time and content of these communications may be essential.

10. In the event of a medication error, you must notify the physician and document the occurrence in a factual way in the medical record. You must also document your observation of the patient and his or her condition and the fact that the physician was notified. Although an incident report or quality assurance monitoring form should be completed, do not refer to these documents in the record.

Minimum Documentation in the Catheterization Laboratory

1. Identifying information
2. Date and time of admission and discharge
3. Vital signs
4. Weight of patient when applicable
5. Time of last meal
6. Last menstrual period when applicable
7. Allergy status
8. Current medications, including what medications taken in the last 24 hours
9. Previous health history
10. Laboratory and x-ray tests (PT, PTT, hemoglobin, K^+, BUN, creatinine)
11. All medications and IVs administered
12. Response to medications
13. Mode of arrival and departure
14. Notification of the physician and the actual time of arrival
15. Discharge assessment

16. Discharge instructions
17. Disposition of patient
18. RN on duty
19. Patient consent when applicable
20. The use of an interpreter when applicable and the name of that individual

Charting Recommendations for Outpatient Catheterization

1. A complete assessment of the patient on admission to the outpatient catheterization unit, including vital signs
2. The identity of anyone who accompanied the patient and the arrangements made to transport the patient home upon discharge
3. Allergies
4. Consent forms that have been completed properly; in the event the patient indicates he or she has not been fully informed and has additional questions, the physician should be contacted immediately and documentation should be made to that effect
5. Information about procedure treatments, preparations, or medications administered and the response of the patient
6. Patient history and physical and preoperative diagnosis data, which must be on the chart before any procedure
7. Completed reports or necessary laboratory tests; document notification to the physician of abnormal lab values
8. Information about the patient's compliance with pre-procedure instructions and details of notification to the physician if the patient states otherwise
9. A completed catheterization laboratory record required as part of the in-patient medical record
10. Complete postcatheterization assessments and vital signs plus pertinent observations recorded to indicate that the patient is alert and without postoperative complications before discharge
11. If discharge criteria are used to determine that the patient is stable for discharge, documentation of observations that the criteria have been met
12. Written after-care instructions given to the patient; the patient should sign a written statement that he or she has received a copy of the instructions and understands them

13. The full name of the person who accompanied the patient upon discharge and an indication of by what method the patient departed

14. A discharge note that includes a thorough assessment of the physical and psychosocial status of the patient

15. Any complications that occurred during or after the procedure, documented in a factual, objective manner; an incident report or quality assurance monitoring form should be completed, but no mention should be made of such reports in the medical record

16. Details of any arrangements made for transfer to inpatient status, including the method of transfer plus the names and titles of the persons accompanying the patient during transfer

17. Documentation of notification to the physician during the recovery period, to include details of the patient's condition reported, the response or lack of response of the physician, as well as steps taken through the chain of command to obtain help for the patient if the physician does not respond or is not available.

Documentation for Medical Treatment Problems or Complications: Events Requiring an Incident Report

Each facility should have a policy outlining the requirement of incident or occurrence reporting. Generally, an incident or occurrence in an unanticipated or unexpected event involving a patient that resulted in, or may have resulted in, an injury to the patient. The following lists several examples of events that will likely require proper reporting.

1. Cardiac/respiratory arrest during or after a procedure
2. Delayed treatment resulting in patient deterioration
3. Failure to diagnose
4. Delayed diagnosis
5. Incorrect diagnosis
6. Hospital-acquired infection
7. Unanticipated death
8. Adverse reaction to medication, blood or blood products, or other substances
9. Neurosensory, functional, or cognitive deficit not present on admission
10. Organ failure not present on admission

11. Acute cardiac dysfunction, MI, or cerebrovascular accident (CVA) following treatment or procedure
12. Unanticipated return to laboratory
13. Unplanned procedure
14. Excessive blood loss requiring transfusion
15. Intubation problem
16. Unintended foreign body retention
17. Any situation where a patient or his or her representative/guardian makes an accusation of wrongdoing.

Techniques for Preventing Medication Errors

1. Calculate dosages on paper, not in your head.
2. Give what you pour and pour what you give.
3. Be alert to drug name similarities. For example, quinine and quinidine, Maalox and Marax, Dilantin and Dilaudid, meperedine and Methergine.
4. Know the dosage ranges of the drugs you administer.
5. Confirm drug names when taking telephone orders—spell them back to the physician.
6. Do not become distracted when preparing medications.
7. Listen to your patients. If they question the route, time, or medication you are administering to them, double check the physician's order.
8. Know the most recent package insert data for drugs used.
9. Always check expiration date.
10. Do not stock "look-alike" medications on the same shelf (i.e., potassium chloride, sodium chloride).
11. Use needles that are the appropriate size for the drug to be administered and for the size of the patient.

PRODUCT LIABILITY ISSUES IN THE CARDIAC CATHETERIZATION LABORATORY

In light of recent publicity surrounding Food and Drug Administration approval of newly developed medical devices and generic drugs, discussion of product liability issues in the catheterization laboratory is appropriate. Several areas have serious medicolegal implications, including equipment/device failure, adverse reactions to contrast media or medication, reuse of equipment, and product recalls.

Equipment Failure

Under the most ideal conditions, equipment can malfunction, devices can fail, and dye or drugs may cause adverse reactions. The result is often immediate or eventual harm to the patient. When such events occur, the first responsibility, of course, is appropriate intervention to address the effects of the event on the patient. In the aftermath of the crisis, there are other steps that must be taken in the interests of professional responsibility and potential liability. Essential to the entire process is careful and complete documentation of the occurrence, the effect on the patient, the treatment, and the response of treatment.

Hospitals are responsible for reporting adverse incidents caused by or attributed to a medical device's failure or malfunction pursuant to the Safe Medical Devices Act of 1990 (SMDA) (Public Law 101-629, 104 Stat. 4511 [1990]; and 21 U.S.C. 3601 [1990]). The SMDA requires that hospitals report certain device-specific and patient-specific information to the manufacturer of a device that caused or contributed to the serious illness, serious injury, or death of a hospital patient. In some situations, this information must be reported to the FDA. The SMDA requires that a hospital conduct an investigation of such incidents to determine the cause of the incident (i.e., whether the incident was caused by or was attributable to device malfunction or failure or some combination of the above and user error) and to identify the specific patient and device involved. The hospital is required to establish policies and procedures for implementing the requirements of the SMDA and to identify an individual who will be responsible for coordinating incident investigation, incident reporting, and in-service training and to serve as facility liaison with manufacturers, the FDA, and any other agencies involved in incident reporting. The hospital's risk manager and, in some cases, attorney(s) should be notified and consulted in the event of a device-related incident.

Apart from the requirements of the SMDA, it is advisable to record equipment or substance descriptions along with such identifiers as serial or lot numbers to facilitate identification of devices or substances that may cause adverse incidents at a later time.

In the case of a device-related incident or equipment failure or malfunction not involving a patient, the equipment must be immediately removed from use, sequestered in a safe place, reported to the supervisor, and assessed by a reputable outside specialist as to cause of malfunction or failure. Prior to or during assessment, the device should not be repaired or altered. It is essential that the device is not altered until a full investigation of the incident is conducted and the device manufacturer or FDA has had an opportunity to conduct any investigation these entities may require. Therefore, it is advisable to not surrender or release the device to any third party, even an outside specialist or the device manufacturer, without the express agreement that the device will be maintained in the condition in which it was received.

If a piece of equipment has been serviced, maintained, and/or calibrated according to the manufacturer's instructions and if it was being used properly for the purpose for which it was intended, the liability for the consequences of failure or malfunction is attributable to the manufacturer rather than the health-care provider. Needless to say, records must be maintained to prove the above.

Intravascular Device Failure

When there are problems with *catheters* and other *intravascular devices,* such as separation or breakage, all portions should be saved in a secure place. Where feasible, immediate contact with the manufacturer or distributor should be made to determine whether the device in question was contained in a defective lot or batch or whether a flaw in design or production may have caused or contributed to the devices failure or malfunction. If time and the situation allow, a different lot of the same make or a different manufacturer's product should be obtained for use until it has been determined that it is safe to use the same type that caused the incident.

Medication Reactions

Reactions to *contrast media* or medication require notation of lot numbers and other identifying information as well as contact with the manufacturer or distributor. Similarly, use of another lot or brand should be standard protocol, when possible, until the problem is clearly identified. It is good practice to routinely include the lot numbers of products such as contrast media in the catheterization laboratory record routinely, because adverse effects are not always immediate; without that information in the record, it is often impossible to determine the source of the problem. The hospital should also be familiar and in compliance with any state and federal law that requires the reporting of adverse incidents related to the use of the products.

It is the conscientious reporting of product hazards and deficiencies that enables the FDA and other agencies and services to identify problems and issue warnings and recalls that ultimately protect other patients from injury and death. These agencies have a duty to observe certain standards of confidentiality regarding patient-identifiable information that may be contained in such reports.

Hand in hand with the responsibility for reporting goes the responsibility for responding effectively to reports received regarding product warnings and recalls. In all too many organizations, such reports are either ignored or erroneously routed, and the information never reaches the areas or individuals affected.

The hospital must establish and follow policies and procedures that designate an individual as responsible for coordinating the investigation and reporting of devices and other product's adverse incidents pursuant to existing law for communicating warning and recall information and for assuring that appropriate action is taken in response to such information. Continued use of a product after a warning or recall has been issued exposes health-care professionals and the organization to liability for adverse outcomes.

Catheter Reuse

A matter of concern recently addressed by several catheterization laboratory professionals is the reuse of catheters and other intravascular lines. Some individuals are being asked or required to do so by administrators or physician directors in the interest of cost containment. This equipment is very expensive and reimbursement continually is being reduced by both government and private payors.

The dangers inherent in this practice cannot be overemphasized. First, if the packaging states "single use only" or similar wording, any reuse is contrary to manufacturer's instructions. Repeated use is likely unsafe and if an adverse event occurs subsequent to such use, the user and hospital may be exposed to liability for negligence, exacerbated by the very fact of reuse.

Although one may argue that a manufacturer's instruction regarding single patient use may be based on a profit motive, one must assume that the directive is based on the fact that it is neither safe nor prudent to reuse equipment so labeled. Amid both the fact and the myth of this situation, it is ill advised, if not foolhardy, to reuse catheters and other devices that, by definition, come in prolonged contact with human blood.

Another significant contraindication for reuse is the potential for transmission of acquired immunodeficiency syndrome and other infectious diseases.

SUMMARY

Professionals must recognize that comprehensive documentation is the most reliable means of demonstrating that every effort is being made to provide the patient the requisite quality care delivered, not only with extraordinary skill and expertise, but also with the safest and most effective diagnostic and therapeutic equipment as part of the catheterization laboratory procedure.

GLOSSARY

Aberrant ventricular conduction. The temporarily abnormal intraventricular conduction of a supraventricular impulse, usually associated with a change in cycle length.

Accelerated idionodal rhythm. An automatic AV rhythm, controlling only the ventricles, at a rate between 60 and 100 bpm.

Accelerated idioventricular rhythm. An automatic ectopic ventricular rhythm, controlling only the ventricles, at a rate between 50 and 100 bpm.

Aneurysm. A saclike bulging of the wall of an artery or vein.

Aorta. The great vessel arising from the left ventricle, from which all other arteries originate, except the pulmonary artery.

Aortography. X-ray examination of the aorta by means of contrast injection.

Artery. A vessel through which the blood passes away from the heart to various parts of the body.

Atheroma. An abnormal mass of fatty material that deposits in and on the inside of the arterial wall.

Atherosclerosis. A condition in which atheromas form in and on the inside of the arteries, causing degeneration and "hardening of the arteries."

Atrial capture. Retrograde conduction to the atria, from AV junction or ventricles, after a period of AV dissociation.

Automaticity. The property inherent in all pacemaking cells that enables them to form new impulses spontaneously.

Automatic beat or rhythm. A beat or rhythm arising in a spontaneously beating center, independent of the dominant sinus (or other) rhythm.

AV dissociation. Independent beating of atria and ventricles.

Bifurcation. A division into two branches, as in an artery or vein.

Bicuspid valve. A valve that is formed by two cusps, as in the mitral valve. An anomaly when associated with the aortic valve.

Block. Pathological delay or interruption of impulse conduction.

Bradycardia. Any heart (or chamber) rhythm having an average rate under 60 bpm.

Bruit. A sound or murmur caused by turbulent flow that can be heard on auscultation.

Capture(d) beat. A conducted beat following a period of AV dissociation.

Cardiac output. The amount of blood pumped by the heart, usually expressed in liters per minute.

Cardiac tamponade. Acute compression of the heart caused by fluid in the pericardium or blood in the pericardium from rupture of the heart.

Chordae tendineae. The tendinous strings that support the valves between the atria and ventricle.

Commissurotomy. The stretching or tearing of a stenotic heart valve by surgical means or with the use of a balloon catheter.

Concealed conduction. Conduction of an impulse within the conduction system, recognizable only by its effect on the subsequent beat or cycle.

Contrast (commonly called a dye). A clear solution containing iodine, which shows up on x-ray. This solution is injected through the catheter in order to visualize the heart and its blood vessels and is eliminated by the kidneys and passed in the urine.

Coronary arteries. Two large arteries that branch from the aorta to supply the heart muscle with blood.

Cor pulmonale. Enlargement of the right ventricle secondary to increased pulmonary resistance to blood flow.

Coupling interval. The interval between an extrasystole and the beat preceding it.

Dextrocardia. Location of the heart on the right side of the thorax.

Diastole. The period of relaxation of the atria and ventricle during the cardiac cycle.

Distal. Farther away from a specific point of reference.

Ductus arteriosus. A small tubular connection (duct) between the aorta and pulmonary artery through which blood circulates to the lungs during fetal circulation. The duct normally closes at birth. If the duct remains open after birth, it is referred to as a *patent ductus arteriosus.*

Dyspnea. Difficult or labored breathing.

Ectopic beat. A beat arising in any focus other than the sinus node.

Ectopy. Ectopic impulse formation.

Embolism. Any substance such as blood clot, air, plaque, fat, etc., which travels in the bloodstream, causing partial or total obstruction of a blood vessel.

Escape(d) beat. An automatic beat ending a cycle longer than the dominant cycle and able to appear only because of a slowing or interruption of the dominant rhythm.

Extrasystole. A premature ectopic beat, dependent upon and coupled to the preceding beat.

Fibrillation. Unsyncronized, unorganized cardiac contractions.

Fibrin. A protein formed from fibrinogen by the action of thrombin in the clotting of blood. The essential portion of a blood clot.

Fibrinolysis. The dissolution of fibrin.

Fibrinolytic. Having the ability to dissolve blood clots.

Fistula. An abnormal communication between two structures, as in an abnormal arterial/venous communication.

Fluoroscopy. Real time viewing of x-ray images of structures within the body.

Foramen ovale. A hole between the right and left atrium that allows blood to bypass the pulmonary circuit in fetal circulation. The foramen ovale normally closes after birth. If it remains open, it is referred to as a *patent foramen ovale.*

Fusion beat. A beat resulting from the simultaneous spread of more than one impulse through the same myocardial territory (either ventricles or atria).

Groin. The area located below the abdomen and above the thigh.

Heparin. An anticoagulant that inhibits clotting by preventing the conversion of prothrombin to thrombin during the clotting cascade.

Hypertrophy. The enlargement of an organ or tissue.

Idioventricular rhythm. A rhythm arising in and controlling only the ventricles.

Intima. The inner lining of the arterial wall.

Ischemia. A term used to describe a condition of receiving inadequate blood supply, often caused by partial or total obstruction of the blood vessel supplying that tissue.

Isorhythmic dissociation. AV dissociation with atria and ventricles beating at the same or almost the same rate.

Left ventricle. The thick, muscular chamber of the heart that pumps oxygenated blood through the aorta to all the tissues and cells of the body.

Lumen. The channel within a tubular structure. The inside passageway of a blood vessel is referred to as the *lumen.*

Myocarditis. Inflammation of the heart muscle.

Murmur. An abnormal heart sound caused by the turbulent flow of blood through cardiac structures.

Myocardial infarction. An injury to the heart muscle resulting from loss of blood supply from a coronary artery.

Palpation. The act of examination by feeling or touch.

Patent. Open and unobstructed.

Pericarditis. Inflammation of the sac (pericardium) surrounding the heart.

Pericardiocentesis. The placement of a needle or small tube into the space between the pericardial sac and the epicardium and removal of accumulated fluid.

Plaque. Another term for localized buildup of cholesterol and fatty material.

Pressure transducer. A device that converts mechanical energy to an electrical signal.

Pulse pressure. The difference between the systolic pressure and the diastolic pressure.

Preexcitation. Activation of a ventricle earlier than its activation would be expected via the normal conducting pathways.

Premature beat. An ectopic beat, dependent upon and coupled to the preceding beat, and occurring before the next expected dominant beat; extrasystole.

Shunt. Passage of blood between normally isolated structures.

Stroke volume. The amount of blood that is ejected from the left ventricle with each contraction.

Syncope. A fainting episode.

Systole. The period of contraction of the atria and ventricles during the cardiac cycle.

Tachyarrhythmia. Any disturbance of rhythm resulting in a heart or chamber rate over 100 bpm.

Tachycardia. Any heart (or chamber) rhythm having an average rate over 100 bpm.

Thrombus. A clot within a blood vessel or cavity of the heart.

Tranquilizer. A medication that produces calming or quieting effects without causing unconsciousness.

Valsalva's maneuver. In this maneuver the patient is instructed to take a deep breath in and force exhalation against a closed glottis in order to increase intrapulmonic pressure.

Ventricular aberration. Aberrant ventricular conduction.

Ventricular capture. Conduction to the ventricles after a period of AV dissociation.

I

PATIENT RECORDS, ORDERS, AND DIAGRAMS

PHYSICIAN'S ORDER SHEET

USE BALL POINT PEN ONLY AND PRESS FIRMLY

	1358798	☐ STAT	☐ NEW	☐ DISCHARGE
	DATE TIME WRITTEN A.M. P.M. TIME IN TIME OUT			

PLEASE GROUP PHARMACY ORDERS IN TOP PORTION OF ORDER SET.

1) Remain on bedrest over night p cath; BRP p initial 8 hrs.

2) B/P, P, & pedal pulses q 30 min. X 2 hrs., and q 1 hr. X 3.

3) If bleeding or hematoma occurs apply pressure over the puncture site. **LOSS** of pedal pulses or ischemia may occur. If any of these problems occur call

GROUP GENERAL ORDERS IN BOTTOM PORTION OF ORDER SET.

Dr.   at: **STAT.**

4) Call MD STAT for B/P <90 sys. or HR <60

5) ECG on day of discharge.

NURSES SIGNATURE   DOCTOR   M.D.   BNDD NUMBER

	1358799	☐ STAT	☐ NEW	☐ DISCHARGE
	DATE TIME WRITTEN A.M. P.M. TIME IN TIME OUT			

PLEASE GROUP PHARMACY ORDERS IN TOP PORTION OF ORDER SET.

6) Tylenol 1000mg po q 4 hr. for pain prn.

7) Dalmane 30mg po hs prn: may repeat in 1 hr.

8) Remove bandage the day after procedure.

9) Resume previous diet and medications.

10) IV @D5½NS @   cc/hr. for   hrs.

GROUP GENERAL ORDERS IN BOTTOM PORTION OF ORDER SET.

11) Discharge date:

NURSES SIGNATURE   DOCTOR   M.D.   BNDD NUMBER

	1358800	☐ STAT	☐ NEW	☐ DISCHARGE
	DATE TIME WRITTEN A.M. P.M. TIME IN TIME OUT			

PLEASE GROUP PHARMACY ORDERS IN TOP PORTION OF ORDER SET.

GROUP GENERAL ORDERS IN BOTTOM PORTION OF ORDER SET.

NURSES SIGNATURE   DOCTOR   M.D.   BNDD NUMBER

Illustrations on pp. 559–563 courtesy of St. Louis University Hospital.

TIME	CATHETERS/PROCEDURE NOTES (Continued)

POST-CATH DATA

		INITIALS	TIME		INITIALS
I:I/C.Arm Ht: ____ Table Ht: ____				Sheath removal	
Fluoro time: ____ min				Drsg applied: ( ) band-aid ( ) pressure	
Arterial time: ____ min				Sandbag: ( )Yes ( ) No	
Contrast agent: ____ Amt: ____ ml				BP: __/__ HR: ____ Rhythm:	
Total IV fluid intake: ____ ml				Insertion site:	
Urine Output in lab: ____ ml					

PULSES	R	L
Dorsalis Pedis		
Posterior Tibial		

Patient instructions given:	
Report given:	
Patient transferred:	

___/___
Initials/PRIMARY NURSE SIGNATURE   ___/___ Initials/SIGNATURE   ___/___ Initials/SIGNATURE

KEY FOR INVASIVE SITES:

					KEY FOR CATH LAB:
#1 (R) hand	#6 LU arm	#11 (R) jugular	#16 (L) fem artery	#21 (L) brachial artery	JR Judkins right
#2 (L) hand	#7 (R) antecubital	#12 (L) jugular	#17 swan sheath	#22 (R) wrist	JL Judkins left
#3 RL arm	#8 (L) antecubital	#13 PA port	#18 (R) radial artery	#23 (L) wrist	AMR Amplatz right
#4 LL arm	#9 (R) subclavian	#14 RA port	#19 (L) radial artery	#24 (R) fem vein	AML Amplatz left
#5 RU arm	#10 (L) subclavian	#15 (R) fem artery	#20 (R) brachial artery	#25 (L) fem vein	PT Pigtail

FORM C2.14 05/88

PRE-CATH DATA

DATE: _____ CINE # _____ ID BAND: _____
Height _____ Weight _____ Age _____ dob _____
Allergies: _____ Chest Diameter _____ BP _____ / _____ HR _____ Rhythm _____
Hgb _____ creat. _____ Pro time _____ PTT _____ T&S _____
Premed on floor: (type/time) _____ Consents: _____

PULSES	R	L
Dorsalis Pedis		
Posterior Tibial		

TIME		
	Arrival to lab	
	Transfer into Room	
	Prepped and draped	
	Physician scrubbed	
	Local Anesthesia:	

TIME	VESSEL ACCESS	SITE	SHEATH SIZE
	( ) Arterial		
	( ) Arterial		
	( ) Venous		
	( ) Venous		

TIME	MEDICATIONS	ROUTE	COMMENT

TIME	CATHETERS/PROCEDURE NOTES

I.V. FLUIDS

TIME	INITIALS	FLUIDS	NEEDLE	SITE	RATE	COMPLETION TIME	AMT. INFUSED	INITIALS

_____/_____ Initials/PRIMARY NURSE SIGNATURE   _____/_____ Initials/SIGNATURE   _____/_____ Initials/SIGNATURE

KEY FOR INVASIVE SITES:

#1 (R) hand   #6 LU arm   #11 (R) jugular   #16 (L) fem artery   #21 (L) brachial artery
   (L) hand   #7 (R) antecubital #12 (L) jugular   #17 swan sheath   #22 (R) wrist
#3 RL arm   #8 (L) antecubital #13 PA port   #18 (R) radial artery   #23 (L) wrist
#4 LL arm   #9 (R) subclavian #14 RA port   #19 (L) radial artery   #24 (R) fem vein
#5 RU arm   #10 (L) subclavian #15 (R) fem artery #20 (R) brachial artery #25 (L) fem vein

KEY FOR CATH LAB:
JR   Judkins right
JL   Judkins left
AMR Amplatz right
AML Amplatz left
PT   Pigtail

FORM C2.14 05/88

Previous CABG: ____YES ____NO
Previous PTCA: ____YES ____NO

1. Stable Angina: _____
   CHC   I   II   III   IV

2. Unstable Angina: _____

3. Acute MI: _____

THIS IS A PRELIMINARY ESTIMATE _____
FROM THE TV SCREEN.
A FINAL FILM ANALYSIS WILL FOLLOW.

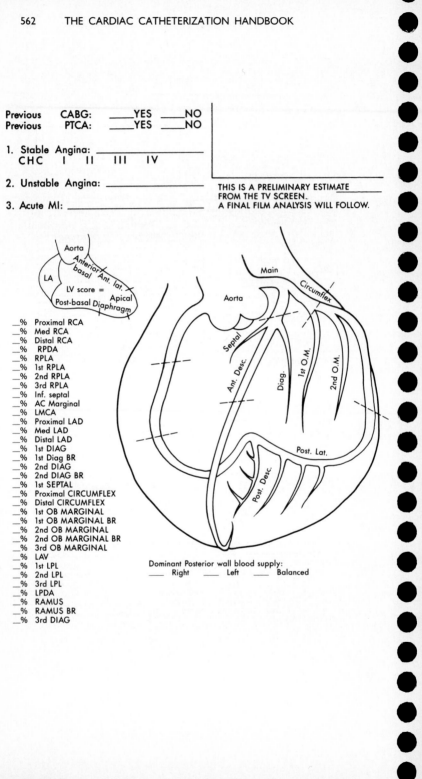

__% Proximal RCA
__% Med RCA
__% Distal RCA
__% RPDA
__% RPLA
__% 1st RPLA
__% 2nd RPLA
__% 3rd RPLA
__% Inf. septal
__% AC Marginal
__% LMCA
__% Proximal LAD
__% Med LAD
__% Distal LAD
__% 1st DIAG
__% 1st Diag BR
__% 2nd DIAG
__% 2nd DIAG BR
__% 1st SEPTAL
__% Proximal CIRCUMFLEX
__% Distal CIRCUMFLEX
__% 1st OB MARGINAL
__% 1st OB MARGINAL BR
__% 2nd OB MARGINAL
__% 2nd OB MARGINAL BR
__% 3rd OB MARGINAL
__% LAV
__% 1st LPL
__% 2nd LPL
__% 3rd LPL
__% LPDA
__% RAMUS
__% RAMUS BR
__% 3rd DIAG

Dominant Posterior wall blood supply:
____ Right   ____ Left   ____ Balanced

Name ....   Date ....
Age   ....   Cath # ....
Wt.   ....
Ht.   ....
Hb.   ....

II

FUNCTIONAL ANATOMY OF THE HEART

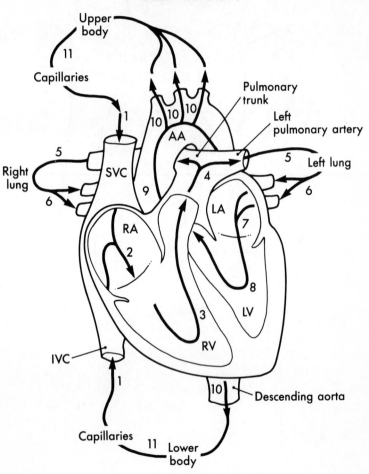

For legend, see bottom of page 565.

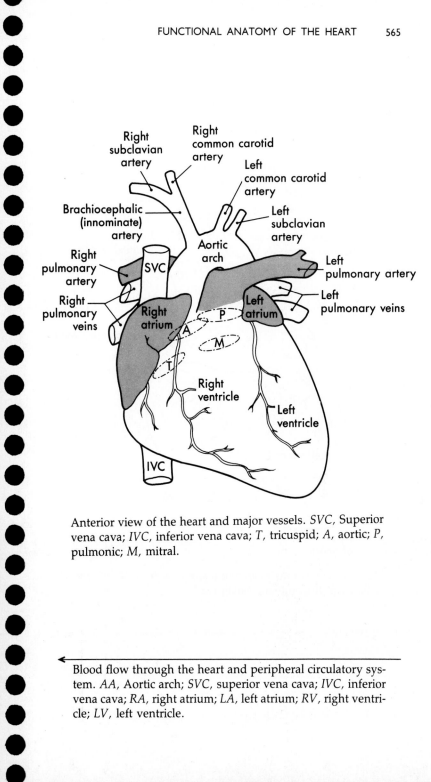

Anterior view of the heart and major vessels. *SVC,* Superior vena cava; *IVC,* inferior vena cava; *T,* tricuspid; *A,* aortic; *P,* pulmonic; *M,* mitral.

Blood flow through the heart and peripheral circulatory system. *AA,* Aortic arch; *SVC,* superior vena cava; *IVC,* inferior vena cava; *RA,* right atrium; *LA,* left atrium; *RV,* right ventricle; *LV,* left ventricle.

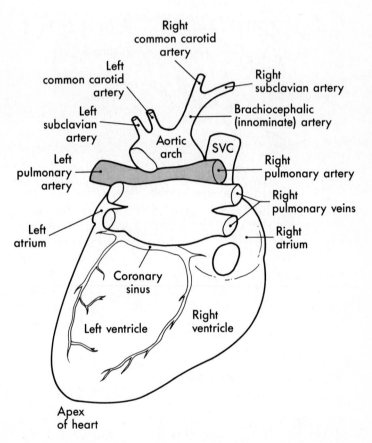

Posterior view of the heart and major vessels. *SVC*, Superior vena cava; *IVC*, inferior vena cava.

CORONARY ARTERY ANATOMY AND PHYSIOLOGY

The average heart beats about 42 million times a year and approximately 525,000 gallons of blood pass through it. The heart is also the most compact form of muscle tissue in the body. The coronary arteries originate from the sinuses of Valsalva, pouches or pockets that are just above the aortic cusps. The left coronary artery arises from the posterior sinus and the right coronary artery arises from the anterior sinus. During ventricular diastole the sinuses distend and fill with blood, resulting in blood flow to the right and left coronary arteries. This accounts for two thirds of the coronary blood supply. The other third occurs during ventricular systole. Blood returns to the heart via the cardiac veins, which empty into the right atrium.

ANATOMY OF THE ARTERIAL WALL

The arterial wall of the coronary arteries is made of three layers: the intima, media, and adventitia. These structures provide the strength and flexibility needed for the high-pressure arterial system. The arterial walls are capable of vasoconstriction and vasodilation, depending on the demands of the body or external stimuli received.

1. The *intima* is the innermost layer of the artery. It is composed of a thin layer of endothelial cells that are supported by connective tissue. The intimal layer is semipermeable, which allows the transport of oxygen and nutrients into the arterial wall. Endothelial cells prevent thrombus formation by regenerating quickly when injured and by secreting chemicals that resist platelet aggregation.

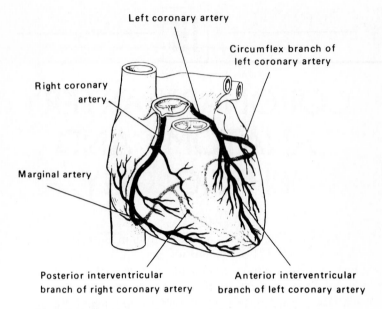

(From Langley LL and others: *Dynamic anatomy and physiology,*
ed 5, New York, 1980, McGraw-Hill, p. 423.)

2. The *media* is the middle muscular layer of the artery. Smooth muscle cells and collagens are the primary constituents of the medial layer. Collagens, which are secreted by smooth muscle cells, are a form of connective tissue. The smooth muscle cells are covered by a thin fibrous network called the internal and external elastic lamina.

3. The *adventitia* is the outer layer of the arterial wall. It is made up of connective tissue, occasional smooth muscle cells, and the vasovasorum. The vasovasorum is an arteriole network that supplies blood to the adventitia and the outer half of the media.

CONFIGURATION OF LESIONS

Lesions tend to vary in their length and their inner luminal circumference. The degree of circumferential arterial wall involvement is categorized as either eccentric or concentric.

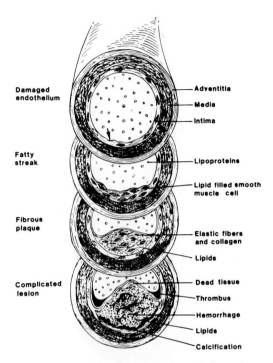

Damaged endothelium

Fatty streak

Fibrous plaque

Complicated lesion

Adventitia
Media
Intima
Lipoproteins
Lipid filled smooth muscle cell
Elastic fibers and collagen
Lipids
Dead tissue
Thrombus
Hemorrhage
Lipids
Calcification

(From Lewis SM, Collier IC: *Medical-surgical nursing: assessment and management of clinical problems,* New York, 1987, McGraw Hill, Inc.)

Eccentric Lesions

Eccentric lesions constitute approximately 70% of lesions. Part of the inner luminal circumference is free of disease in the eccentric lesion. Arterial walls dilate, constrict, and engage in spasm, depending on the stimulus. The eccentric lesion will have variable changes in the luminal diameter. Vasodilatation and vasoconstriction will have a profound effect on blood flow through the artery.

Concentric Lesions

The other 30% of lesions are concentric. The entire circumference of the arterial lumen is diseased. The diameter is fixed. Vasodilation and vasoconstriction at the site of disease will not change the inner luminal diameter.

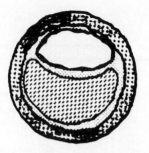

(From Brown BG, Bolson EL, Dodge HT: Dynamic mechanism in human coronary stenosis, *Circulation* 70:917, 1984.)

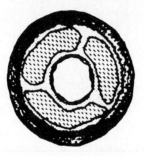

(From Brown BG, Bolson EL, Dodge HT: Dynamic mechanism in human coronary stenosis, *Circulation* 70:917, 1984.)

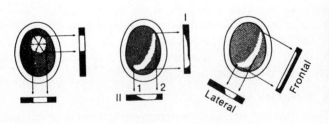

Diagrams of eccentric vessel narrowings that produce circular or crescent-shaped lumina, and their projections in two orthogonal views. Coronary artery disease produces a concentric or eccentric lumen, depending on whether the atheroma involves the circumference of the vessel evenly or unevenly. The concentric lumen is over the central axis of the artery and its shape is almost circular. The eccentric lumen is lateral to the vessel's central axis, and its shape may be circular or slitlike or crescentic. The black bars indicate the width that the shadow of the normal vessel should have on the film in two orthogonal views. The white portion in each bar indicates the shadow that the narrowed lumen projects. The depth of the white notch indicates the density that the shadow reaches on the film. When the notch is the entire width of the bar, the narrowed lumen is seen to be as white as a normal vessel. If the white notch is less than the full width of the bar, the shadow of the vessel is less dense (has a gray hue).

Circular lumen. All the diameters of a circular lumen have the same length (see *arrows* inside the lumen). It is readily apparent that any radiological view permits precise knowledge of the true degree of narrowing. It is not even necessary to have two orthogonal views. Furthermore there is no difference between concentric or eccentric disease as long as the narrowed lumen is more or less circular. Conversely an eccentric crescent-shaped lumen causes severe underestimation of the degree of pathologic change in coronary angiography.

Crescent-shaped lumen. Even with two orthogonal views there may be severe underestimation of the degree of narrowing of the vessel's diameter, but indirect evidence of severe disease is present. In view *I* the x-rays encounter different widths of contrast media; thus the vascular shadow will show irregular density in the angiogram. In view *II* the x-rays at 2 encounter a thick layer of contrast media, so that the shadow of the artery forms a sharp border, but progressing toward the other border the shadow of the vessel becomes progressively gray, as the layer of contrast material thins out and merges smoothly with the dark background, giving this arterial border an unsharp or out-of-focus appearance.

When the plane of the film is parallel to the long axis of the lumen (frontal or AP view), underestimation of the narrowing is maximal, but the density of the shadow on the film is diminished (rarefaction). On the other hand, when the long axis is perpendicular to the film (lateral view of the lumen), the narrowing is correctly estimated.

From Pujadas G: *Coronary angiography in the medical and surgical treatment of ischemic heart disease*, New York, 1980, McGraw-Hill.

NORMAL HEMODYNAMIC VALUE TABLES

TABLE IV-I. Normal left ventriculogram ejection phase indexes

	Average	SE	Range
Sinus beat			
Ejection fraction*	0.71	0.01	0.64–0.77
Ejection fraction†	67.3	1.0	62–72
Ejection vector*	1.19	0.03	1.28–1.07
End diastolic volume (ml/m²)	70.4	3.9	54–89
End systolic volume (ml/m²)	20.3	0.7	17–24
Postextrasystolic potentiation beat			
Ejection fraction*	0.82	0.01	0.76–0.85
Ejection fraction†	69.9	1.9	64–79
Ejection vector*	1.39	0.03	1.26–1.50
End diastolic volume (ml/m²)	78.5	3.2	68–90
End systolic volume (ml/m²)	14.2	0.7	11–17

From Pujadas G: *Coronary angiography in the medical and surgical treatment of ischemic heart disease,* New York, 1980, McGraw-Hill.
*As fraction of end-diastolic volume.
†Percentage of total stroke output is 50.

TABLE IV-2. Oxygen consumption per body surface area in (ml/min)/m^2 by sex, age, and heart rate

Age (yr)	Heart rate (bpm)												
	50	60	70	80	90	100	110	120	130	140	150	160	170
Male patients													
3				155	159	163	167	171	175	178	182	186	190
4			149	152	156	160	163	168	171	175	179	182	186
6		141	144	148	151	155	159	162	167	171	174	178	181
8		136	141	145	148	152	156	159	163	167	171	175	178
10	130	134	139	142	146	149	153	157	160	165	169	172	176
12	128	132	136	140	144	147	151	155	158	162	167	170	174
14	127	130	134	137	142	146	149	153	157	160	165	169	172
16	125	129	132	136	141	144	148	152	155	159	162	167	
18	124	127	131	135	139	143	147	150	154	157	161	166	
20	123	126	130	134	137	142	145	149	153	156	160	165	
25	120	124	127	131	135	139	143	147	150	154	157		
30	118	122	125	129	133	136	141	145	148	152	155		
35	116	120	124	127	131	135	139	143	147	150			
40	115	119	122	126	130	133	137	141	145	149			
Female patients													
3				150	153	157	161	165	169	172	176	180	183
4			141	145	149	152	156	159	163	168	171	175	179
6		130	134	137	142	146	149	153	156	160	165	168	172
8		125	129	133	136	141	144	148	152	155	159	163	167
10	118	122	125	129	133	136	141	144	148	152	155	159	163
12	115	119	122	126	130	133	137	141	145	149	152	156	160
14	112	116	120	123	127	131	134	138	143	146	150	153	157
16	109	114	118	121	125	128	132	136	140	144	148	151	
18	107	111	116	119	123	127	130	134	137	142	146	149	
20	106	109	114	118	121	125	128	132	136	140	144	148	
25	102	106	109	114	118	121	125	128	132	136	140		
30	99	103	106	110	115	118	122	125	129	133	136		
35	97	100	104	107	111	116	119	123	127	130			
40	94	98	102	105	109	112	117	121	124	128			

From LaFarge CG, Miettinen OS: The estimation of oxygen consumption, *Cardiovasc Res* 4:23, 1970.

TABLE IV-3. Normal values for cardiac output and related measurements by the Fick method

Measurements	Units	±SD
O$_2$ uptake	143 ml/min/m^2	14.3
Arteriovenous O$_2$ difference	4.1 vol%	0.6
Cardiac index	3.5 L/min/m^2	0.7
Stroke index	46 ml/beat/m^2	8.1

From Barratt-Boyes R, Wood EH: Cardiac output and related measurements and pressure values in the right heart and associated vessels, together with an analysis of the hemodynamic response to the inhalation of high oxygen mixtures in healthy subjects, *J Lab Clin Med* 51:72, 1958.

UNITS OF MEASURE

TABLE V-I.   Dimensions and units of some commonly used physical quantities

Physical quantity	Definition	Common units	Dimensions
Mass	Not defined	gram (g)	M
Length	Not defined	centimeter (cm)	L
Time	Not defined	second (sec)	T
Area	Length squared	cm^2	L^2
Volume	Length cubed	cm^3	L^3
Density	Mass per unit of volume	g/cm^3	ML^{-3}
Velocity	Length per unit of time	cm/sec	LT^{-1}
Acceleration	Velocity per unit of time	cm/sec^2	LT^{-2}
Flow	Volume per unit of time	cm^3/sec	L^3T^{-1}
Force	Mass times acceleration	dyne or gcm/sec^2	MLT^{-2}
Pressure	Force per unit of area	$dyne/cm^2$ or $g/cm/sec^2$	$ML^{-1}T^{-2}$
Resistance to flow	Pressure drop across a hydraulic segment per unit of flow	$dyne\ sec\ cm^{-5}$	$ML^{-5}T$
Work	Force times distance	erg or dyne cm or $g\ cm^2/sec^2$	ML^2T^{-2}
Power	Work per unit of time	dyne cm/sec or $g\ cm^2/sec^3$	ML^2T^{-3}

From Yang SS: *From cardiac catheterization data to hemodynamic parameters*, ed 3, Philadelphia, 1987, Davis.

CONVERSION FACTORS AND CONSTANTS
Decimal Factors

Multiples	Designation	Symbol	Submultiples	Designation	Symbol
10^{12}	tera-	T	10^{-12}	pico-	p
10^{9}	giga-	G	10^{-9}	nano-	n
10^{6}	mega-	M	10^{-6}	micro-	μ
10^{3}	kilo-	K	10^{-3}	milli-	m
10^{2}	hecto-	h	10^{-2}	centi-	c
10		dk	10^{-1}		d

LENGTH

1 meter (m) = 10 decimeters = 100 centimeters (cm) = 1000 millimeters (mm) = 1.0936 yards (yd) = 3.2808 feet (ft) = 39.37 inches

1 kilometer (km) = 1000 meters (m) = 0.6214 mile (mi)

1 centimeter (cm) = 0.3937 inch (in)

1 inch (in) = 2.54 centimeters (cm)

1 foot (ft) = 30.48 cm = 0.3048 m

1 mile (mi) = 1.6093 km = 1609.3 m = 1760 yd = 5280 ft

1 micron (μ) = 0.000001 m = 10^{-6} m

1 millimicron (mμ) = 0.000000001 m = 10^{-9} m

PRESSURE

$$1 \text{ atmosphere} = 760 \text{ mm Hg}$$
$$= 14.6 \text{ pounds/in}^2$$

TABLE V-2. Normal pressures in heart and great vessels*

Pressure (mm Hg)	Average	Range
Right atrium		
Mean	2.8	1–5
a wave	5.6	2.5–7
z point	2.9	1–5.5
c wave	3.8	1.5–6
x wave	1.7	0–5
v wave	4.6	2–7.5
y wave	2.4	0–6
Right ventricle		
Peak systolic	25	17–32
End-diastolic	4	1–7
Pulmonary artery		
Mean	15	9–19
Peak systolic	25	17–32
End-diastolic	9	4–13
Pulmonary artery wedge		
Mean	9	4.5–13
Left atrium		
Mean	7.9	2–12
a wave	10.4	4–16
z point	7.6	1–13
v wave	12.8	6–21
Left ventricle		
Peak systolic	130	90–140
End-diastolic	8.7	5–12
Brachial artery		
Mean	85	70–105
Peak systolic	130	90–140
End-diastolic	70	60–90

*Reference level = 10 cm above the spine of the recumbent subject.

VI

VENTRICULAR VOLUME AND MASS

MEASUREMENT OF VENTRICULAR VOLUME

The following will provide measurements of ventricular volume calculation of left ventricular mass, wall stress, and regional wall motion (see Chapter 6).

Calculation of ventricular volume assumes a shape of elipsoid of revolution (a football). The volume may be calculated by

$$V = \frac{4}{3} \times \frac{L}{2} \times \frac{D_1}{2} \times \frac{D_2}{2}$$
$$= \frac{LD_1D_2}{6}$$

where L is the major axis and D_1 and D_2 are minor axes.

Biplane Cineangiography

Biplane techniques (Sandler and Dodge) determine LV volume using the longest length in either view ($_{AP}$ or $_{LAT}$) and determined the transverse diameters in each plane (D_{AP}, D_{LAT}) by the area-length method. Tracings were made of the ventricular silhouettes and A_{LAT} and A_{AP} (areas) were obtained by planimetry as shown on p. 578.

L from the original volume of an ellipse equation will be the longer L from the two silhouettes (usually the AP). Then

$$V = \frac{\pi}{6} \times L_{MAX} \times D_{AP} \times D_{LAT}$$

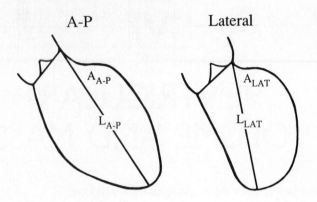

where

$$D = \frac{4\,\text{AREA}}{L}$$

simplified

$$V = \frac{8\,\text{AREA}_{AP} \times \text{AREA}_{LAT}}{3\,L_{MIN}}$$

L_{MAX} cancels out, leaving L_{MIN} (usually L_{LAT}) in the denominator. In most laboratories, the 30° RAO/60° LAO planes are used. This equation then becomes

$$V = \frac{8A_{RAO}A_{LAO}}{3\,L_{MIN}}$$

Correction Factors

To obtain absolute volumes, correction must be made for distortion caused by the divergence of the x-ray beams and the magnification of the image during projection of the film. Correction factors are obtained from a grid of square centimeters filmed at the level of the patient's heart during the procedure in both RAO and LAO projections. Utilizing the planimetered area of the projected grids, a linear correction factor (CF) for each plane is calculated:

$$CF = \frac{Aa}{Ap}$$

where Aa is the actual area and Ap is the planimetered area.

All three axes of the ventricle (L_{MAX}, D_{RAO}, D_{LAO}) must be multiplied by their respective correction factor. Thus,

$$V = \frac{8A_{RAO}A_{LAO}}{3\,L_{MIN}} \times CF_{MAX} \times CF_{RAO} \times CF_{LAO}$$

Single-Plane Cineangiography

When biplane is compared with single-plane measurements, chamber radii D_1 and D_2 do not differ significantly. Therefore a prolate spheroid (soccer ball) viewed in a single plane would be an adequate representation of the LV chamber.

$$V = \frac{\pi}{6}L \times D_1D_2 \text{ and } D_1 = D_2 = D_{RAO}$$

then

$$V = \frac{\pi}{6}L(D_{RAO})^2$$

because

$$D_{RAO} = \frac{4A}{L}$$

then

$$V = \frac{\pi}{6}L\frac{(4A)_2}{L} = \frac{8A^2}{3\,L}$$

Corrected: finally

$$V = \frac{8A^2}{3\,L} = (CF_{RAO})^3$$

LV Mass

Total volume of the LV chamber and wall can be determined by adding the wall thickness (h) to end-diastolic dimensions. By subtracting the chamber volume from this value, the myocardial volume is obtained. Multiplication by the specific gravity of muscle (1.050) yields LV mass in grams (for single-plane angiogram):

LV mass = [V chamber + V wall] − V chamber

$$= \left(\frac{\pi4}{3}\left[\frac{L = 2h)}{2}\frac{(D_{RAO} + 2h)}{2}\frac{(D_{LAO} + 2h)}{2}\right] - V\right)(1.050)$$

Normal Values

See Table VI-1.

TABLE VI-I. Normal average values for left ventricular parameters by angiocardiography

Angiographic method	Number of patients	Age group	End-diastolic volume (ml/m²)	End-systolic volume (ml/m²)	Ejection fraction	Wall thickness (mm)
Biplane modified Arvidsson	3	Adults	95	36	0.63	7.7
Biplane Dodge area-length	16	Adults	70	24	0.67	10.9
Biplane Dodge area-length	6	Adults	79	29	0.67	8.5
Biplane modified Dodge	6	Adults	71	30	0.58	
Single plane cineangiogram (right anterior oblique)	5	Adults	104	31	0.70	
Biplane Arvidsson	9	Children	88	32	0.64	
Biplane cineangiographic	19	Children less than 2 yr	42		0.68	
Biplane cineangiographic	37	Children older than 2 yr	73		0.63	

RADIOGRAPHIC IDENTIFICATION OF PROSTHETIC VALVES

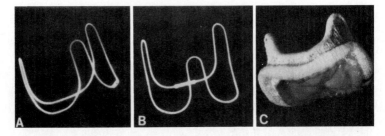

Fig. VII-1.   Carpentier-Edwards SupraAnnular Bioprosthesis. Aortic position: **A,** posterioanterior radiograph; **B** and **C,** left lateral view radiograph and photograph. One continuous narrow wireform outlines each of the three stents and that portion of the base ring between stents. Although superficially similar to the radiographic silhouettes of the Carpentier-Edwards Bioprosthesis, in the SupraAnnular model the change of shape of the wireform as it shifts from base ring to stent is more gradual, giving the wire a gently curving appearance rather than a right-angle appearance.

From Mehlman DJ: A guide to the radiographic identification of prosthetic heart valves: an addendum, *Circulation* 69:102, 1984. By permission of the American Heart Association, Inc.

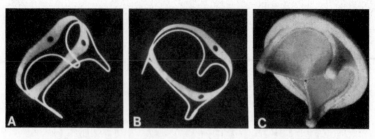

Fig. VII-2.   Carpentier-Edwards pericardial valve prosthesis. Mitral position: **A,** posterioanterior radiograph; **B** and **C,** left lateral radiograph and photograph. The base ring is marked by a flattened circular ring with three holes. The flattened ring does not extend into the stents as is seen in the Ionescu-Shiley xenograft. In addition, a narrow wireform outlines each of the three stents and the base ring between the stents. The wire curves gently between stent and base ring, similar to the Carpentier-Edwards SupraAnnular Bioprosthesis.

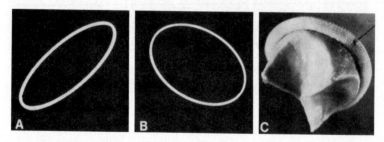

Fig. VII-3.   Hancock pericardial heart valve. Mitral position: **A,** posterioanterior radiograph; **B** and **C,** left lateral radiograph and photograph. The base ring is a narrow, circular, wirelike form. The remainder of the valve is radiolucent. The radiographic silhouette is similar to that of the Hancock porcine xenograft.

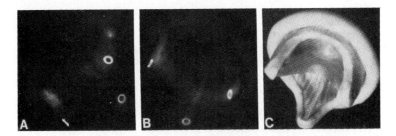

Fig. VII-4. Hancock II porcine xenograft. Mitral position: A, posterioanterior radiograph; B and C, left lateral radiograph and photograph. The base ring and stents are radiolucent. Three tiny circular rings mark the distal external aspects of the three stents.

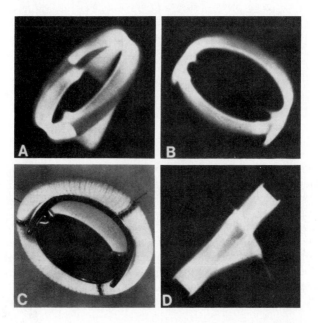

Fig. VII-5. Omniscience prosthetic heart valve. Mitral position: A, posterioanterior radiograph; B and C, left lateral radiograph and photograph; D, oblique radiograph demonstrating disc on edge. Emerging from the wide base ring are two low profile struts that are fastened to the base ring along their length. Although reminiscent of the silhouette of the Lillehei-Kaster prosthesis, the struts are shorter and form a much lower profile. On routine chest radiographs the disc is likely to be radiolucent. The disc of the Omniscience prosthesis (unlike the Lillehei-Kaster) is radiopaque when viewed on edge.

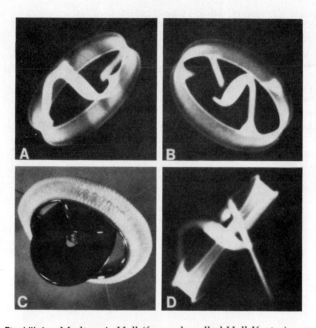

Fig. VII-6.   Medtronic Hall (formerly called Hall-Kaster) prosthetic heart valve. Mitral position: **A**, posterioanterior radiograph; **B** and **C**, left lateral radiograph and photograph; **D**, oblique radiograph demonstrating disc on edge. Four projections emerge from the base ring toward the center of the ring. Two short straight projections of equal size are on opposing sides of the base ring. A longer straight projection is perpendicular to the short projections. A large hooklike projection is opposite the long straight projection. On routine chest radiographs, the disc is likely to be radiolucent. When viewed on edge, the disc is radiopaque.

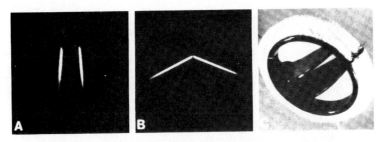

Fig. VII-7.   St. Jude Medical cardiac valve. Mitral position:
A, oblique radiograph demonstrating both discs on edge in
the open position; **B,** oblique radiograph demonstrating both
discs on edge in the closed position; **C,** left lateral photograph.
On routine chest radiographs the St. Jude Medical Valve is
likely to be radiolucent. When viewed on edge, the discs are
radiopaque. The base ring is radiolucent.

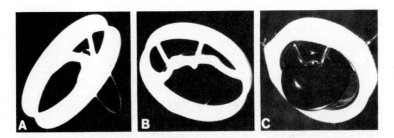

Fig. VII-8.   Bjork-Shiley cardiac valve prosthesis with Convex-
oconcave disc. Mitral position: **A,** posterioanterior radiograph; **B** and **C,** radiograph and photograph. The radiographic silhouette is essentially the same as the Bjork-Shiley
prosthesis with straight disc and incorporated disc marker.
The flattened base ring is encircled by a groove. Emerging
from the base ring toward its center are two eccentrically
located U-shaped structures of unequal size. The radiolucent
disc contains a narrow circular radiopaque disc marker that
is seen from any projection.

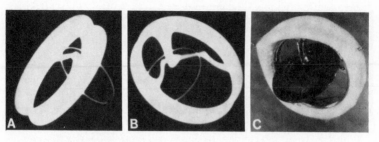

Fig. VII-9. Bjork-Shiley integral monostrut cardiac valve prosthesis. Mitral position: **A**, posterioanterior radiograph; **B** and **C**, left lateral radiograph and photograph. The radiographic silhouette is similar to that of the Bjork-Shiley Convexo-Concave and Straight disc valves. The flattened base ring is encircled by a groove. Emerging from the base ring toward its center is a wide U-shaped structure. Perpendicular to the flattened portion of the U is a short straight projection with a very small hook or bulge on its end. The radiolucent disc contains a narrow circular radiopaque disc marker that is seen from any projection.

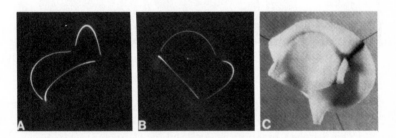

Fig. VII-10. Ionescu-Shiley low profile pericardial xenograft. Mitral position: **A**, posterioanterior radiograph; **B** and **C**, left lateral radiograph and photograph. The base ring consists of three narrow wireform arcs, each length approximately one-third the circumference of the base ring. Adjoining arcs are separated by small radiolucent areas. The stents are radiolucent.

VIII

PTCA AND OTHER INTERVENTIONAL EQUIPMENT SPECIFICATIONS

Because of the proliferation of coronary angiography procedures, balloon and guiding catheters and guidewires are available in a wide variety of configurations for general and specific applications. The following tables in this section provide different specifications and a partial list of available PTCA and other interventional device equipment.

TABLE VIII-1. PTCA balloon catheter specifications

System		Type	Shaft Prox	Shaft Dis	1.5	2.0	2.5	3.0	3.5	4.0	Max gw (in)	Balloon Material	Nominal (atm)	RBP (atm)
							Balloon Size (mm)							
Over-The-Wire														
Cordis	Sleek	OTW	3.2F	2.5F	.025	.027	.028	.030	.031	—	.014	DURALYN	8	10
	Sleuth	OTW	3.5F	3.0F	—	.031	.031	.032	.033	.035	.018	DURALYN	8	8
	Olympix	OTW	3.5F	3.0F	—	.030	.031	.031	.033	.035	.018	DURALYN	8	10
	Olympix Long	OTW	3.5F	3.0F	—	.030	.031	.031	.033	.035	.018	DURALYN	8	10
ACS	ACX II	OTW	3.3F	3.3F	.029	.031	.032	.034	.035	.037	.014	PE600	6	6
	Omega	OTW	2.9F	2.9F	.022	.023	.025	.028	.030	.034	.010	VERBATIM	6	6
	Pinkerton .018	OTW	3.6F	3.6F	—	.035	.037	.039	.040	.042	.018	PE600	6	6
	Prism	OTW	3.3F	3.3F	.029	.031	.032	.034	.035	.037	.014	VERBATIM	6	6
	RX .014	RX	3.3F	3.3F	—	.032	.034	.037	.039	-	.014	PE600	6	6
	RX .018	RX	3.7F	3.7F	—	.035	.038	.040	.042	.046	.018	PE600	6	6
	RX Alpha .014	RX	2.3F	3.3F	.029	.030	.031	.033	.034	.035	.014	PE600	6	8
	RX Perfusion	RX	3.7F	4.2F	—	.053	.054	.055	.056	.059	.018	PE600	6	6
	RX Streak	RX	2.3F	3.3F	.029	.030	.031	.033	.034	.035	.014	VERBATIM	6	8

Brand	Product	Type										Material		
	RX Flowtrack 40	RX	2.3F	3.5F	—	.048	.049	.050	.051	.052	.018	PE 600	6	6
	Stack	OTW	3.9F	4.5F	—	.056	.057	.058	.060	.062	.018	PE600	6	6
	Stack 40-S	OTW	3.9F	4.5F	—	—	.052	.053	.054	.055	.018	PE600	6	8
	Ten	OTW	2.8F	2.8F	.024	.026	.027	.028	.030	.033	.010	PE600	6	6
Baxter	Slinky	OTW	3.2F	3.0F	—	.028	.031	.032	.036	—	.014	POC	6	6-9
	Reach	OTW	3.2F	2.9F	.028	.030	.032	.035	.037	.039	.014	POC	6	6-8
Mansfield	Nitech	OTW	2.9F	2.9F	—	.029	.033	.035	.039	—	.014	HDPE	6	10
	Slider .014	OTW	3.4F	3.4F	—	.035	.036	.040	.044	.045	.014	HDPE	6	10
	Slider .018	OTW	3.4F	3.4F	—	.037	.038	.042	.044	.048	.018	HDPE	6	10
	Slider ST	OTW	2.7F	2.7F	—	.029	.033	.035	.039	—	.014	HDPE	6	10
	Synergy	RX/OTW	2.9F	2.9F	—	.029	.033	.035	.039	.040	.014	HDPE	6	10
	Synergy	RX/OTW	2.9F	2.9F	—	.032	.035	.039	.041	.044	.018	HDPE	6	10
Medtronic	14K	OTW	2.9F	2.9F	.026	.030	.033	.036	.041	—	.014	PE	6	8
	18K	OTW	3.5F	3.5F	—	.032	.036	.038	.040	—	.018	PE	5	6
Schneider	Piccolino	RX	3.0F	3.2F	.025	.027	.029	.031	.034	.036	.014	PET	10	16
	Piccolino Forte	RX	3.0F	3.2F	.025	.027	.028	.031	.034	.036	.014	PET	10	16
	Speedy	RX	3.0F	3.3F	.030	.031	.032	.034	.036	.039	.016	PET	5	10

Continued on pages 590–591.

TABLE VIII-1. *Continued from pages 588–589.* PTCA balloon catheter specifications

System	Type	Shaft		Balloon Size (mm)						Max gw (in)	Balloon Material	Nominal (atm)	RBP (atm)
		Prox	Dis	1.5	2.0	2.5	3.0	3.5	4.0				
Microsoftrac XLP	OTW	3.5F	3.0F	.025	.027	.029	.031	.034	.035	.014	PET	4	16
Magnum-Meier	OTW	4.5F	4.5F	—	.039	.041	.043	.044	.047	.021	PET	N/A	16
Mongoose	RX	3.2F	3.1F	.027	.029	.029	.032	.034	.038	.014	PET	N/A	16
SciMed													
Cobra 10	OTW	2.8F	2.5F	.027	.029	.031	.033	.034	—	.010	POC	6	9
Cobra 14	OTW	3.0F	2.7F	.030	.031	.033	.037	.039	.042	.014	POC	6	9
Express	RX	1.8F	2.7F	.028	.029	.031	.035	.039	.040	.014	POC	6	9
Mirage	OTW	3.6F	2.9F	.032	.034	.035	.038	.040	.044	.018	POC	6	9
NC Shadow	OTW	3.6F	2.7F	—	.031	.032	.036	.040	.043	.014	TRIAD	6	16
SC Shadow	OTW	3.6F	2.7F	.030	.031	.033	.037	.039	.042	.014	POC-8	8	9
Shadow	OTW	3.6F	2.7F	.030	.031	.033	.037	.039	.042	.014	POC	6	9
Skinny .014	OTW	3.5F	3.0F	.028	.031	.033	.037	.040	.042	.014	POC	8	9
Skinny .018	OTW	3.5F	3.0F	.031	.034	.037	.039	.040	.044	.018	POC	8	9

USCI	Force	OTW	3.5F	3.5F	—	.031	.033	.034	.036		.018	PET	5	12
	Solo	OTW	3.0F	3.0F	.028	.030	.030	.032	.034	.035	.014	PET	5	12
	Sprint	OTW	3.5F	3.5F	—	.031	.033	.035	.037	.039	.018	PET	5	12
Fixed-Wire														
Cordis	Orion	FW	2.4F	1.8F	—	.024	.028	.030	.032		FW	DURALYN	8	12
	Lightning	FW	2.4F	1.8F	—	.024	.027	.030	.032		FW	DURALYN	8	12
ACS	Slalom	FW	2.5F	2.0F	—	.023	.025	.029	.033		FW	PE600	6	8
SciMed	Ace	FW	1.8F	1.8F	.020	.022	.030	.032	.036		FW	POC	7	8
USCI	Probe III	FW	1.7F	1.7F	—	.019	.021	.026	—	—	FW	PET	5	10.6

Shaft/RBP specifications are for 3.0 mm catheters.
(Courtesy of Cordis Corporation, Miami, FL.)

TABLE VIII-2. PTCA guiding catheters

| Company | Product name | French size | I.D. | Construction | | | Radiopaque tip marker | Metal curve support |
				Top coat	Braid type	Lumen surface		
ACS	Powerguide	7	.070"	Polyurethane	Kevlar	FEP	Yes	Yes
	Powerguide	8	.080"	Polyurethane	Kevlar	FEP	Yes	Yes
Baxter	Marathon	7	.070"	Pebax	Stainless steel	Silicone	No	No
	Marathon	8	.078"	Pebax	Stainless steel	Silicone	No	No
	Marathon Gold	8	.082"	Pebax	Stainless steel	Silicone	No	No
Cordis	Petite Brite Tip	6	.062"	Nylon blends	Stainless steel	PTFE	Yes	Yes
	Brite Tip	7	.072"	Nylon blends	Stainless steel	PTFE	Yes	Yes
	Brite Tip Large Lumen	8	.078"	Polyurethane	Stainless steel	PTFE	Yes	No
	New XL Brite Tip	8	.084"	Nylon blends	Stainless steel	PTFE	Yes	Yes
	Vista Brite Tip	9	.098"	Nylon blends	Stainless steel	PTFE	Yes	Yes
	Vista Brite Tip	10	.110"	Nylon blends	Stainless steel	PTFE	Yes	Yes
DVI	DVI	9.5	.104"	Polyurethane	Stainless steel	PTFE	Yes	No
	DVI	10	.104"	Polyurethane	Stainless steel	PTFE	Yes	Yes
	DVI	11	.111"	Polyurethane	Stainless steel	PTFE	Yes	Yes
Mansfield	Proformer	8	.081"	Polyur./Teflon	Stainless steel	Polyur./Teflon	No	Yes

Company	Model							
Medtronic	Sherpa	6	.057"	Polyurethane	Stainless steel	FEP	No	No
	Sherpa	7	.070"	Polyurethane	Stainless steel	FEP	No	No
	Sherpa Peak Flow	7	.072"	Polyurethane	Stainless steel	FEP	No	No
	Sherpa	8	.079"	Polyurethane	Stainless steel	FEP	No	No
	Sherpa Peak Flow	8	.083"	Polyurethane	Stainless steel	FEP	Yes	No
	Giant Lumen	9	.088"	Polyurethane	Stainless steel	FEP	No	No
	Sherpa	9	.092"	Polyurethane	Stainless steel	FEP	No	No
	Sherpa	10	.108"	Polyurethane	Stainless steel	FEP	No	No
	Sherpa 10Firm	10	.108"	Polyurethane	Stainless steel	FEP	No	No
Schneider	Solid 7	7	.072"	Polyurethane	Stainless steel	PTFE	No	No
	Superflow	7	.072"	Polyurethane	Stainless steel	PTFE	No	No
	Stamina	8	.079"	Polyurethane	Stainless steel	PTFE	No	No
	Superflow	8	.082"	Polyurethane	Stainless steel	PTFE	No	No
	Superflow	9	.092"	Polyurethane	Stainless steel	PTFE	No	No
	Superflow	10	.107"	Polyurethane	Stainless steel	PTFE	No	No
SciMed	Triguide—Elite	6	.060"	Nylon	Stainless steel	FEP	Yes	Yes
	Triguide—Lite	7	.072"	Nylon	Stainless steel	FEP	Yes	Yes
	Triguide—Standard	8	.079"	Nylon	Stainless steel	FEP	Yes	Yes
	Triguide—Intermediate	8	.080"	Nylon	Stainless steel	FEP	Yes	Yes
USCI	Super 7	7	.070"	Nylon	Kevlar	PTFE	Yes	Yes
	Illumen 8	8	.080"	Nylon	Kevlar	PTFE	Yes	Yes
	Super 9	9	.092"	Nylon	Kevlar	PTFE	Yes	Yes

TABLE VIII-3. Atherectomy, ultrasound imaging catheters, and stents

Manufacturer	Intracoronary device	Outer diameter*		French	Recommended minimum guide (in.)
		mm	In.		
Atherectomy systems					
Device for vascular intervention	Simpson Coronary Atherocath*	2.3	0.091	5.0	0.105
		2.5	0.099	6.0	0.105
		2.8	0.110	7.0	0.105
Heart technology	Rotoblator	1.25	0.049	3.75	0.076
		1.50	0.059	4.50	0.076
		1.75	0.068	5.25	0.079
		2.00	0.079	6.00	0.092
		2.15	0.084	6.45	0.092
		2.25	0.088	6.75	0.107
		2.50	0.098	7.50	0.107
		2.75	0.107	8.25	0.115
Interventional Technologies	Tec	1.83	0.071	5.5	0.092
		2.00	0.079	6.0	0.092
		2.20	0.086	6.5	0.092
		2.30	0.091	7.0	0.100
		2.50	0.098	7.5	0.107

594

Intracoronary imaging devices

CVIS	"Insight" imaging catheters	1.43	0.056	4.3	0.072
		1.67	0.065	5.0	0.079
Diasonics	Sonicath	1.60	0.062	4.8	0.082
			0.014 (guidewire)		
Endosonics	Visions	1.00	0.039	3.0	0.063
		1.67	0.065	5.0	0.076
		1.83	0.071	5.5	0.078
Intertherapy	Interpret	1.37	0.054	4.1	0.076
		1.63	0.064	4.9	0.079
Stents[†]					
Cook	Gianturco-Roubin	2.0		4.4	0.077
	FlexStent	2.5		4.4	0.077
		3.0		4.4	0.077
		3.5		4.4	0.089
		4.0		4.4	0.089
Johnson-Johnson Interventional Systems	Palmaz-Schatz	1.67	0.066	5.0	0.079
		2.00	0.079	6.0	0.092

*The dimensions here are based on the following: French size outer diameter refers to the cutter housing diameter, and the millimeter and inch outer-diameter dimensions refer to the crossing profile of the balloon when deflated.

[†]The dimensions are based on the following: All stents are deployed with a 4.4 balloon catheter manufactured by Cook, Inc. and the millimeter outer-diameter measurements are for expanded outer diameters of the stent.

TABLE VIII-4. Surgical procedures for congenital heart disease

Name	Procedure	Objective	Mechanism
Blalock-Hanlon	Surgical removal of atrial septum	Palliative	Increases mixing of blood for TGA
Blalock-Taussig	Subclavian artery to pulmonary artery anastomosis	Palliative	Increases pulmonic flow
Brock	Closed pulmonary valvotomy and infundibulectomy	Palliative	Increases pulmonic flow
Fontan	Anastomosis or conduit (may be valved or nonvalved) between the right atrium and pulmonary artery	Partial correction	Increases pulmonic flow (for univentricular morphology or tricuspid atresia)
Glen	Superior vena cava to pulmonary artery anastomosis	Palliative	Increases pulmonic flow
Arterial switch	Aorta and pulmonary artery moved to the proper ventricle (for TGA); coronaries are reimplanted	Corrective	Creates normal relationship between ventricles and great arteries
Mustard	Atrial switch with intraatrial baffle made of pericardium	Corrective	Re-establish proper flow sequence to pulmonary artery and aorta for TGA

PDA ligation	Ties off a patent ductus arteriosus (usually with silk suture)	Corrective	Closes a left-to-right shunt at the ductal level
Potts (AKA Potts-Smith shunt)	Descending aorta to pulmonary artery shunt	Palliative	Increases pulmonic flow
PA band	Constrictive band around the main pulmonary artery	Palliative	Decreases pulmonary flow
Rashkind	Atrial septostomy with balloon catheter	Palliative	Increases mixing of blood for TGA or truncus
Rastelli	Valved conduit from right ventricle to pulmonary artery and VSD closure	Corrective	Increases pulmonic flow and reestablish proper flow sequence of Ao/PA
Senning	Atrial switch with intraatrial baffle (utilizes atrial wall flaps)	Corrective	Re-establish flow sequence to pulmonary artery and aorta for TGV
Waterston shunt	Ascending aorta to right pulmonary artery	Palliative	Increases pulmonic flow

TGA, transposition of great arteries; PDA, patent ductus arteriosus; AKA, also known as; PA, pulmonary artery; VSD, vesicular septal defect; AoPA, aortic-pulmonary communication.

ELECTRO-CARDIOGRAPHY IN THE CARDIAC CATHETERIZATION LABORATORY

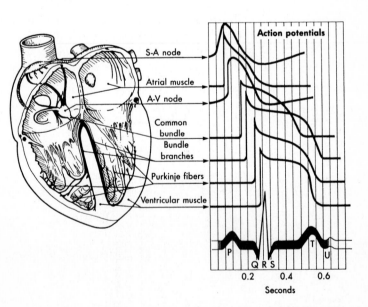

Fig. AIX-1. Genesis of electrocardiogram and pathways through the heart. (Adapted from the CIBA Collection of Medical Illustrations, Vol. 5.)

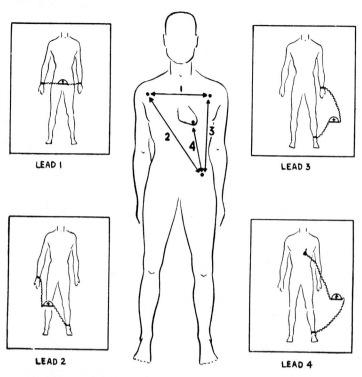

Fig. AIX-2.   Standard limb leads and 1 precordial lead. (From Marriott HLJ: *Practical electrocardiography,* ed 7, Baltimore, 1983, Williams and Wilkins.)

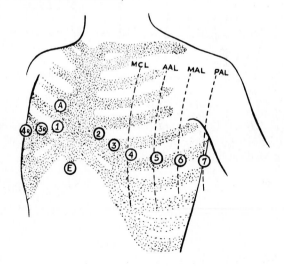

Fig. AIX-3.   Precordial points for chest leads. (From Marriott HLJ: *Practical electrocardiography,* ed 7, Baltimore, 1983, Williams and Wilkins.)

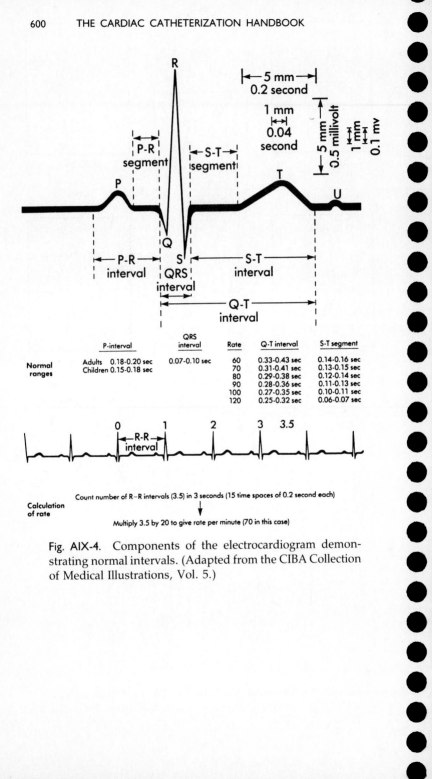

Fig. AIX-4. Components of the electrocardiogram demonstrating normal intervals. (Adapted from the CIBA Collection of Medical Illustrations, Vol. 5.)

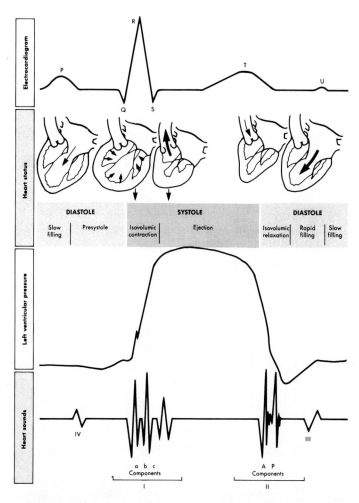

Fig. AIX-5.   Electrical and mechanical activity sequence of the heart. (Adapted from the CIBA Collection of Medical Illustrations, Vol. 5.)

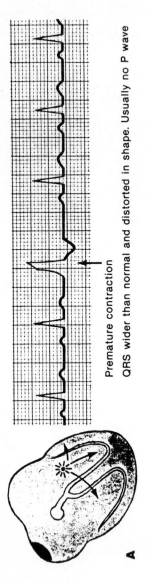

Premature contraction

QRS wider than normal and distorted in shape. Usually no P wave

Rate >120: ventricular tachycardia

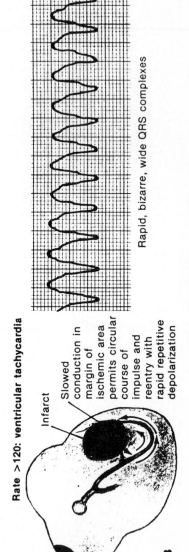

Infarct

Slowed conduction in margin of ischemic area permits circular course of impulse and reentry with rapid repetitive depolarization

Rapid, bizarre, wide QRS complexes

Fig. AIX-6. *Continued on page 603.*

602

Ventricular fibrillation

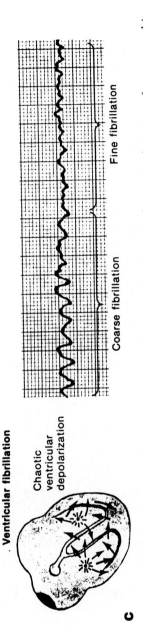

Chaotic
ventricular
depolarization

C

Coarse fibrillation

Fine fibrillation

Fig. AIX-6. Continued. A, Rhythm strip demonstrating a run of monomorphic ventricular tachycardia. **C,** Rhythm strip demonstrating ventricular fibrillation. (Adapted from Scheidt S: *Clinical Symposia* 35(2):37, 1983; 36(6):29, 1984.)

Infarction

1. Injury = elevated ST segment

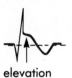

elevation

- Signifies an acute process, ST returns to baseline with time.
- If T wave is also elevated off baseline, suspect pericarditis.
- Location of injury may be determined similar to infarction location.
- If ST depression, suspect digitalis effect or subendocardial infarction.

2. Ischemia = inverted T wave

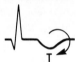

T

- Inverted T wave is symmetrical.
- T waves are usually upright in leads, I, II, and V_2-V_6, so check these leads for T wave inversion.

3. Infarction = Q wave

Q

- Small Qs may be normal in V_5 and V_6.
- Abnormal Q must be one small square *(.04 sec)* wide.
- Also abnormal if Q wave depth is greater than $1/3$ of QRS height in lead III.

Anterior infarction

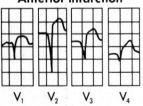

V_1 V_2 V_3 V_4

1. ST elevation with/without abnormal Q wave.

2. Usually associated with occlusion of the left anterior descending branch of the left coronary artery.

Fig. AIX-7.   ECG changes seen during myocardial injury, ischemia, and infarction. (Courtesy of Genentech, Inc., South San Francisco, CA.)

Inferior infarction

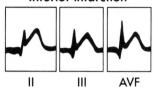

II   III   AVF

1. ST elevation with/without abnormal Q wave.

2. Usually associated with right coronary artery (RCA) occlusion.

Lateral infarction

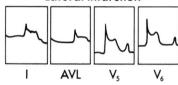

I   AVL   V₅   V₆

1. ST elevation with/without abnormal Q wave.

2. May be a component of a multiple site infarction.

3. Usually associated with obstruction of left circumflex artery.

Posterior infarction

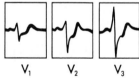

V₁   V₂   V₃

1. Tall R wave and ST depression in V₁ and V₂ (reciprocal changes).

2. May be a component of a multiple site infarction.

3. Usually associated with obstruction of RCA and/or left circumflex coronary artery.

Fig. AIX-8.   ECG changes in which acute inferior, lateral, and posterior infarction are demonstrated. (Courtesy of Genentech, Inc., South San Francisco, CA.)

INDEX

Page numbers in italics indicate pages with figures.

Abdominal aorta, angiography, 327
Ablation, 243–259
    accessory pathway, 253–256, *254, 255*
    atrial fibrillation, 245–246, *250,* 250–251
    atrial flutter, 246, 251
    atrioventricular nodal reentrant tachycardia, 252–253, *253*
    atrioventricular reciprocating tachycardia, 246, 251–252
    ectopic atrial tachycardia, 246, 251–252
    indications, 243–247
    technical aspects, 247–259, *248, 249*
    ventricular tachycardia, 247, 256–259, *258*
Accessory pathway, ablation, 253–256, *254, 255*
Acetylcholine, 367
Adenosine, 367, 470
Adult complex congenital heart disease, 441–442
Adventitia, 568
Allergic reaction, premedication, 13–15
Amplatz-type catheter, 95, *97*
Amyl nitrate, 408
Angiography, 266–374
    blood flow techniques, 399–400
    cardiac output, measurement, 137–138
    cardiac shunt, 148–149
    catheter, 364
    common coronary anomalies, 298–303
    contrast media, 358–364
        selection, 360–364, *361, 362–363*
    digital (subtraction) angiography system, compared, 351–352, *352*
    equipment, 355–364
    image distortion, 336–340
    left main coronary artery stenosis, 294–298, *295, 297*
    lower extremities, 327–329, *329, 330, 331*
    magnification, 336, *338*
    medications, 364–370, *365–366*
    pacemaker, 370–374
    poor opacification, 293
    power injector, 355–358, *356*
    rare anomalies of aortic coronary origin, 303–304, *305*
    reasons for poor, *268*
    spasm, 293–294
    total occlusion, 293
    vessel overlap, 293
Anticoagulation, stent, 536
Aortic pressure, hemodynamic data, *173*
Aortic regurgitation, hemodynamic data, 180, *181, 182, 183*
Aortic stenosis
    catheter, 126

Aortic stenosis—cont'd
  hemodynamic data, 176–178,
    177, 178
  valve resistance, 123–130, *125*
Aortic valve
  gradient, 122
  guidewire, 126–127
Aortic valve flow, 120
Arrhythmia
  cardiopulmonary resuscitation,
    457, *462, 463*
  cardioversion, 456, *458–459,*
    460–461
  defibrillation, 456, *458–459,*
    460–461
  management, 452–470
  primary prevention, 455–456
Arterial access, 45
  brachial approach, 60–69
  equipment, 83–106
  nurse, 81–83
    baseline vascular assessment,
      81–82
    obese patient, 83
    patient positioning, 82–83
    precatheterization assess-
      ment, 81
  pain control, 45
  percutaneous femoral ap-
    proach, 46–60
  problems, 69–81
  site selection, 45, *46*
  technician, 81–83
    baseline vascular assessment,
      81–82
    obese patient, 83
    patient positioning, 82–83
    precatheterization assess-
      ment, 81
  type, 45
  ultrasound, 55
Arterial wall, anatomy, 567–568
Ascending aortography, 318–320
  radiographic projections, 319
  technique, 319–320, *320, 321*
Atherectomy, equipment, *594–595*
Atrial fibrillation, 468–470
  ablation, 245–246, *250,* 250–251
Atrial flutter, ablation, 246, 251

Atrial pressure, hemodynamic
    data, pathological changes,
    171–172
Atrioventricular block, types, *237*
Atrioventricular conduction disor-
    ders, electrophysiologic
    study, 237–238
Atrioventricular nodal function,
    electrophysiologic study, *227,*
    227–228
Atrioventricular nodal function
    curve, electrophysiologic
    study, 228–230, *229, 230, 231*
Atrioventricular nodal reentrant
    tachycardia, ablation,
    252–253, *253*
Atrioventricular reciprocating
    tachycardia, ablation, 246,
    251–252
Atropine, 368, 456, 467

Balloon catheter
  percutaneous transluminal coro-
    nary angioplasty, 489–497,
    588–591
  right heart catheterization,
    103–105
Beta blocker, 470
Bjork-Shiley cardiac valve prosthe-
    sis, *585*
Bjork-Shiley integral monostrut
    cardiac valve prosthesis, *586*
Blood, 31
Blood product, measurement,
    382–384
Bloodborne virus, 31
Body fluids, 31
Brachial artery cutdown tech-
    nique, *63–64,* 63–67
  arterial localization, 63
  arteriotomy, 65–67
  artery control, 65
  blunt dissection, 65
  skin entry, 63
Brachial catheter, 98–102
Brachial venous cutdown, 67–68
Brachial ventriculography cathe-
    ter, Sones catheter, 100–102,
    102

Bradycardia, 459–463
Bretylium tosylate, 466
Bypass graft, problems, 74–80, *75, 76*

Calcium channel blocker, 366–367
Cardiac index, 118
Cardiac output
    angiography, measurement, 137–138
    computations of valve areas, 119–123
    Douglas bag method, 133–134
    Fick (O_2 consumption) method, 117–118
    Fick principle, 131, 134
    indicator dilution technique, 135–137
    measurement techniques, 131–206
        differences, 138–139
    polaragraphic method, 131–133, *132*
Cardiac shunt
    angiography, 148–149
    dye dilution method, 148
    hemodynamic data, 139–149, *141, 142, 143*
    locations, *140*
    oximetry, 143–148
    radioactive tracer, 149
Cardiac support device, 470–479
Cardiopulmonary resuscitation, arrhythmia, 457, *462, 463*
Cardiovascular technologist. *See also* Technician
    area of practice, 27–29
    definition, 26
    equipment, 29–31
    life support techniques, 29
    safety, 31
    training, 26–41
Cardioversion, arrhythmia, 456, *458–459, 460–461*
Carpentier-Edwards pericardial valve prosthesis, *582*
Carpentier-Edwards SupraAnnular Bioprosthesis, *581*

Catheter
    angiography, 364
    aortic stenosis, 126
    electrophysiologic study, 213–216, *215*
        positioning, 218–220, *219*
    failure, 552
    femoral arterial technique, 88–90, 88–106, *89*
    multipurpose, 95
        femoral ventriculography, 98
    reuse, 553–554
    right heart angiography, 105–106
    right heart catheterization, 102–103, *103*
Catheterization
    complications, *4, 5, 6*
    complications management, 445–450, *446–449*
    contraindications, *4, 5*
    exercise, 400–411
    heart transplant patient, 439–441
    indications, 1–5, *3*
    patient preparation, 6–13
    postcatheterization checkup, 12
    radiation, 36–40, *355*
    sterile preparations, 11–12
    team approach, 17–20
    as urgent procedure, 5
Catheterization laboratory, 1–42
    employer responsibility, 35–36
    equipment, 22–26, *23, 24, 25*
        safety, 34–35
    hazards, 31–40, *32*
    instruction, 20–22
    professional attitude, 7–9
    protection methods, 31–35, *33*
    radiation safety, 36–40, *355*
    suite preparations, 10–11
Catheterization order, 9
    in-lab preparations, 9–10
Catheterization team
    nurse viewpoint, 19–20
    physician viewpoint, 17–18
    technicinan viewpoint, 19–20

Central aortic pressure, hemodynamic data, normal, 167–171, *169, 170*
Certification, physician, 41–42
Chemical sterilization, 26
Circumflex coronary artery, anomalous origin, 301–302, *302*
Circumflex vein graft, 76–77
Cold pressor testing, 407
Communication, 7, 8, 541
  angiogram review, 12–13
Concentric lesion, 569, *569, 570–571*
Congenital heart disease, surgical procedures, *596–597*
Constrictive pericarditis, hemodynamic data, 191–192, *192, 193, 194, 195*
  right atrial pressure, 192, *196*
Contrast media, 568
  anaphylactoid reactions, *17*
  angiography, 358–364
    selection, 360–364, *361, 362–363*
  reactions, 13–15, *14, 17,* 552–553
  renal failure, 15
Contrast power injector, 24, *24*
Cook Flexstent, 536, *537*
Coronary angiographic catheter, 90–100, *91, 92*
Coronary angioplasty, high-risk, 481–482
Coronary arteriography, *267,* 267–304
  coronary stenosis, 289–292, *290, 291, 292*
  left coronary artery, 285–288
  nomenclature, *272–273, 272–284, 274, 275–283, 284–285*
  right coronary artery, 288–289
  techniques, 269–272, *270, 273*
  views, 272
Coronary artery, anatomy, 567–568, *568*
Coronary atherectomy, 530
Coronary cannulation, Sones catheter, 98–100, *99*

Coronary flow reserve, Doppler coronary flow velocity techniques, 393
Coronary sinus catheterization, 384–385, 429–430
  indications, 429
  techniques, 429–430
Coronary stenosis, coronary arteriography, 289–292, *290, 291, 292*
Crash cart, 24

Dagger effect, 88
Defibrillation, arrhythmia, 456, *458–459, 460–461*
Defibrillator, 24
Diabetes, 15–17
Diagnostic saturation run, oximetry, 143–148
Digital angiography, 345–351, *346*
Digital fluoroscopy aid, 349
Digital (subtraction) angiography system, 345–348, *347*
  angiography, compared, 351–352, *352*
Digitalis, 470
Direct transthoracic left ventricle puncture, 421–422
  complications, 422
  indications, 421–422
Directional coronary atherectomy, 530–534, *531*
Dobutamine, 369, 411
Dopamine, 369
Doppler catheter, types, 385–389, *389*
Doppler coronary flow velocity techniques, 385–393
  characteristics, 391, *392, 394–395*
  coronary flow reserve, 393
  problems, 393
  setup, 389–390
  translesional velocity, 391–393
  uses, *390,* 391
Douglas bag method, cardiac output, 133–134
Dye dilution method, cardiac shunt, 148
Dynamic exercise, 404–405

Eccentric lesion, 569, *569*, *570*
Ectopic atrial tachycardia, ablation, 246, 251–252
Electrocardiography
  abnormal rhythm, 261
  catheterization laboratory
    changes, 261–264
  components, 260–264
  electrode placement, 259–260
  fundamentals, 259–264
Electrocardiography amplifier,
    physiologic recorder, *152*,
    152–153
Electromechanical dissociation,
    467–468
Electronic radiography, 349
Electrophysiologic study, 208–243
  atrioventricular conduction disorders, 237–238
  atrioventricular nodal function,
    227, 227–228
  atrioventricular nodal function
    curve, 228–230, *229*, *230*,
    231
  catheter, 213–216, *215*
    positioning, 218–220, *219*
  clinical applications, 210
  complications, 220–221
  conduction interval measurement, *222*, 222–224, *223*
  equipment, *211*, 211–213, *213*,
    214
  evaluation, 216, *217*, *221*
  His Purkinje system function,
    227, 227–228
  ICD, 239
  patient preparation, 216, *217*,
    221
  procedures, 216–235
  programmed electrical stimulation, 224–225
  refractory periods, 228, *228*
  sequence of activation, 224, *225*
  sinus node, 225–226, *226*
  sinus node disease, 235
  study protocol, 221, *221*
  supraventricular tachycardia,
    240–243, *241*, *245*
  syncope of unknown etiology,
    239–240, *240*

  technical aspects, 209–216
  venous access, 216–218
  ventricular arrhythmia, 238
  ventricular stimulation,
    230–235, *233*, *234*, *236*
  wide complex tachycardia,
    238–239
Endomyocardial biopsy, 422–429
  biopsy devices, *423*, 423–424,
    424
  contraindications, 423
  femoral approach, 424–425
  indications, *422*, 423
  internal jugular approach
    echocardiographic guidance,
      425–429, *426*, *428*
    fluoroscopic guidance, 429
  technique, 424–429
Environmental safety, 31–40
Epinephrine, 369
Equipment
  angiography, 355–364
  arterial access, 83–106
  atherectomy, *594–595*
  cardiovascular technologist,
    29–31
  catheterization laboratory,
    safety, 34–35
  electrophysiologic study, *211*,
    211–213, *213*, *214*
  failure, 551–552
  hemodynamic data, 149
  percutaneous transluminal coronary angioplasty, 486–499,
    489
  preventive maintenance, *344*
  stent, *594–595*
  ultrasonography, *594–595*
  venous access, 83–106
  vessel tortuosity, 70–71
Ergonovine, 368
Ethylene oxide sterilization, 26
Exercise
  cardiac catheterization, 400–411
  measurements of response,
    405–406

Femoral angiography catheter,
    special purpose, 95–97

Femoral arterial pressure, hemo-
dynamic data, normal,
167–171, *169, 170*
Femoral artery, anatomy, *331*
Femoral artery pseudoan-
eurysm, *72*
Femoral ventriculography cathe-
ter, 97–98
Fick principle, cardiac output,
131, 134
Film processing, 342–345
Fixed core guide, 87
Fixed-wire angioplasty balloon
catheter, 494–496, *495*
Fluoroscope, 22
Foreshortening, *339, 339*–340

Guidewire, *85,* 86–87
aortic valve, 126–127
core wire, 86
distal tip, 86
proximal tip, 86

Hall-Kaster prosthetic heart valve,
584
Hancock II porcine xenograft, *583*
Hancock pericardial heart valve,
582
Heart
electrical system, 259
functional anatomy, 564–566
pressure wave, 108–112
Heart transplant patient, cardiac
catheterization, 439–441
Hemodynamic data, 108–205
aortic pressure, *173*
aortic regurgitation, 180, *181,
182, 183*
aortic stenosis, 176–178, *177,
178*
artifact, 192–203, *196, 197, 198,
199, 200, 201, 202, 203, 204,
205*
atrial pressure, pathological
changes, *171–172*
cardiac shunt, 139–149, *141,
142, 143*
central aortic pressure, normal,
167–171, *169, 170*

computations, 116–123
constrictive pericarditis, 191–
192, *192, 193, 194, 195*
right atrial pressure, 192, *196*
equipment, 149
femoral arterial pressure, normal, 167–171, *169, 170*
left atrial pressure, simultaneous transseptal and right
heart catheterization, 167,
169
left ventricle gradient, below
aortic valve, *179,* 179–180,
180
mitral regurgitation, 182, *184,
185*
mitral stenosis, 182–187, *185,
186, 187, 188*
mixed, 188, *189*
right ventricle-left ventricle
pressure differences,
189–190, *190, 191*
normal, *110, 111*
normal right atrial pressure
waves, 161, *162*
normal right ventricle pressure
waves, 161, *162*
normal values, 572–573
PCW tracing, large v waves,
174–176, *175, 176*
pulmonary artery pressure, *173*
recording techniques, 157–161
right atrial pressure
atrioventricular dissociation,
165–167, *166, 168*
normal, 161, *162*
tricuspid regurgitation,
161–164, *163, 164, 165,
166*
ventricular pressure, pathological changes, *172–173*
wide aortic pulse pressure,
173–174
Hemostasis
percutaneous brachial artery
puncture, 62–63
percutaneous femoral artery
puncture, 56–59
Heparin, 69

Hepatitis B, 31
High-fidelity micromanometer-tip pressure measurement, 378–379
  indications, 378–379
  setup, 379
  ventricular function, 379, *380*
High-frequency two-dimensional coronary ultrasound imaging, 393, *399*
High-risk cardiac catheterization, 444–482
His Purkinje system function, electrophysiologic study, *227*, 227–228
Human immunodeficiency virus, 31
Hyperventilation, 408
Hypotension, management, 450–452

ICD, electrophysiologic study, 239
Image intensifier, 336, *337*
Incident report, 543–544
Indicator dilution technique, cardiac output, 135–137
Informed consent, 6–7
Insulin, 15–17
Internal mammary artery graft, 77–80, *78*, *79*
Intima, 567
Intraaortic balloon counterpulsation placement
  contraindications, *472*
  indications, *472*
Intraaortic balloon placement, 470–479, *471*
  technique, 471–478, *474*, *475*, *476–477*
Intravascular device, failure, 552
Intravascular foreign body retrieval, 434–438, *439–440*
Intravascular imaging, 393–397
Ionescu-Shiley low profile pericardial xenograft, *586*
Isometric exercise, 406
Isoproterenol, 369, 408–411

J-curve guidewire, *85*, 88
Judkins catheter, *84*
Judkins-type coronary catheter, 90–95, *93*, 95
Junctional rhythm, 461

Laboratory management personnel, 40–41
Lead apron, 39–40, *40*
Lead eyeglasses, *37*, 37–38
Left anterior descending artery, anomalous origin, 302–303, *304*
Left anterior descending artery vein graft, 76
Left atrial pressure, hemodynamic data, simultaneous transseptal and right heart catheterization, 167, *169*
Left coronary artery
  coronary arteriography, 285–288
  problems, 72–73
Left heart catheterization, *109*
  protocol, 115, *115–116*
Left main coronary artery, 299, *300*
  anomalous origin, 298–299, *299*
  anterior free wall course, 298–303
  interarterial course, 300–301, *301*
  retroaortic course, 299–300, *300*
Left main coronary artery stenosis, angiogram, 294–298, *295*, *297*
Left ventricle gradient, hemodynamic data, below aortic valve, *179*, 179–180, *180*
Left ventricular contractility, measurements, 316
Left ventriculography
  indications, 305, *306*
  left ventricle dysfunction, 308
Lesion, configuration, 568–569
Lidocaine, 368–369
Life support techniques, cardiovascular technologist, 29
Long tapered core wire, 88

Magnification, 336, *338*

Manometer, transducer, *154*, 155–157

Medical malpractice, 541

Medical record, 542–550, 559–563
  complications, 543–544
  guidelines, 542–546
  incident report, 543–544
  medication, 546
  medication error, 550
  minimum documentation, 547–548
  outpatient catheterization, 548–549

Medication
  infusion methods, *453*
  infusion rate conversion, *454*
  medical record, 546
  quick Millerau method, *454*
  reactions, 552–553
  ventricular tachycardia, 466–468

Medication error
  medical record, 550
  prevention, 550

Medtronic Hall prosthetic heart valve, *584*

Mitral regurgitation, hemodynamic data, 182, *184*, *185*

Mitral stenosis, hemodynamic data, 182–187, *185*, *186*, *187*, *188*
  mixed, 188, *189*
  right ventricle-left ventricle pressure differences, 189–190, *190*, *191*

Mitral valve area, calculation, *127*, 127–129

Mitral valve flow, 120

M-mode echocardiography, 400

Moveable core guide, 87

Muller maneuver, 407

Myocardial blood flow, research techniques, 381–382, *383*

Myocardial metabolism, research techniques, 382–384

Nitroglycerin, 408

Nitroprusside, 370

Nurse
  arterial access, 81–83
    baseline vascular assessment, 81–82
    obese patient, 83
    patient positioning, 82–83
    precatheterization assessment, 81
  cineangiography preparations, 340–343
  research techniques, 411
  venous access, 81–83
    baseline vascular assessment, 81–82
    patient positioning, 82–83
    precatheterization assessment, 81

Omniscience prosthetic heart valve, *583*

Over-the-wire angioplasty balloon catheter, 491–493, *492*, *493*

Oximetry
  cardiac shunt, 143–148
  diagnostic saturation run, 143–148

Oxygen consumption measurement, 131–134

P wave, 260

Pacemaker, angiography, 370–374

Papaverine, 367

Paroxysmal supraventricular tachycardia, 468–470

Patient education, 20–22

PCW tracing, hemodynamic data, large v waves, 174–176, *175*, *176*

Percutaneous balloon aortic valvuloplasty, 510–514, *511*, *513*

Percutaneous balloon mitral valvuloplasty, 514–520, *517*, *518*, *519*

Percutaneous balloon valvuloplasty, 510–520

Percutaneous brachial artery puncture, 60–63
  anesthesia, 61
  artery puncture, 61–62

brachial artery location, 61
catheter selection, 62
catheter sheath introduction, 62
guidewire introduction, 61–62
hemostasis, 62–63
heparin, 62
needle sheath removal, 62
sheath selection, 62
skin entry, 62
skin preparation, 62
Percutaneous brachial vein puncture, 63
Percutaneous cardiopulmonary support, 478–482
elective, 479–480, 481–482
emergency, 480–481
technique, 479–482
Percutaneous femoral artery puncture, 46–59
arterial puncture, 49–51, *50*
artery location, *47*, 47–48
guidewire insertion, 51–53
hemostasis, 56–59
local anesthesia, 48–49
pain, 54–55
postprocedure care, 59
sheath, 53–54, *54*, 56–57
skin entry, 49
subcutaneous tunnel, 49
ultrasound, 55
vagal reaction, 54–55
Percutaneous femoral vein puncture, 59–61
femoral vein location, 59
skin entry, 59
vein puncture, 59–60
Percutaneous transluminal coronary angioplasty, 393, 394–399, *397*, 484–503
balloon catheter, 489–497, *588–591*
clinical procedure, 499–503
complications, 486
contraindications, 486
equipment, 486–499, *489*
guiding catheter, 487–489, *490, 491, 592–593*
indications, 485–486
inflation device, 497

long sheath, 497–499
mechanisms, 485
steerable guidewire, 497, *498*
torque (tool) device, 497
translesional pressure
equipment, 502
technique, 502–503, *504, 505, 506, 507*
Y connector, 497
Pericardiocentesis, 430–434
indications, 430
positioning, 430–431
procedure, 430–434
puncturing pericardium, 431–434, *432, 433, 435, 436–437, 438*
route to pericardium, 430, *431*
setup, 430–431
Peripheral arterial balloon angioplasty, 503–509, *508*
complications, 508–509
contraindications, 506
indications, 506
technique, 506–508
Peripheral vascular angiography, 325–329
Personnel, 209–211
Pharmacologic stress, 408–411
Physician
certification, 41–42
training, 41–42
Physiologic maneuvers, 400–411
Physiologic recorder, 22, *151*, 151–157
electrocardiography amplifier, *152*, 152–153
pressure amplifier, *153*, 153–155
Pigtail catheter, *97*, 97–98
Polaragraphic method, cardiac output, 131–133, *132*
Power injector, angiography, 355–358, *356*
Premedication, allergic reaction, 13–15
Pressure amplifier, physiologic recorder, *153*, 153–155
Pressure gradient, *119*
anatomic variables, 119
artifactual variables, 119

Pressure gradient—cont'd
    computations of valve areas,
        119–123
Pressure manifold, 149–151, *150*
Pressure wave, heart, 108–112
Procainamide, 467
Product liability issues, 551–554
Propranolol, 470
Prosthetic valve, radiographic
    identification, 581–586
Protamine
    reaction, 15
    reaction treatment, 56
Provider-patient relationship, 541
Pulmonary angiography, 321–325
    technique, 322–325, *324, 326*
Pulmonary arteriolar resistance,
    118
Pulmonary artery catheterization,
    complications, *104*
Pulmonary artery pressure, hemo-
    dynamic data, *173*
Pulmonary valvuloplasty,
    520–522, *521*
Pulmonary wedge pressure,
    114–115
Pulmonic valve stenosis, 130, *130*

QRS complex, 260
Quantitative coronary angiogra-
    phy, 349–351
Quantitative ventriculography,
    379–380, *381*
    technique, 313–317

Radiation
    catheterization, *355*
    dose limitation, 38–39
    safety, 352–355, *354*
        catheterization laboratory,
            36–40
        personal radiation protection,
            353–355
Radiation badge, 38
Radiation safety policy, 37
Radiation unit, definitions, 38
Radioactive tracer, cardiac shunt,
    149

Rapid-exchange (monorail) angi-
    oplasty balloon catheter,
        493–494, *495*
Regurgitant fraction, 317, *318*
Renal arteriography, 325–327
Renal balloon angioplasty,
    509–510
    complications, 510
    contraindications, 509
    indications, 509
    postprocedural care, 510
    technique, 509
Renal failure, contrast media, 15
Research techniques, 376–411
    myocardial blood flow,
        381–382, *383*
    myocardial metabolism,
        382–384
    nurse, 411
    technician, 411
Right atrial pressure, hemody-
    namic data
    atrioventricular dissociation,
        165–167, *166, 168*
    normal, 161, *162*
    tricuspid regurgitation,
        161–164, *163, 164, 165,*
        166
Right coronary artery
    anomalous origin, 302, *303*
    coronary arteriography,
        288–289
    problems, 73–74
Right heart angiography, cathe-
    ter, 105–106
Right heart catheterization, *109*
    balloon catheter technique,
        103–105
    catheter, 102–103, *103*
    complications, 113–114, *114*
    indications, 112
    protocol, *112–113*
Right heart pressure, normal in
    catheter pullback, 174
Right internal mammary artery
    graft, 80
Right ventriculography, indica-
    tions, 306
Road mapping, 349, *350*

Rotablator, *534*, 534–535
Rotational atherectomy, *534*, 534–535

Safety, radiation, 36–40, 352–355, *354*
  personal radiation protection, 353–355
Safety ribbon, 86–87
Second degree atrioventricular block, 461
Seldinger technique, *50–51*
Sinus node, electrophysiologic study, 225–226, *226*
Sinus node disease, electrophysiologic study, 235
Sinus rhythm, 461
Sones catheter, 98–102
  brachial ventriculography catheter, 100–102, *102*
  coronary cannulation, 98–100, *99*
Spring guide, 86
Spring wire, 87
St. Jude Medical cardiac valve, *585*
ST segment, 260–261
Stent, 535–539
  anticoagulation, 536
  equipment, *594–595*
  implantation, 536–538
  postprocedural care, 538–539
Streptokinase, 525
Stroke index, 118
Stroke volume, 118
Stroke work, 118
Supraventricular arrhythmia, 468–470
Supraventricular tachycardia, electrophysiologic study, 240–243, *241*, *245*
Syncope of unknown etiology, electrophysiologic study, 239–240, *240*
Synthetic graft conduit, vascular access, 68–69
Systemic vascular resistance, 118

T wave, 260–261
Tapered core wire, 87–88
Team autoclave sterilization, 26
TEC atherectomy, 535, *536*
Technician. *See also* Cardiovascular technologist
  arterial access, 81–83
    baseline vascular assessment, 81–82
    obese patient, 83
    patient positioning, 82–83
    precatheterization assessment, 81
  cineangiography preparations, 340–343
  research techniques, 411
  venous access, 81–83
    baseline vascular assessment, 81–82
    obese patient, 83
    patient positioning, 82–83
    precatheterization assessment, 81
Third degree atrioventricular block, 461–463
Thoracic aorta, angiography, 327
Thrombolytic therapy, 522–526, *523*, *524*
  complications, 526
  indications, 522–523
  technique, 525–526
Thyroid shield, *37*, 40
Total pulmonary resistance, 118
Training, 26–42
  cardiovascular technologist, 26–41
  physician, 41–42
Transducer
  calibration, *154*, 155–157
  manometer, *154*, 155–157
Translesional pressure, percutaneous transluminal coronary angioplasty
  equipment, 502
  technique, 502–503, *504*, *505*, *506*, *507*
Translesional velocity, Doppler coronary flow velocity techniques, 391–393

Transseptal heart catheterization, 414–421
  contraindications, 415
  indications, 414, 415
  risks, 420–421
  techniques, 415–420, 416, 417, 419
Tricuspid valve gradient, 130, 185
Two-dimensional echocardiography, 400

Ultrasound
  arterial access, 55
  equipment, 594–595
  venous access, 55
Units of measure, 574–576
Urokinase, 525

Valsalva maneuver, 402, 406–407, 409
Valve area, calculation, 119–123
Valve resistance
  aortic stenosis, 123–130, 125
  formula, 124
Valvuloplasty, 510–526
Vascular access, 68, 68–69
  problems, 69–81
  site, 11
  synthetic graft conduit, 68–69
Vascular tracing, 349, 350
Vasovagal reaction, 459
Venous access, 45
  brachial approach, 60–69
  electrophysiologic study, 216–218
  equipment, 83–106
  nurse, 81–83
    baseline vascular assessment, 81–82
    patient positioning, 82–83
    precatheterization assessment, 81
  pain control, 45
  percutaneous femoral approach, 46–60
  problems, 69–81
  site selection, 45, 46
  technician, 81–83
    baseline vascular assessment, 81–82

obese patient, 83
patient positioning, 82–83
precatheterization assessment, 81
type, 45
ultrasound, 55
Ventricular arrhythmia, electrophysiologic study, 238
Ventricular fibrillation, 463–465, 464
Ventricular mass, 579, 580
Ventricular pressure, hemodynamic data, pathological changes, 172–173
Ventricular stimulation, electrophysiologic study, 230–235, 233, 234, 236
Ventricular tachycardia
  ablation, 247, 256–259, 258
  medication, 466–468
  nonsustained, 465–466
Ventricular volume, measurement, 577–579, 580
Ventriculography, 304–317, 306, 318. See also Specific type
  complications, 310
  regional left ventricle wall motion, 310–313, 312
  technique, 307–309
  views, 309–310, 310, 311
Verapamil, 469–470
Vessel tortuosity, 70–72
  arterial access complications, 71–72
  equipment, 70–71
Videodensitometry, 399–400
  limitations, 399–400
  technique, 399
Videotape recorder, 340

Wall motion, 379–380, 381
Wide aortic pulse pressure, hemodynamic data, 173–174
Wide complex tachycardia, electrophysiologic study, 238–239

X-ray generator, 330–333
X-ray tube, 333, 333–335, 334